GAIT ANALYSIS

Normal and Pathological Function

GAIT ANALYSIS

Normal and Pathological Function

Jacquelin Perry, MD
Chief of Pathokinesiology
Rancho Los Amigos Medical Center
Downey, CA

Illustrated by
Bill Schoneberger, PT
Yorba Linda, CA

SLACK Incorporated, 6900 Grove Road, Thorofare, NJ 08086-9447

SLACK International Book Distributors

In Japan
Igaku-Shoin, Ltd.
Tokyo International P.O. Box 5063
1-28-36 Hongo, Bunkyo-Ku
Tokyo 113
Japan

In Canada
McGraw-Hill Ryerson Limited
300 Water Street
Whitby, Ontario
L1N 9B6

In all other regions throughout the world, SLACK professional reference books are available through offices and affiliates of McGraw-Hill, Inc. For the name and address of the office serving your area, please correspond to

McGraw-Hill, Inc.
Medical Publishing Group
Attn: International Marketing Director
1221 Avenue of the Americas —28th Floor
New York, NY 10020
(212)-512-3955 (phone)
(212)-512-4717 (fax)

Editorial Director: Cheryl D. Willoughby
Publisher: Harry C. Benson

Printed in the United States of America

Library of Congress Catalog Card Number: 90-050830

ISBN: 1-55642-192-3

Published by: SLACK Incorporated
               6900 Grove Road
               Thorofare, NJ 08086-9447

Last digit is print number: 10   9   8   7   6   5   4   3   2

Contents

Expanded Contents

Acknowledgments

The development of a systematic means of observational gait analysis was a collaborative effort with Rancho Los Amigos physical therapy supervisors and instructors, Downey, California. Membership of this group has changed sufficiently over the 12 years of the program's evolution that I cannot name all the contributors. A thank-you for your help is extended to each person. In addition, I particularly wish to acknowledge the help of Jaqueline Montgomery and Maureen Rodgers, who continue their involvement in the gait project.

For extensive assistance in the final preparation of this book, very special thanks go to JoAnne K. Gronley and Bill Schoneberger. JoAnne, physical therapist and associate director of clinical research in Pathokinesiology, has provided the monumental task of critiquing the entire book, finalizing all the references and creating all the EMG illustrations. Bill, a physical therapist and computer artist, was a major design consultant as well as producer of the computer artwork. Special appreciation also is extended to Dr. Mary Ann Keenan for providing an orthopedist's critique of the material, and Ernie Bontrager, associate director of engineering research in Pathokinesiology, for technical assistance with the section on gait analysis systems.

Introduction

Walking is the body's natural means of moving from one location to another. It also is the most convenient means of traveling short distances. Functional versatility allows the lower limbs to readily accommodate stairs, doorways, changing surfaces, and obstacles in the path of progression. Efficiency in these endeavors depends on free joint mobility and muscle activity that is selective in timing and intensity. Energy conservation is optimal in the normal pattern of limb action. Because of the numerous advantages of walking, patients strive to retain this capability even in the presence of severe impairment. As the various types of pathology alter mobility and muscular effectiveness, the patients substitute wherever possible, yield when they must, and accept compensatory reactions of adjacent segments as they occur. The resulting walking pattern is a mixture of normal and abnormal motions that differ in significance. Energy costs are increased and functional versatility is compromised.

At the other extreme, athletes push normal function to its limit. This results in greater forces and motion arcs being experienced. Substitutive actions and trauma are not infrequent occurrences. Generally, there are therapeutic measures that can lessen the magnitude of the disability and the impediment to walking it creates. To be effective, however, the corrective measures must be directed to the primary deficit and not toward compensatory actions that happen to be more conspicuous. Ligamentous strain may mask a critical insufficiency of strength. The area of maximum motion may be a bone's length away from the origin of the pathological dysfunction.

When poliomyelitis and amputations in otherwise healthy, young persons were the primary causes of gait abnormalities, it was sufficient to memorize a few key action patterns. Now the clinical concerns relate to a far broader scope of pathology. Stroke, spinal cord injury, brain trauma, cerebral palsy, myelodysplasia, muscular dystrophy, geriatric amputation, degenerative joint disease, rheumatoid arthritis, multiple sclerosis, and complex patterns of mixed trauma comprise a representative but not exhaustive list.

Identification of such patients' dysfunction requires an ability to recognize the subtle as well as obvious events and the knowledge of how to interpret the observations. The most convenient sensor is the trained eye of the practicing clinician. This permits assessment of the problem at any time and in any environment. Assessment of the more complex situations, however, necessitates laboratory measurements. They add greater precision, provide information that cannot be obtained by eye and facilitate correlation of multiple factors.

Currently such analysis is time consuming and the data complex. Progress in data integration and advanced instrumentation is making comprehensive examination of the patient's walking ability more available. These gains will permit better management of the difficult patient. Laboratory gait analysis thus provides a consultative service to solve the more difficult problems. Observation remains the basic technique for daily patient management. Each professional involved in the treatment of patients with gait deficits (physicians, physical therapists, orthotists, prosthetists, engineers) must have this skill. In addition, they must know the normal mechanics of walking and the changes that can be induced by pathology.

To meet this complex of needs, a systematic method of gait analysis and interpretation has been devised.[1] Included is a generic terminology that is equally appropriate for normal performance and for the gait of amputees or patients disabled by paralysis, arthritis or trauma. Walking is a complex activity because it is dependent on a series of interactions between two multisegmented lower limbs and total body mass. Significant information about the person's ability to walk, therefore, can be obtained by several different levels of analysis. These include gross body function, reciprocal relationships between the two limbs, interaction of the segments within the limb, and individual joint action.

In analyzing pathological gait, normal function is the model against which disability is judged. Deviations from the normal pattern define the functional error needing correction. Forty-eight gait abnormalities have been identified as common occurrences by the Rancho Los Amigos Pathokinesiology and physical therapy staffs.[1] These errors include all segments from the toes to the trunk and are applicable to all types of pathology.

In this text the basic descriptions of motion and posture will relate to that which is observable. As even a trained eye is unlikely to differentiate changes of less than 5°, this will be the gradient used. In addition to the descriptions of normal and pathological function, a representative group of clinical examples has been included to facilitate the interpretation of the identified gait deviations. A final section will discuss the techniques of instrumented gait analysis and the reference data so obtained.

Reference

1. Pathokinesiology Department, Physical Therapy Department: *Observational Gait Analysis Handbook*. Downey, CA, The Professional Staff Association of Rancho Los Amigos Medical Center, 1989.

About the Author

Preparation for her current interest in gait began in college (UCLA). Her major in physical education (1935-1940) introduced her to anatomy and provided a strong background in kinesiology with application to both sports and corrective therapy for the disabled. Part of this experience was her attendance at the Physical Therapy Clinic of the Los Angeles Children's Hospital where she began her exposure to disability. Subsequently she became a physical therapist (Walter Reed Army Hospital, 1941) which expanded her knowledge of anatomy, kinesiology and disability.

Although her physical therapy experience was in army hospitals during World War II, the clinical exposure was very broad (1941-1945). In addition to working with a regular flow of trauma patients, she spent two years at a center that had army programs for poliomyelitis and rheumatoid arthritis. All three clinical areas involved a great deal of informal observational gait analysis as one sought to improve the patient's ability to walk. During most of this time she was also an instructor at two of the

Army schools of physical therapy (Hot Springs, AR and Denver, CO). There she taught anatomy, kinesiology and therapeutic exercise as well as the modalities. Both normal and disabled gait were strong elements of this program.

After the war ended, she used her GI bill to go to medical school (UC San Francisco, 1946-1950) for the specific purpose of becoming an orthopaedic surgeon. This led her to a residency in orthopaedic surgery (UCSF, 1951-1955) during the period when poliomyelitis and reconstructive surgery were strong clinical programs. Observational gait analysis and experience in correcting disabled gait became daily practice.

Her next move was in 1955 to join the staff of The Rancho Los Amigos Medical Center where she is currently Chief of Pathokinesiology. In 1955, poliomyelitis was the entire program. Disability of lower limbs, spine and arms were all major concerns while bracing and reconstructive surgery received equal emphasis. Working with this program further expanded her knowledge of muscle function and gait disability. Also, her experience in observing polio patients has exposed her to a number of different gait patterns as the type of paralysis resulting from this disease varies from patient to patient.

Following the introduction of the Salk vaccine, polio was conquered so Dr. Perry and her colleagues redirected their attention to other types of chronic impairment. This change was the beginning of their intensive rehabilitation program for spinal cord injury, hemiplegia, arthritis and children's disorders (primarily muscular dystrophy, myelodysplasia and cerebral palsy). Subsequently, amputees became a part of the program. At first the program was for general rehabilitation. Then as the patient groups became large, they formed separate clinical categories with a ward for each (1961). While continuing the polio spine surgery program, Dr. Perry also developed a stroke unit.

Responsibility for persons disabled by a stroke forced her to expand her analysis process as the functional pathology of the hemiplegic is much more complex than that of polio. Because the standard clinical examination findings correlated poorly with the gait dysfunctions, they initiated a system of observational gait analysis. Developed in conjunction with a group of knowledgeable and dedicated physical therapists, the Rancho Los Amigos Observational Gait Analysis System became highly organized. For the first time there was a means of cataloging the multiple dysfunctions that occur with the various types of pathology. For the past 15 plus years, they have taught this program nationwide. It is this program on which the organizational background of this book is based.

A second development was the gait laboratory (1968). Its initial purpose was to document the improvement resulting from reconstructive surgery in patients who could not be returned to normal. This system was designed to help ascertain whether or not surgery actually was the better alternative for these patients. Out of this beginning was developed a functional diagnostic system to be used for planning the reconstructive surgery of spastic patients. The emphasis of the program was, and still is, kinesiology electromyography because the primary disability of spastic patients is inappropriate muscle action (errors in timing and intensity). Footswitches were developed to define the patient's stride characteristics, and an electrogoniometer, that accommodated for braces, was also developed. Clinical service and research have had equal emphasis from the beginning. Another novel emphasis has been on energy cost analysis of walking. An outdoor court was designed where habitual gait could be studied (Dr. Waters spearheaded this). Today, the laboratory is fully equipped with automated motion analysis (Vicon™) and force plates, and force sensing walking aids are being added.

All types of disability have been studied over the years and continue to be seen as the clinical need increases (cerebral palsy, hemiplegia, spinal cord injury, post polios, arthritis, joint replacement, amputees, myelodysplasia, and muscular dystrophy). At the Rancho Los Amigos Medical Center, current gait research is related to the effect of the new "energy storing" prosthetic feet for amputees.

Thus, Dr. Perry continues her lifelong dedication to the research and clinical application of gait. This publication encompasses the extensive work of Dr. Perry and her successful years as a therapist and a surgeon renowned for her expertise in human gait.

Tables

Illustrations

Chapter 15: Clinical Examples

Chapter 16: Gait Analysis Systems

Chapter 17: Motion Analysis

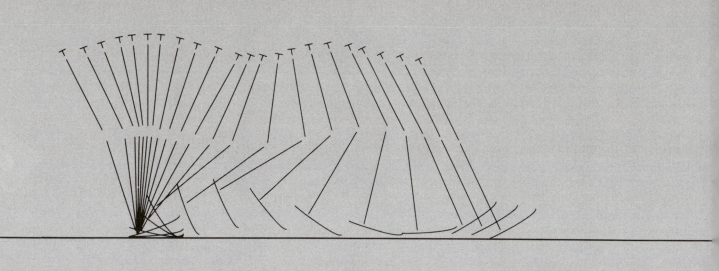

Section One

Fundamentals

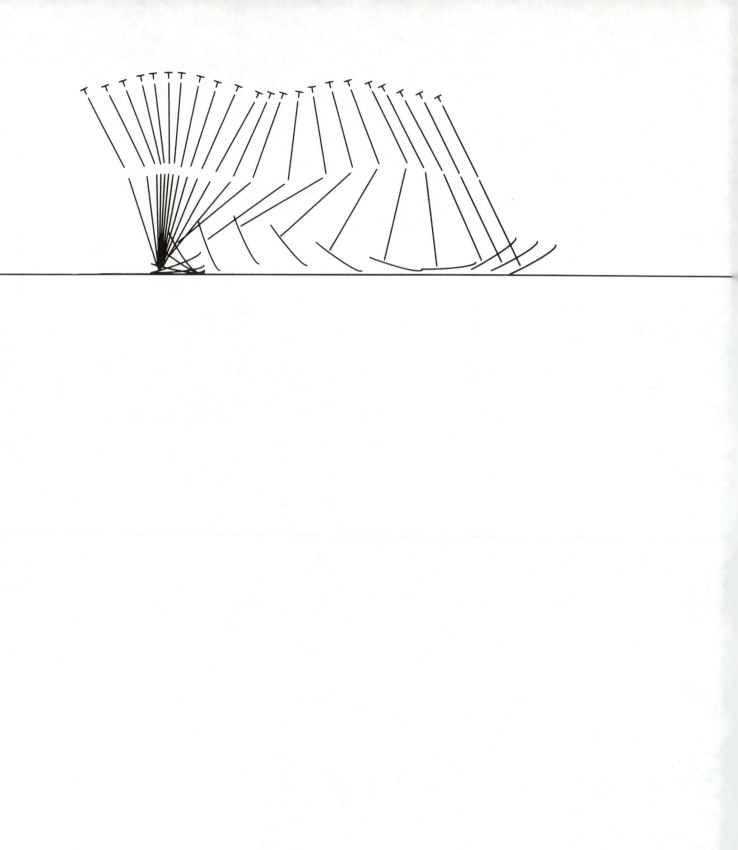

Chapter 1

Gait Cycle

W alking uses a repetitious sequence of limb motion to move the body forward while simultaneously maintaining stance stability. Because each sequence involves a series of interactions between two multisegmented lower limbs and the total body mass, identification of the numerous events that occur necessitates viewing gait from several different aspects. There are three basic approaches. Of these, the simplest system subdivides the cycle according to the variations in reciprocal floor contact by the two feet. A second method uses the time and distance qualities of the stride. The third approach identifies the functional significance of the events within the gait cycle and designates these intervals as the functional phases of gait.

Reciprocal Floor Contact Patterns

As the body moves forward, one limb serves as a mobile source of support while the other limb advances itself to a new support site. Then the limbs reverse their roles. For the transfer of body weight from one limb to the other, both feet are in contact with the ground. This series of events is repeated by each limb with reciprocal timing until the person's destination is reached.

A single sequence of these functions by one limb is called a *gait cycle* (GC).[3] With one action flowing smoothly into the next, there is no specific starting or ending point. Hence, any event could be selected as the onset of the gait cycle. Because the moment of floor contact is the most readily defined event, this action generally has been selected as the start of the gait cycle. Normal persons initiate floor contact with their heel (i.e., heel strike). As not all patients have this capability, the generic term *initial contact* (IC) will be used to designate the onset of the gait cycle.[5]

Cycle Divisions

Each gait cycle is divided into two periods, stance and swing. These often are called gait phases. In this book the phases will identify the functional subdivisions of total limb activity within the gait cycle.

Stance is the term used to designate the entire period during which the foot is on the ground. Stance begins with initial contact (Figure 1.1). The word *swing* applies to the time the foot is in the air for limb advancement. Swing begins as the foot is lifted from the floor (toe-off).

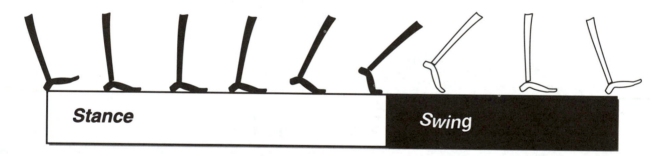

Figure 1.1 Divisions of the gait cycle. Clear bar represents the duration of stance. Shaded bar is the duration of swing. Limb segments show the onset of stance with initial contact, end of stance by roll-off of the toes, and end of swing by floor contact again.

Stance is subdivided into three intervals according to the sequence of floor contact by the two feet (Figure 1.2). Both the start and end of stance involve a period of bilateral foot contact with the floor (*double stance*), while the middle portion of stance has one foot contact (Figure 1.2).

Initial double stance begins the gait cycle. It is the time both feet are on the floor after initial contact. An alternate term is double limb support. This designation is to be avoided, however, as it implies an equal sharing of body weight by the two feet, which is not true during most of the double stance interval.

Single limb support begins when the opposite foot is lifted for swing. In keeping with the terminology for the double contact periods, this should be (and often is) called *single stance*. To emphasize the functional significance of

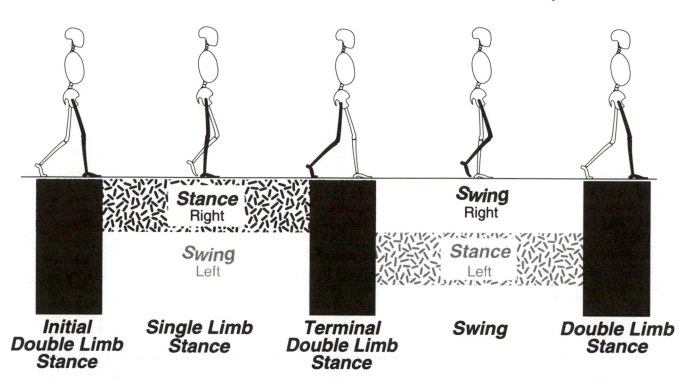

Figure 1.2 The subdivisions of stance and their relationship to the bilateral floor contact pattern. Vertical dark bars are the periods of double limb stance (right and left feet). Horizontal shaded bar is single limb support (single stance). Total stance includes three intervals: the initial double stance, single limb support and the next (terminal) double stance. Swing is the clear bar that follows terminal double stance. Note that right single limb support is the same time interval as left swing. During right swing there is left single limb support. The third vertical bar (double stance) begins the next gait cycle.

floor contact by just one foot, the term *support* is preferred. During the single limb support interval the body's entire weight is resting on that one extremity. The duration of single stance is the best index of the limb's support capability.

Terminal double stance is the third subdivision. It begins with floor contact by the other foot (contralateral initial contact) and continues until the original stance limb is lifted for swing (ipsilateral toe-off). The term terminal double limb support has been avoided, as weight bearing is very asymmetrical.

Timing. The gross normal distribution of the floor contact periods is 60% for stance and 40% for swing[3] (Table 1.1). Timing for the phases of stance is 10% for each double stance interval and 40% for single limb support. Note that single limb support of one limb equals swing of the other, as they are occurring at the same time (Figure 1.2).

The precise duration of these gait cycle intervals varies with the person's walking velocity.[1,4] At the customary 80m/min rate of walking, the stance and swing periods represent 62% and 38% of the gait cycle respectively. The duration of both gait periods shows an inverse relationship to walking speed. That is, both total stance and swing times are shortened as gait velocity increases. The change in stance and swing times becomes progressively greater

Table 1.1

Floor Contact Periods

Stance		60%
Initial Double Stance	10%	
Single Limb Support	40%	
Terminal Double Stance	10%	
Swing		40%

as speed slows. Among the subdivisions of stance a different relationship exits. Walking faster proportionally lengthens single stance and shortens the two double stance intervals.[4] The reverse is true as the person's walking speed slows. This pattern of change also is curvilinear.

Having an interval when both feet are in contact with the ground for the limbs to exchange their support roles is a basic characteristic of walking. When double stance is omitted, the person has entered the running mode of locomotion.[2]

Stride and Step

The gait cycle also has been identified by the descriptive term *stride*.[3] Occasionally the word *step* is used, but this is inappropriate (Figure 1.3).

Stride is the equivalent of a gait cycle. It is based on the actions of one limb.

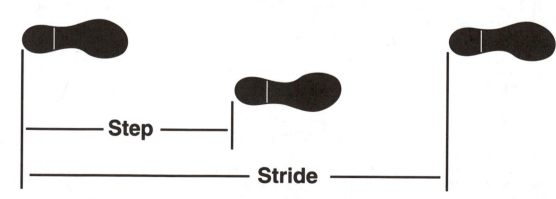

Figure 1.3 A step versus a stride. Step length is the interval between initial contact of each foot. Stride length continues until there is a second contact by the same foot.

The duration of a stride is the interval between two sequential initial floor contacts by the same limb (i.e., right IC and the next right IC).

Step refers to the timing between the two limbs. There are two steps in each stride (or gait cycle). At the midpoint of one stride the other foot contacts the ground to begin its next stance period. The interval between an initial contact by each foot is a step (i.e., left and then right). The same offset in timing will be repeated in reciprocal fashion throughout the walk.

References

1. Andriacchi TP, Ogle JA, Galante JO: Walking speed as a basis for normal and abnormal gait measurements. *J Biomech* 10(4):261-268, 1977.
2. Mann R: Biomechanics. In Jahss MH (Ed): *Disorders of the Foot.* Philadelphia, W. B. Saunders Company, 1982, pp. 37-67.
3. Murray MP, Drought AB, Kory RC: Walking patterns of normal men. *J Bone Joint Surg* 46A(2):335-360, 1964.
4. Otis JC, Burstein AH: Evaluation of the VA-Rancho gait analyzer, Mark I. *Bull Prosthet Res* 18(1):21-25, 1981.
5. Pathokinesiology Department, Physical Therapy Department: *Observational Gait Analysis Handbook.* Downey, CA, The Professional Staff Association of Rancho Los Amigos Medical Center, 1989.

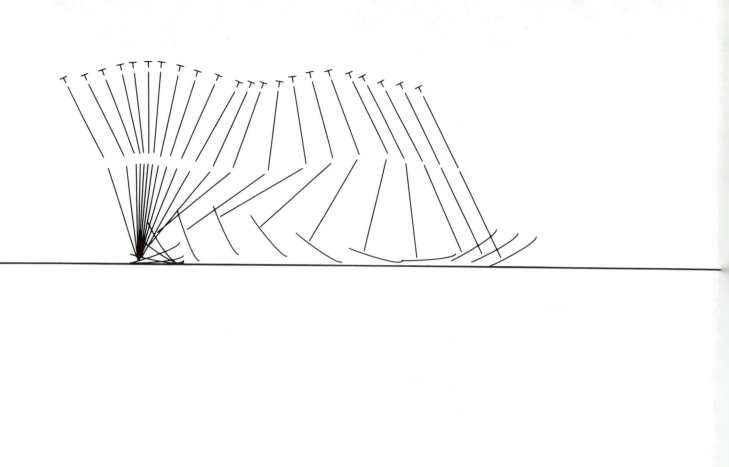

Chapter 2

Phases of Gait

In order to provide the basic functions required for walking, each stride involves an ever-changing alignment between the body and the supporting foot during stance and selective advancement of the limb segments in swing. These reactions result in a series of motion patterns performed by the hip, knee and ankle. Early in the development of gait analysis the investigators recognized that each pattern of motion related to a different functional demand and designated them as the phases of gait. Further experience in correlating the data has progressively expanded the number of gait phases identified. It now is evident that each stride contains eight functional patterns. Technically these are sub phases, as the basic divisions of the gait cycle are stance and swing, but common practice also calls the functional intervals *phases*.

In the past it has been the custom to use normal events as the critical actions separating the phases. While this practice proved appropriate for the amputee, it often failed to accommodate the gait deviations of patients impaired by paralysis or arthritis. For example, the onset of stance customarily has been called *heel strike;* yet the heel of a paralytic patient may never contact the ground or do so much later in the gait cycle. Similarly initial floor contact may be by the whole foot (*foot flat*), rather than having forefoot contact occur later, after a period of heel-only support. To avoid these difficulties and other areas of confusion, the Rancho Los Amigos gait analysis committee developed a generic terminology for the functional phases of gait.[1]

Analysis of a person's walking pattern by phases more directly identifies the functional significance of the different motions occurring at the individual joints. The phases of gait also provide a means for correlating the simultaneous actions of the individual joints into patterns of total limb function. This is a particularly important approach for interpreting the functional effects of disability. The relative significance of one joint's motion compared to the other's varies among the gait phases. Also, a posture that is appropriate in one gait phase would signify dysfunction at another point in the stride, because the functional need has changed. As a result, both timing and joint angle are very significant. This latter fact adds to the complexities of gait analysis.

Each of the eight gait phases has a functional objective and a critical pattern of selective synergistic motion to accomplish this goal. The sequential combination of the phases also enables the limb to accomplish three basic tasks. These are weight acceptance (WA), single limb support (SLS) and limb advancement (LA) (Table 2.1). Weight acceptance begins the stance period and uses the first

Table 2.1

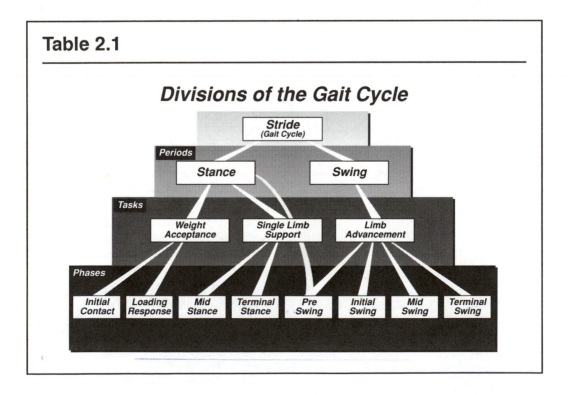

Divisions of the Gait Cycle

two gait phases (initial contact and loading response). Single limb support continues stance with the next two phases of gait (mid stance and terminal stance). Limb advancement begins in the final phase of stance (pre-swing) and then continues through the three phases of swing (initial swing, midswing and terminal swing).

Task A: Weight Acceptance

This is the most demanding task in the gait cycle. Three functional patterns are needed: shock absorption, initial limb stability and the preservation of progression. The challenge is the abrupt transfer of body weight onto a limb that has just finished swinging forward and has an unstable alignment. Two gait Phases are involved, initial contact and loading response (Table 2.1).

Phase 1—Initial Contact

Interval: 0-2% GC
> This phase includes the moment when the foot just touches the floor (Figure 2.1). The joint postures present at this time determine the limb's loading response pattern.

Objective:
> The limb is positioned to start stance with a heel rocker.

Phase 2—Loading Response

Interval: 0-10% GC
> This is the initial double stance period (Figure 2.2). The phase begins with initial floor contact and continues until the other foot is lifted for swing.

Objectives:
> Shock absorption
> Weight-bearing stability
> Preservation of progression

Task B: Single Limb Support

Lifting the other foot for swing begins the single limb support interval for the stance limb. This continues until the opposite foot again contacts the floor. During the resulting interval, one limb has the total responsibility for supporting body weight in both the sagittal and coronal planes while progression must be continued. Two phases are involved in single limb support: mid stance and terminal stance. They are differentiated primarily by their mechanisms of progression.

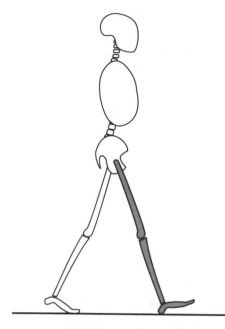

Initial Contact

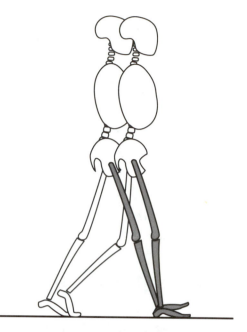

Loading Response

Figure 2.1 Initial Contact. The hip is flexed, the knee is extended, the ankle is dorsiflexed to neutral. Floor contact is made with the heel. Shading indicates the reference limb. The other limb (clear) is at the end of terminal stance.

Figure 2.2 Loading Response. Body weight is transferred onto the forward limb (shaded). Using the heel as a rocker, the knee is flexed for shock absorption. Ankle plantar flexion limits the heel rocker by forefoot contact with the floor. The opposite limb (clear) is in its pre-swing phase.

Phase 3—Mid Stance

Interval: 10-30% GC

This is the first half of the single limb support interval (Figure 2.3). It begins as the other foot is lifted and continues until body weight is aligned over the forefoot.

Objectives:

Progression over the stationary foot

Limb and trunk stability

Phase 4—Terminal Stance

Interval: 30-50% GC

This phase completes single limb support (Figure 2.4). It begins with heel rise and continues until the other foot strikes the ground. Throughout this phase body weight moves ahead of the forefoot.

Objective:

Progression of the body beyond the supporting foot

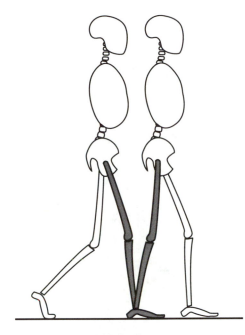

Mid Stance

Figure 2.3 Mid Stance. In the first half of single limb support, the limb (shaded) advances over the stationary foot by ankle dorsiflexion (ankle rocker) while the knee and hip extend. The opposite limb (clear) is advancing in its mid swing phase.

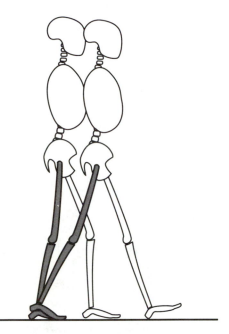

Terminal Stance

Figure 2.4 Terminal Stance. During the second half of single limb support, the heel rises and the limb (shaded) advances over the forefoot rocker. The knee increases its extension and then just begins to flex slightly. Increased hip extension puts the limb in a more trailing position. The other limb (clear) is in terminal swing.

Task C: Limb Advancement

To meet the high demands of advancing the limb, preparatory posturing begins in stance. Then the limb swings through three postures as it lifts itself, advances and prepares for the next stance interval. Four gait phases are involved: pre-swing (end of stance), initial swing, mid swing and terminal swing.

Phase 5—Pre-Swing

Interval: 50-60% GC

> This final phase of stance is the second (terminal) double stance interval in the gait cycle (Figure 2.5). It begins with initial contact of the opposite limb and ends with ipsilateral toe-off.
>
> *Weight release* and *weight transfer* are other titles some investigators give to this phase. While the abrupt transfer of body weight promptly unloads the limb, this extremity makes no active contribution to the event.
>
> Instead, the unloaded limb uses its freedom to prepare for the rapid demands of swing. All the motions and muscle actions occurring at this

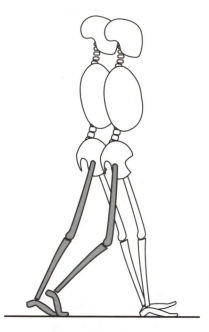

Pre-Swing

Figure 2.5 Pre-Swing. Floor contact by the other limb (clear) has started terminal double support. The reference limb (shaded) responds with increased ankle plantar flexion, greater knee flexion and loss of hip extension. The opposite (clear) limb is in Loading Response.

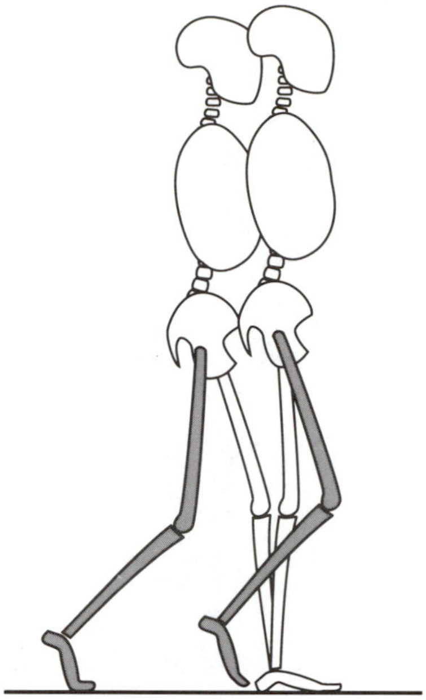

Initial Swing

Figure 2.6 Initial Swing. The foot is lifted and limb advanced by hip flexion and increased knee flexion. The ankle only partially dorsiflexes. The other limb (clear) is in early mid stance.

time relate to this latter task. Hence, the term *pre-swing* is more representative of its functional commitment.

Objective:

Position the limb for swing

Phase 6—Initial Swing

Interval: 60-73% GC

This first phase is approximately one-third of the swing period (Figure 2.6). It begins with lift of the foot from the floor and ends when the swinging foot is opposite the stance foot.

Objectives:

Foot clearance of the floor

Advancement of the limb from its trailing position

Phase 7—Mid Swing

Interval: 73-87% GC

This second phase of the swing period begins as the swinging limb is opposite the stance limb (Figure 2.7). The phase ends when the swinging limb is forward and the tibia is vertical (i.e., hip and knee flexion postures are equal).

Objectives:

Limb advancement

Foot clearance from the floor

Phase 8—Terminal Swing

Interval: 87-100% GC

This final phase of swing begins with a vertical tibia and ends when the foot strikes the floor (Figure 2.8). Limb advancement is completed as the leg (shank) moves ahead of the thigh.

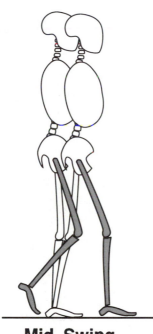

Mid Swing

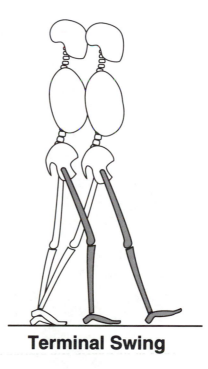

Terminal Swing

Figure 2.7 Mid Swing. Advancement of the limb (shaded) anterior to the body weight line is gained by further hip flexion. The knee is allowed to extend in response to gravity while the ankle continues dorsiflexing to neutral. The other limb (clear) is in late mid stance.

Figure 2.8 Terminal Swing. Limb advancement is completed by knee extension. The hip maintains its earlier flexion, and the ankle remains dorsiflexed to neutral. The other limb (clear) is in terminal stance.

Objectives:
  Complete limb advancement
  Prepare the limb for stance

Reference

1. Pathokinesiology Department, Physical Therapy Department: *Observational Gait Analysis Handbook*. Downey, CA, The Professional Staff Association of Rancho Los Amigos Medical Center, 1989.

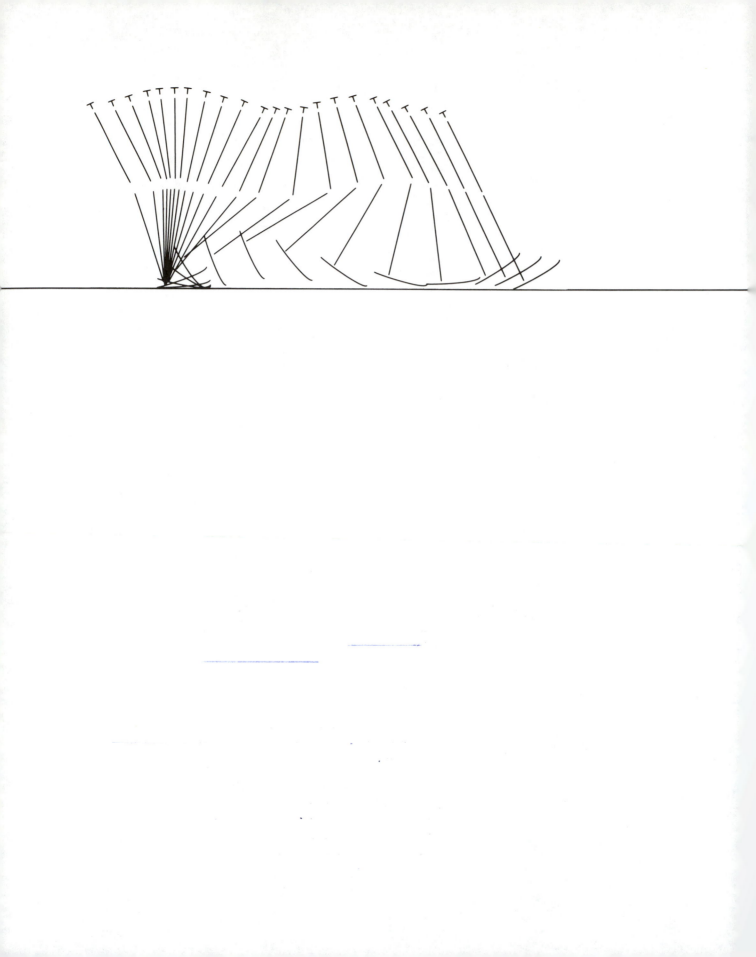

Chapter 3

Basic Functions

W alking forward on level ground is the basic locomotor pattern. A change in direction increases the requirements. Stairs and rough terrain further the demand. Running and the various sports present even greater needs. Despite these variations in complexity, there are underlying functional patterns common to all.

Body Subdivisions

During walking the body functionally divides itself into two units, passenger and locomotor (Figure 3.1). While there is motion and muscle action occurring in each, the relative intensity of these functions is markedly different in the two units. Basically, the passenger unit is responsible only for its own postural integrity. Normal gait mechanics are so efficient that the demands on the passenger unit are reduced to a minimum, making it virtually a passive entity that is carried by the locomotor system. Alignment of the passenger unit over the limbs, however, is a major determinant of muscle action within the locomotor system.

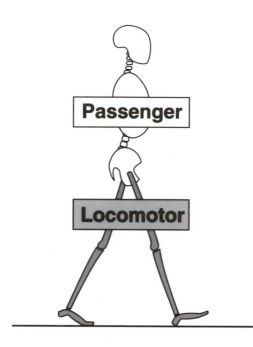

Figure 3.1 Functional division of the body. During walking, the upper body is a relatively passive passenger unit that rides on a loco- motor system.

Passenger Unit

The head, neck, trunk and arms are grouped as a passenger unit, because they are carried rather than directly contributing to the act of walking. Elftman introduced the term *HAT* to represent this mass, that is, a structure on top of the locomotor apparatus.[7]

Muscle action within the neck and trunk serves only to maintain neutral vertebral alignment with minimal postural change occurring during normal gait. Arm swing involves both passive and active elements, but the action does not appear essential to the normal gait pattern. Experimental restraint of the arms registered no measurable change in the energy cost of walking.[19]

The structures comprising the HAT form a large and heavy mass that represents 70% of body weight (Figure 3.2a).[6] Within this composite mass, the center of gravity (C/G) is located just anterior to the tenth thoracic vertebra.[10] This presents a long lever that is 33cm (12in) above the level of the hip joints in an average height man (184cm) (Figure 3.2b).[6] As a result, balance of the passenger unit is very dependent upon the instantaneous alignment of the lower limbs to move the base of support under the HAT's momentary center of gravity.

Locomotor Unit

The two lower limbs and pelvis are the anatomical segments that form the locomotor system. Eleven articulations are involved: lumbosacral, bilateral hip, knee, ankle, subtalar, and metatarsophalangeal joints (Figure 3.3). Timeliness

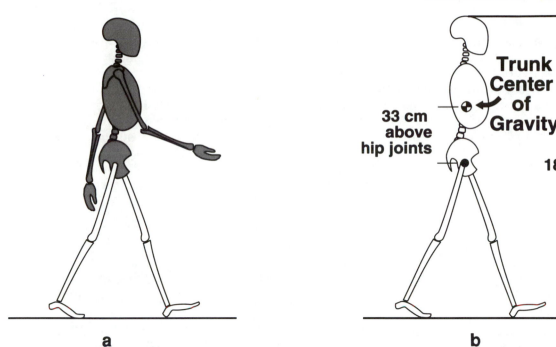

a   **b**

Figure 3.2 The passenger unit. (a) Components are the head, neck, arms, trunk and pelvis. This is called the *HAT* unit. (b) The center of gravity of the HAT lies just anterior to the tenth thoracic vertebra (T_{10}). In a man of average height (184cm) this point is 33cm above the hip joint.

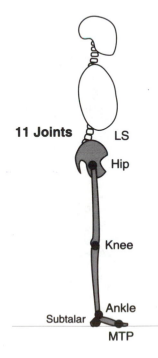

Figure 3.3 The locomotor system includes the pelvis and both lower extremities. This means the pelvis is dually considered a part of the passenger unit and the locomotor system. Between the base of the spine and the toes, 11 joints are involved (lumbosacral and both hips, knees, ankles, subtalars, and metatarsophalangeal groups).

and magnitude of motion in each limb is controlled by 57 muscles acting in a selective fashion. The bony segments (pelvis, thigh, shank, foot and toes) serve as levers.

As a multisegmented unit, each limb alternately assumes the responsibility to support the passenger unit in a manner that also carries it forward (Figure 3.4). Then, after being relieved of body weight, the limb rapidly swings itself forward to a new position and prepares to provide progressional support again (Figure 3.5).

The pelvis has a dual role. As part of the locomotor system it is a mobile link between the two lower limbs (Figure 3.6). In addition, the pelvis serves as the bottom segment of the passenger unit that rides on the hip joints.

Locomotor Functions

As the locomotor unit carries the body to its desired location each weight-bearing limb accomplishes four distinct functions. (1) A propulsive force is generated. (2) Upright stability is maintained, despite an ever-changing posture. (3) The shock of floor impact at the onset of each stride is minimized. (4) Energy is conserved by these functions being performed in a manner that reduces the amount of muscular effort required (Table 3.1). The accomplishment of each function depends on a distinct motion pattern. Each represents a complex series of interactions between the body mass and the two multisegmented lower limbs. During walking these blend into a single, three-dimensional pattern.

Standing Stability

Stability in the upright position is determined by the functional balance between the alignment of the body and muscle activity at each joint. Each body segment is a weight that will fall toward the ground (through the pull of gravity) unless it is restrained. Within each segment there is a point, the center

---

Table 3.1

Locomotor Functions

Propulsion
Stance Stability
Shock Absorption
Energy Conservation

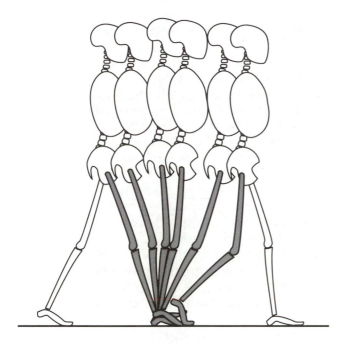

Figure 3.4 During stance, the supporting limb (shaded) provides an advancing base that rolls forward over the foot.

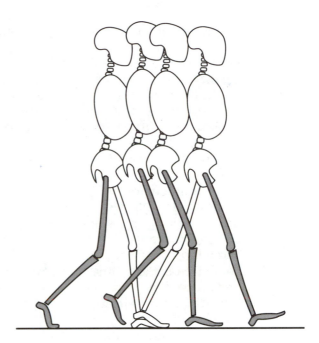

Figure 3.5 During swing, the limb (shaded) advances itself to its next position for weight acceptance.

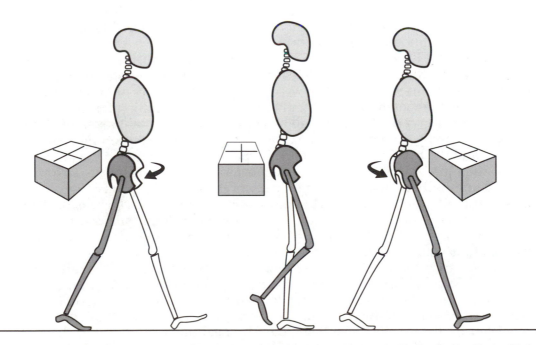

Figure 3.6 Pelvic mobility: Rotation of the pelvis with the swing limb adds to step length. The boxes identify the relation of the pelvis to the reference limb (terminal stance, mid swing, terminal swing).

of gravity (C/G), that is representative of the weight of that mass. There is passive stability when the C/G of the upper segment is aligned directly over the center of the supporting joint. The security of this position depends on the quality of the supporting surface and the nature of any external forces.

In the body three anatomical situations challenge standing stability. First is the top-heavy relationship between the passenger unit and the locomotor system. Seventy percent (70%) of body weight is resting on a support system that represents only 30% of the body mass. Second is the multisegmented nature of the supporting limbs. The third factor is the contours of the lower limb joints.

Alignment of body weight is the dominant factor. During standing and walking the effect of body weight is identified by the ground reaction force vector (GRFV) or *body vector* (Figure 3.7). That is, as body weight falls toward the floor, it creates a force in the floor of equal magnitude but opposite in direction. This can be captured by appropriate instrumentation and represented as a mean line, the *body vector.* By relating the alignment of the body vector to the joint centers, the magnitude and direction of instability are defined. This indicates the muscle and ligament forces required to establish stability.

The ligamentous skeleton is built for mobility rather than stability. The bones are long and the joint surfaces rounded. Hence, controlling forces are required. If the limb segments were shaped like a cube, force demand would be minimal. The supporting surfaces would be broad and flat and mass center low (Figure 3.8). Stability would be maximal, as the upper segment must tilt more than 45° before its weight line passes beyond that of the supporting base and balance is lost. With less tilt, the mass of the cube would fall back to its usual resting position once the displacing force was relaxed. The normal long, slender shape of the femur and tibia reduces the theoretical tolerance for tilt to less than 9° (Figure 3.9). Even this margin of stability is not available in the normal skeleton, as the rounded joint surfaces of all the bones offer no stabilizing edges (Figure 3.10). Consequently, whenever the segments' centers of gravity are not in line, the upper segment will fall, unless there are controlling forces.

Three forces act on the joints: falling body weight, ligamentous tension and muscular activity. The hip and knee can use a balance between ligamentous tension and the body vector as a source of passive stability when the joints are hyperextended. At the knee there is the posterior oblique ligament. The hip is limited anteriorly by the iliofemoral ligament (Figure 3.11). Hyperextension of these joints allows the body weight line to pass anterior to the center of the knee (and posterior to the hip) joint axis. In this position the joints are locked by two opposing forces: the body weight vector on one side of the joint and ligamentous tension on the other.

At the ankle there is no similar source of passive stability. The ankle and subtalar joints each have a significant range of motion beyond neutral in both directions. Also, the ankle joint is not located at the middle of the foot. It is far closer to the heel than the metatarsal heads (Figure 3.12). Heel length is further restricted by the support area being the calcaneal tuberosities rather than the posterior tip of this bone. The apex of these rounded tuberosities is almost in line with the posterior margin of the ankle joint. Hence, the margin for security

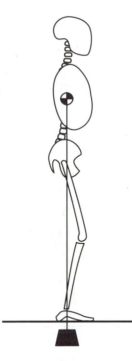

Figure 3.7 Body weight vector: The mean instantaneous alignment of body weight (vertical line) is the sum of the ground reaction forces (GRF) sensed by the force plate (floor weight). The height of the vector is proportional to the magnitude of the GRF. Because the HAT, as the largest body mass, tends to dominate vector alignment, it is customary to locate the 100% body weight at the HAT center of gravity (circle).

is minimal (about 1cm). Anteriorly the mid- and forefoot extend the foot lever to the metatarsal heads, thus providing a much longer segment (about 10cm). The midpoint between the calcaneal tuberosities and metatarsal heads would lie about 5cm anterior to the transverse axis of the ankle. To place the body vector over this spot requires ankle dorsiflexion (5°) accompanied by soleus muscle activity to restrain the forward aligned tibia.

Quiet Standing. With the body erect and weight evenly distributed between

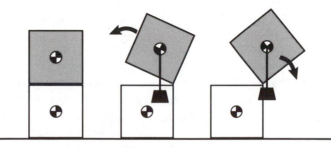

Figure 3.8 Square blocks offer a broad base and low position for the center of gravity (C/G). This allows a large tilt (45°) before an unstable alignment is created by the C/G moving beyond the supporting base.

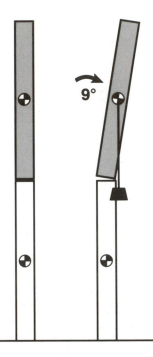

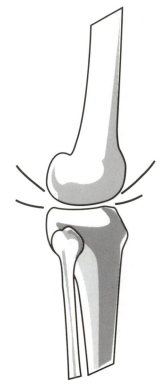

Figure 3.9 Tall rods provide a narrow base and a relatively high center of gravity (C/G). Tilting of just 9° moved the C/G beyond the bases of support, creating an unstable alignment.

Figure 3.10 The rounded surfaces of joint further narrow the width of the base as the margins are curved.

the two feet, the demands for muscle action are minimal, as there is no progression, that is, gait velocity is zero. In theory quiet standing balance can be attained without any muscle action. This necessitates aligning the center of the passenger unit (anterior margin of the eleventh thoracic vertebra) exactly over the axis of the hip, knee, ankle and subtalar joints. Stability, however, is lacking, as none of the joints are locked. Consequently, the slightest sway can unbalance every segment. Even the force of a heart beat might be sufficient.

During quiet standing, balance beam measurements showed the body vector extends downward from the center of the head (ear canal), passes 1cm anterior to the L_4 vertebral body and rests in the foot 1.5 to 5cm anterior to the ankle (Figure 3.13).[2,3] Force plate measurements show 5cm anterior to the ankle axis to be the mean posture.[1,17] The standard deviations of 2cm also confirm considerable variability in the resting location of the center of pressure. Variations in mobility of the ankle and knee, as well as relative strength of the gastrosoleus muscle groups, would determine the different alignments.

With knee extension limited to zero, stable alignment of the body vector requires ankle dorsiflexion. Persons having a range of knee hyperextension can

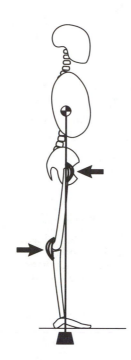

Figure 3.11 During quiet standing, passive stability at the hip and knee is gained by hyperextension. The stabilizing forces are ligamentous tension on one side and the vector on the opposite side of the joint. The ankle lacks passive stability.

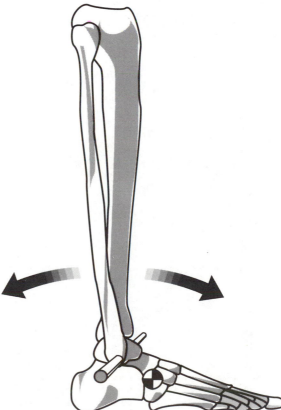

Figure 3.12 The ankle joint is located posterior to the center of the foot (C/G marker). Hence, the heel lever is much shorter than the forefoot lever, which extends to the metatarsal heads.

attain similar balance while the ankle is in neutral or slightly plantar flexed. The normal "easy standing" position uses only a minimal margin of stability, with the body's center of gravity being just 0.6cm posterior to the hip joint axis and anterior to the knee (Figure 3.13).

In the coronal plane the width of the foot support area is determined by the distance between the lateral margins of the feet. The usual 7° of toeing-out by each foot makes the anterior (metatarsal) area wider than that provided by the heels. Mean distance between the centers of the feet averages 3 inches.[15,16]

Equal sharing of body weight would place the body vector through the center of the support area. In reality, the normal quiet standing posture tends to be shifted slightly to the right of midline (0.6cm) (Figure 3.14).[1,17] The average differences in weight bearing by the two limbs have varied with the technic of analysis. Paired scales showed a mean 5.4kg difference, reaching 12.2kg at the 95% confidence level. In contrast, force plate measurements registered a 0.8kg difference in vertical force.

Recordings of postural sway reveal that quiet standing is not totally stationary. In both planes (sagittal and coronal) there is a slow, but continual, shifting of body weight between the two limbs.[16] The rate was four to six cycles per second[17] and the arc small, 5mm laterally and 8mm anteriorly.[7] Two mechanisms contribute to this subtle body instability: cardiac dynamics and the lack of absolute proprioception.[8,17] Normal persons also can use 54% of the length (sagittal plane) and 59% of the width (coronal plane) for voluntary postural deviations and still maintain upright stability.[17] This can be considered a measure of postural versatility.

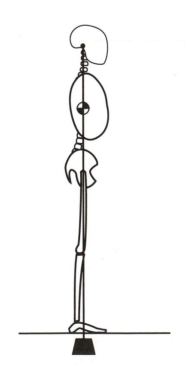

Figure 3.13 During quiet standing, balanced alignment aligns the body weight vector between the ear canal in the head and anterior to the ankle (near the middle of the supporting foot). It passes slightly anterior to the thoracic spine, just anterior to the knee and barely posterior to the hip joint.

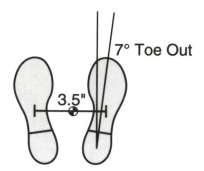

Figure 3.14 During quiet standing, the feet are approximately 3.5 inches apart and toed-out 7°.

Limb posture during quiet standing is similar to that used in mid stance. Hence, the person's ability to stand is a preliminary test of his or her ability to walk. The alignment needed is a functional balance of proprioception, joint mobility and muscle control.

Dynamic Stability. During walking, the body moves from behind to ahead of the supporting foot. At the same time the area of support changes from the heel to flat foot and then the forefoot. These two variables mean that the body lacks passive stability throughout stance. Only in the midpoint of the stance period does body alignment approximate that of a stable quiet standing posture (Figure 3.13).

As the limb is loaded at the beginning of stance, the foot is ahead of the trunk. This places the body vector anterior to the hip and posterior to the knee (Figure 3.15a). A flexion torque is created at both joints, necessitating active extensor muscle response to restrain the fall of body weight. During mid stance the body advances to a position over the supporting foot (Figure 3.15b). This reduces the flexion torques to zero. Continued advancement of the body over the supporting foot gradually introduces passive extension at the hip and knee. At the same time body weight moves ahead of the ankle and thus introduces a new area of postural instability. Now active control by the plantar flexor muscles is needed to restrain the forward fall of body weight (Figure 3.15c). Thus, throughout stance, muscle action is directed toward decelerating the influences of gravity and momentum that create flexion torques at the hip and knee and dorsiflexion torques at the ankle, all of which threaten standing stability.

Faster walking speeds increase the demands on the decelerating muscles, as the body vector becomes greater with acceleration. Conversely, within a limited range, the required intensity of muscular activity can be reduced by walking more slowly. The limitation in this saving is the need for sufficient gait velocity to preserve the advantages of momentum, which is used as a substitute for direct extensor muscle action. An analysis of ankle muscle action demonstrated that during free walking (80m/min) the average intensity of muscle activity was equivalent to grade 3 by manual muscle testing. Fast walking (116m/min) increased the intensity of muscle action to 3+. Walking slowly (60m/min) reduced

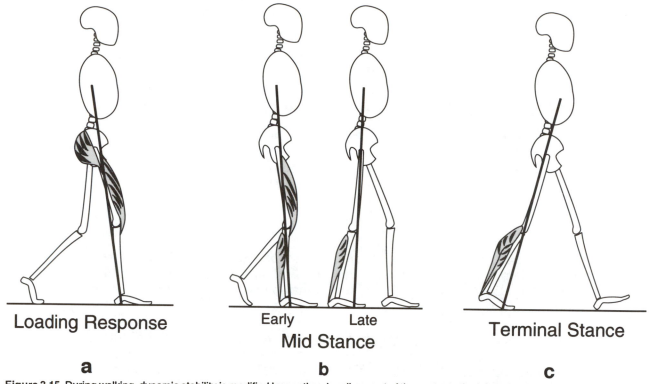

Loading Response

a

Early   Late
Mid Stance

b

Terminal Stance

c

Figure 3.15 During walking, dynamic stability is modified by continual realignment of the vector to the joints. Loading Response: the vector is anterior to the hip and posterior to the knee and ankle. Mid Stance: At the onset of this phase (early) the body weight vector is slightly behind the knee but anterior to the ankle. By the end of the phase (late) the vector has moved forward of the ankle and the knee. At the hip the vector has moved posteriorly. Terminal Stance: The vector is posterior to the hip, anterior to the knee and maximally forward of the ankle.

the effort to grade 3-.[18] By Beasley's quantitated scales, the strength used would be 15%, 40% and 5% of normal.[5]

Single Limb Support. When both feet are in contact with the ground, the trunk is supported on either side (Figure 3.16). As one foot is lifted for swing, this balance is lost abruptly.

Now the center of the HAT is aligned medial to the supporting limb, and the connecting link is a highly mobile hip joint. Two preparatory actions are essential to preserve standing balance over a single limb. These are lateral shift of the body mass and local muscular stabilization of the hip joint to keep the pelvis and trunk erect (Figure 3.17).

During quiet standing the lateral shift places the center of the trunk over the foot. Both foot and knee valgus are used. For walking, less stability is sought since the swinging limb will be prepared to catch the falling body at the onset of the next step and knee valgus is less.

Progression

The basic objective of the locomotor system is to move the body forward from the current site to a new location so the hands and head can perform their

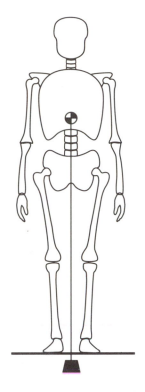

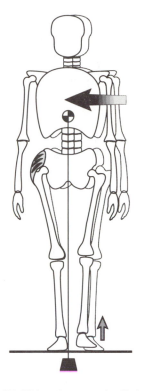

Figure 3.16 In the coronal plane, during quiet standing the body vector (weight line) passes through the middle of the pelvis and between the two feet.

Figure 3.17 Lifting the opposite limb for a step removes the support for that side. Instability is avoided by a shift of the body vector toward the stance limb and strong contraction of the hip abductors to support the unstable pelvis.

numerous functions.

To accomplish this objective of the locomotor system, forward fall of body weight is used as the primary propelling force (Figure 3.18). Mobility at the base of the supporting limb is a critical factor in the freedom to fall forward. Throughout stance, momentum is preserved by a pivotal system created by the foot and ankle. In serial fashion the heel, ankle and forefoot serve as rockers that allow the body to advance while the knee maintains a basically extended posture (Figure 3.19). Progression occurs because the ankle muscles yield as well as restrain the joint.

Forward swing of the contralateral limb provides a second pulling force (Figure 3.20). This force is generated by accelerated advancement of the limb and its anterior alignment. The sum of these actions provides a propelling force at the time residual momentum in the stance limb is decreasing. It is particularly critical in mid stance to advance the body vector past the vertical and again create a forward fall position.

At the end of the step the falling body weight is caught by the contralateral swing limb, which by now has moved forward to assume a stance role. In this

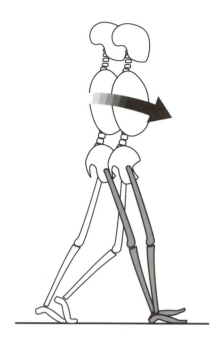

Figure 3.18 For progression, forward fall of body weight (arrow) is the primary force.

manner a cycle of progression is initiated that is serially perpetuated by reciprocal action of the two limbs.

The Initial Step. From a quiet standing posture with weight on both feet, three actions are used to begin walking. The sequence starts with a brief shift of body weight (6% of stance width) toward the limb to be lifted.[1,12] Presumably, this assesses the mass that is to be balanced. Then all weight is transferred laterally to the continuing stance limb. Lastly, weight moves forward on the stance limb as the body is allowed to fall forward and the swing foot is lifted (Figure 3.21).

Ankle control of the supporting limb is modified to allow the forward fall.[12] The exact action pattern depends on the persons's quiet standing position (Figure 3.22). From the common stance posture of slight ankle dorsiflexion, the soleus merely reduces its holding force and the tibia increases its forward tilt. Body weight follows the change in limb alignment.

When the person stands with a hyperextended knee and the ankle is slightly plantar flexed, the pretibial muscles (tibialis anterior and long toe extensors) contract to actively pull the tibia forward. Once the vertical axis has been passed, the limb is in a position to fall passively under soleus control in the usual manner. Hence, regardless of the initial standing posture of the limb, initiation of a step begins with a shift in body weight and anterior displacement at the ankle of the supporting limb. Lifting the swing limb uses the change in body posture for the propulsion. Hip flexion and ankle dorsiflexion lift the swing limb, creating an anterior force that further disturbs standing balance. A more rapid hip flexion adds acceleration that augments the effect.[13,14]

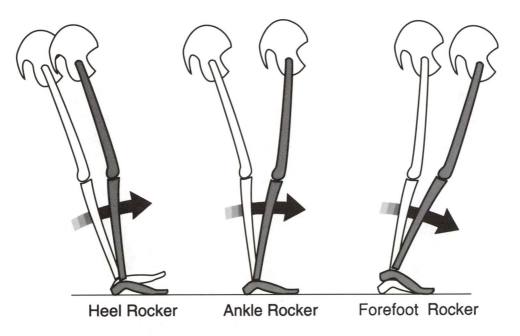

Heel Rocker   **Ankle Rocker**   **Forefoot Rocker**

Figure 3.19 Progression (arrow) over the supporting foot is assisted by the actions of three functional rockers: (1) heel rocker, (2) ankle rocker, (3) forefoot rocker.

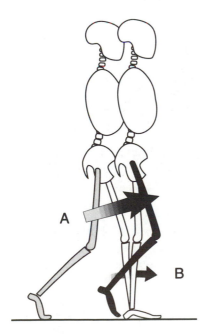

Figure 3.20 A progressional force (arrow) also is provided by the swinging limb (shaded; light to dark).

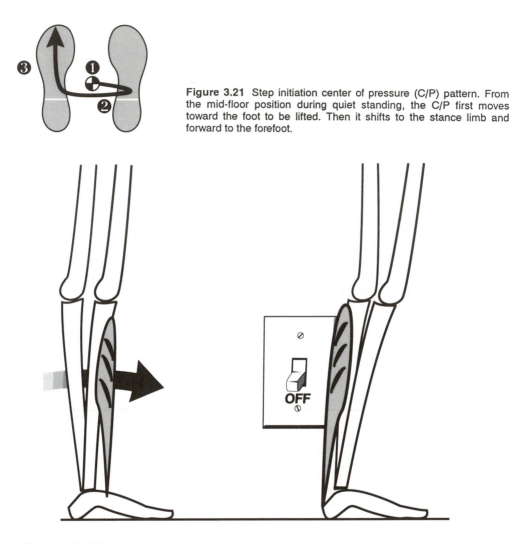

Figure 3.21 Step initiation center of pressure (C/P) pattern. From the mid-floor position during quiet standing, the C/P first moves toward the foot to be lifted. Then it shifts to the stance limb and forward to the forefoot.

Figure 3.22 Tibial posture in quiet standing determines the initial ankle muscle action. With the tibia back and the knee relatively hyperextended, the tibialis anterior (and other pretibial muscles) acts to advance the tibial. If the tibia is forward with the C/P anterior to the ankle, the soleus decreases action (off switch) so passive alignment draws the tibia forward.

The falling body weight is caught by the contralateral limb, which by now has completed its forward swing and is ready to assume a stance (i.e., supporting) role. Floor contact is made with the heel to continue the progression in stance. In this manner a cycle of progression is initiated and then serially perpetuated by reciprocal action of the two limbs.

The Progression Cycle. Advancement of the body depends on stance limb mobility. As body weight is dropped onto the limb, the force is primarily directed toward the floor. Advancement of the body depends on redirecting some of this force in a manner that combines progression and stability. The essential element for progression over the stance limb is rocker action by the foot and ankle. Full ranges of passive extension at the knee and hip are the other critical factors.

Heel rocker. As body weight is dropped onto the stance limb, the momentum generated by the forward fall is preserved by the heel rocker (Figure 3.23). Floor contact is made by the rounded surface of the calcaneal tuberosities. The bony segment between this point and the center of the ankle joint serves as an unstable lever that rolls toward the ground as body weight is dropped onto the foot. Action by the pretibial muscles to restrain the rate of foot drop also creates a tie to the tibia that draws the leg forward. This progressional effect is transferred to the thigh by the quadriceps (Figure 3.24). While acting to restrain the rate of knee flexion, the quadriceps muscle mass also ties the femur to the tibia. In this manner, the heel rocker facilitates progression of the entire stance limb. As a result the force of falling, rather than being totally directed toward the floor, has a significant portion realigned into forward momentum.

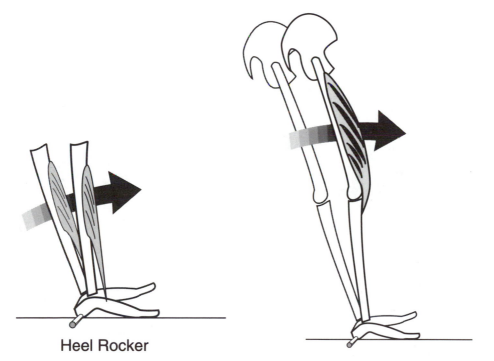

Heel Rocker

Figure 3.23 Heel Rocker: Using the heel as the fulcrum (rod designation motion axis), the foot rolls into plantar flexion. Pretibial muscles, as they decelerate the foot drop, also draw the tibia forward. Limb progression preserved.

Figure 3.24 Quadriceps action extends the progression of the tibia initiated by the heel rocker to advancing the thigh (arrow).

Ankle rocker. Once the forefoot strikes the floor, the ankle becomes the fulcrum for continued progression. With the foot stationary, the tibia continues its advancement by passive ankle dorsiflexion in response to the momentum present (Figure 3.25). During this period the body vector advances along the length of the foot to the metatarsal heads. A critical aspect of the ankle rocker is the yielding quality of the soleus muscle action. As it contracts to make the tibia a stable base for knee extension, the soleus muscle, assisted by the gastrocnemius, also allows tibial advancement. Hence, there is graded intensity of plantar flexor muscle action. This is a prime example of selective control.

Forefoot rocker. As the base of the body vector (center of pressure) reaches the metatarsal heads, the heel rises. The rounded contour of the metatarsals serves as a forefoot rocker (Figure 3.26). Progression is accelerated as body weight falls beyond the area of foot support. This is the strongest propelling force during the gait cycle. The body mass is a passive weight at the end of a long lever, and there is no force restraining the fall. The forefoot rocker also serves as the base for accelerated limb advancement in pre-swing.

Pre-swing knee flexion. An anterior propelling force is created through the

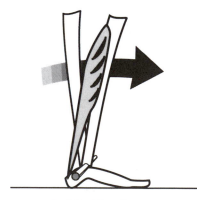

Ankle Rocker

Figure 3.25 Ankle Rocker: With the ankle as the fulcrum (rod designating the axis of motion) the tibia (and whole limb) rolls forward in response to momentum (arrow). The rate of tibial progression is decelerated by the soleus muscle.

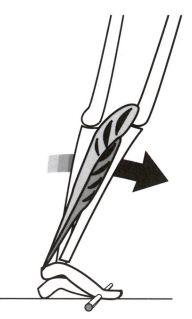

Forefoot Rocker

Figure 3.26 Forefoot Rocker: Tibial progression (arrow) is continued over the forefoot rocker (rod as the axis). Both gastrocnemius and soleus act vigorously to decelerate the rate of tibial advancement.

complex interaction of ankle, knee and hip mechanics that initiates limb advancement in pre-swing (Figure 3.27). The base of the body vector is at the metatarsal heads and then passes through the center of the knee joint, so there no longer are stabilizing forces acting on the foot or knee. Also, the limb is being rapidly unloaded by a transfer of body weight to the other foot. Residual gastrosoleus muscle action pivots the foot about the metatarsophalangeal (MP) joint. The result is simultaneous ankle plantar flexion and knee flexion. At the same time the adductors acting to restrain medial fall of the body also flex the hip. Continued hip flexion in initial swing results in rapid advancement of the thigh, and needed momentum is added to the progressional system.

Swing phase hip flexion. The progressional effect of the forward swinging limb is used by the weight-bearing limb during the early portion of its mid stance phase. At this time an added force is needed to draw the body mass and supporting limb forward and upward from the relatively low loading position acquired in the initial double support interval (Figure 3.20).

Swing phase knee extension. The combination of knee extension and further thigh advancement in mid swing adds tibial weight to the limb mass that is forward of the stance limb axis. This change in swing limb alignment continues the pulling force at a time when the stance limb has minimal intrinsic momentum. Active knee extension in terminal swing completes the contribution of the swing limb to propulsion. Due to the small weight of the shank and

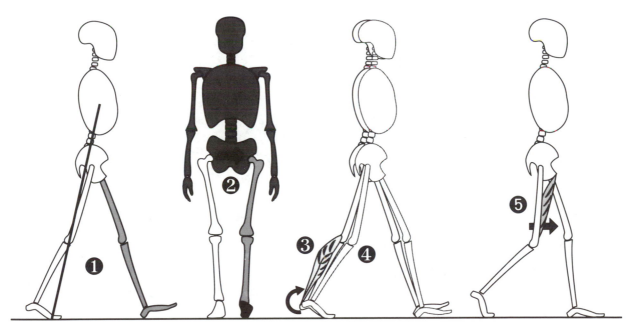

Figure 3.27 Pre-Swing knee flexion continues limb progression. Four factors contribute: (1) ankle is dorsiflexed to allow the vector to lie over the metatarsophalangeal joint (MPJ); (2) the limb is rapidly unloaded by the transfer of body weight to the other limb (shaded areas); (3) residual gastrosoleus muscle action plantar flexes the foot about the forefoot rocker; (4) the resulting tibial advancement flexes the knee; and (5) adductor longus action flexes the hip as it controls coronal plane balance.

foot, the force generated by this action, however, would be much less than from body weight falling forward over the stance limb. By the end of these actions the total advancement of the thigh and tibia results in a limb posture that is appropriate to catch the falling body weight at the onset of the next stance period. A new progressional cycle is begun.

Shock Absorption

Transfer of body weight from the rear to forward foot is a fairly abrupt exchange, even though it occurs during a double stance interval. At the end of the single support period, body weight is significantly ahead of the area of forefoot support. This creates an unbalanced situation with the body falling forward toward the floor. At the same time, the foot of the forward limb, while positioned for stance, still is about 1cm above the floor's surface (Figure 3.28).[16] Hence, for a short period the body is in a free fall. This results in an abrupt loading of the forward limb (60% body weight in 0.02 seconds) (Figure 3.29).

The full intensity of this floor impact is reduced by shock-absorbing reactions at the ankle, knee and hip. All three motion patterns occur during the loading response phase of gait.

Ankle plantar flexion is an immediate reaction to initial floor contact by the heel. Most of the eventual 10° occurs as a brief free foot fall (Figure 3.30).[16] Then pretibial muscle action significantly restrains the motion and delays floor contact by the forefoot until the 8% point in the gait cycle, rather than having it occur immediately. The rate at which falling body weight is transferred onto to the floor is correspondingly reduced.

Knee flexion is the second and greater shock-absorbing mechanism. This motion also is a reaction to the heel rocker initiated by floor contact. As the pretibial muscles act to restrain foot fall, their bony attachments to the tibia and fibula create a tie that causes the leg to follow the falling foot. Forward roll of the tibia reduces the support available to the femur and thus allows the body to drop. This also causes knee flexion, as the joint center is anterior to the body vector. Action by the quadriceps to decelerate the rate of knee flexion transfers some of the loading force to the thigh muscle mass (Figure 3.31). Hence, the intensity of the joint loading force is reduced (floor impact is less). This is reflected by the forceplate as an absence of an initial high impact vertical load (Figure 3.29).

Abrupt loading of the weight acceptance limb similarly unloads the other limb. This removes the support from that side of the pelvis, introducing a contralateral pelvic drop. The HAT resting on the middle of the pelvis also falls. The rate of pelvic drop is restrained by the stance limb's abductor muscles. Again, the impact of limb loading is absorbed by muscular action. As a result the total load experienced by the stance hip joint is reduced (Figure 3.32).

Energy Conservation

The efficiency of doing any activity is the ratio between the work

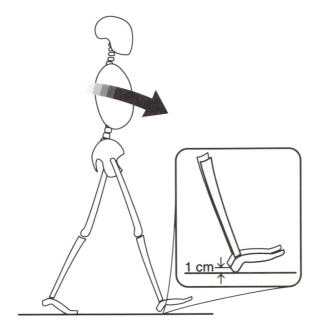

Figure 3.28 Floor contact is abrupt because body weight had a free fall (arrow) for about 1cm (insert). This is the distance between the heel and the floor at the end of terminal swing.

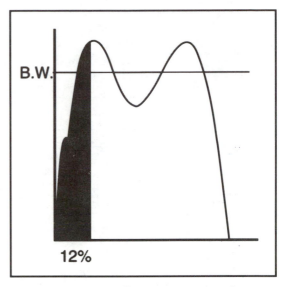

Loading response phase

Figure 3.29 The effect of the terminal swing free fall is an abrupt floor impact (first hump in the vertical floor reaction force curve). Shaded area = loading response.

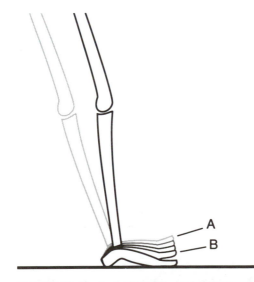

Figure 3.30 The immediate shock-absorbing reaction to floor impact is free ankle plantar flexion following heel contact, before the pretibial muscle action catches it.

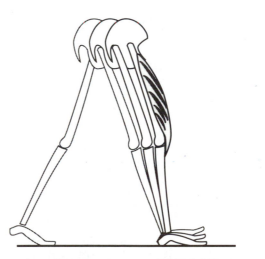

Figure 3.31 Knee flexion restrained by the quadriceps is the second shock-absorbing reaction to floor contact.

accomplished and the energy expended. During walking, preservation of stance stability by selectively restraining falling body weight and advancing the swinging limb as the body progresses along the desired distance constitutes the work being performed. The amount of muscular effort required in these actions determines the energy cost. In the terms of physics, the word *work* indicates controlled motion, that is, kilogram-meters of displacement. Physiologically there are two other concerns. The intensity of the muscular effort as a percent of its capacity indicates the person's capability of performing the task. The amount of energy required by the muscular action indicates the person's endurance.

Unlimited endurance requires the energy cost of walking be below the cardiopulmonary midpoint in a person's maximum energy production capacity.[4,21] This energy threshold is expressed as 50% VO_2 Max. Normal walking at the average speed of 80 meters per minute uses energy at a rate that is 38% of the maximum. Thus, walking is not so effortless as assumed.

To maintain the "low" effort level, the normal stride includes two mechanisms to conserve energy. These are C/G alignment modulation and selective muscular control. Both serve to reduce the intensity and duration of the muscular action involved.

C/G Control. Minimizing the amount that the body's center of gravity is displaced from the line of progression is the major mechanism for reducing the muscular effort of walking and, consequently, saving energy.

The least energy would be used if the weight being carried remained at a constant height and followed a single central path. Then no additional lifting effort would be needed to recover from the intermittent falls downward or laterally. This is equally true for moving the body during walking; displacement should be minimized.

Dependence on reciprocal bipedal locomotion, however, presents two potentially costly situations during each stride. As the right and left limbs alternate their support roles, the body must shift from one side to the other. The limbs also change their vertical alignment between double and single support, causing a change in the height of the pelvis, leading to the body mass moving up and down.

The body is at its lowest point when the limbs become obliquely aligned during the two double support periods (initial and terminal). Then in mid stance the body is raised to its highest position (right or left) when the supporting limb is vertical (Figure 3.33). The potential difference in hip height is approximately 9.5cm. Repeatedly lifting the body this amount would quickly be exhaustive. Potential transverse displacement of the body from side to side could equal the average stride width of 8cm.[15]

Through a mixture of six motion patterns, called *determinants of gait*, the magnitude of these costly vertical and horizontal displacements is reduced to just 2.3cm in each direction for a total arc of 4.6cm (Figure 3.34).[20] This represents more than a 50% improvement. In addition, abrupt changes in direction are avoided, which is another energy-saving maneuver.[9]

Three of the energy-conserving motions relate to changes in alignment of the pelvis. These are contralateral drop, horizontal rotation and lateral displace-

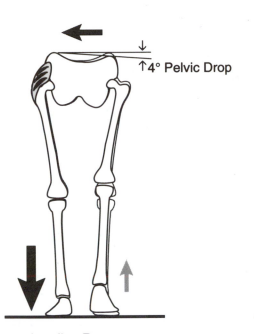

Loading Response

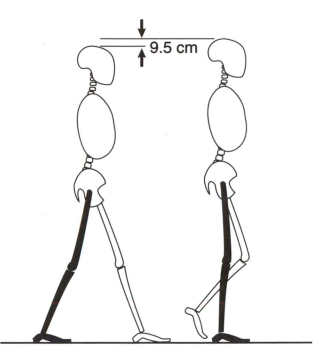

↑4° Pelvic Drop

9.5 cm

Figure 3.32 Contralateral pelvic drop decelerated by the hip abductors provides a third shock-absorbing maneuver. This occurs as weight is rapidly dropped onto the loading limb (large arrow) as the other limb is being lifted (small arrow).

Figure 3.33 The change in body height between double and single limb support would be 9.5cm if no modifying action were performed.

ment (Figure 3.35). The first two actions occur passively as the pelvis follows the swinging limb and average 4° of motion in each plane. Lateral displacement of the pelvis relates to the transfer of body weight onto the limb.

During loading response and early mid stance both vertical and lateral realignment of the body C/G occurs. Contralateral drop of the pelvis lowers the base of the HAT. Shifting weight to the stance limb at the onset of stance removes the support from the swing side of the pelvis, causing a contralateral pelvic drop. Half of this drop is experienced by the body center as it lies at the midpoint of the pelvic width between the two hips.

Lateral displacement of the pelvis with limb loading involves two factors. First is the natural valgus angle between the femur and the tibia. This places the knees (and supporting feet) closer to each other than a vertical line down from the hip joints would provide. Anatomical width between the hip joints approximates 20-25cm. Normal step width is 8cm.[15] As the limb is loaded there is a slight increase in knee abduction that moves the body C/G nearer to the supporting foot.

The third pelvic motion is forward rotation, which occurs as the swing limb advances. This action moves the hip joint of the swing limb anterior to that of the stance limb, placing the width of the pelvis into a relatively sagittal position.

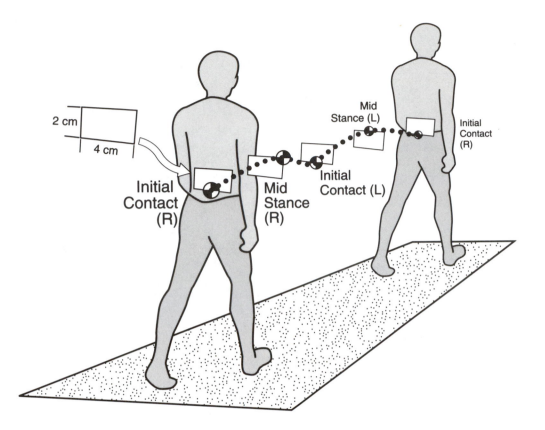

Figure 3.34 The normal path of the body center of gravity (black/white circle) illustrated by a stride beginning with the right foot. From the low, central point in double limb support (right initial contact), the C/G moves upward and laterally (right mid stance), drops to a second central low point (left initial contact), rises to a peak again (left mid stance) and drops once more (second right initial contact). Each deviation is approximately 2cm (up and to each side).

The resulting horizontal segment between the two hips functionally lengthens the limbs by increasing the distance between the points of the floor contact and the base of the trunk. Pelvic rotation also moves the hip joints (and thus the supporting feet) closer to the midline. Both effects reduce the amount of limb obliquity needed to accomplish the desired step length. The effect, greatest in terminal stance, is a decrease in the amount that the body center is lowered during double support.

Limb motions also contribute to smoothing the path of the body's vertical travel. The mechanics vary with the phase of gait. During the double stance intervals, ankle control is critical. Heel rise in terminal stance relatively lengthens the trailing limb by lifting the ankle. Initial contact by the heel similarly adds length to the forward limb (Figure 3.36).

The interchange between ankle and knee motion is a second means of reducing body mass displacement. As the limb is loaded the combination of increasing ankle plantar flexion and knee flexion decreases the rate of body elevation, part of the loading response becomes more vertical by rolling

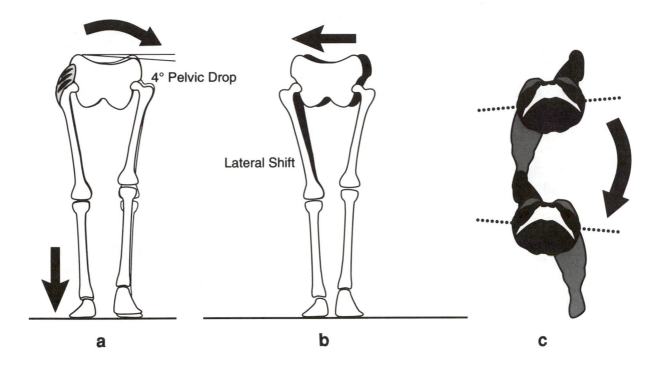

4° Pelvic Drop

Lateral Shift

a

b

c

Figure 3.35 Pelvic maneuver to minimize C/G displacement in a stride. Each motion is approximately 4°. (a) Contralateral pelvic drop. (b) Anterior tilt. (c) Transverse rotation.

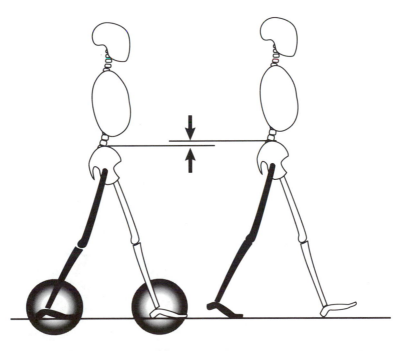

Figure 3.36 Ankle actions to elevate the C/G. Left: No accommodation. Note: The shaded circles identify foot flat bilaterally. Right: Terminal stance heel rise lengthens the trailing limb. Initial contact heel strike increases the length of the forward limb.

forward on the heel. Following forefoot contact with the floor, limb advancement continues as ankle dorsiflexion while the knee increases its flexion. By the time the tibia is fully upright at the end of the loading phase, the knee is flexed 15°. Subsequent blending of progressive dorsiflexion that lowers the tibia and knee extension that elevates the femur continues the avoidance of an abrupt change in the level of the body center during the weight-bearing period (Figure 3.37).

In addition to the anatomical narrowing of step width, the body does not fully align itself over the supporting foot as would occur in quiet standing. The potential imbalance is controlled by inertia. By the time body weight loses its lateral momentum and would fall to the unsupported side, the swing limb has completed its advancement and is prepared to accept the load. Transverse rotation also narrows the distance between the hip joints.

Thus, in summary, vertical lift of the passenger unit during single limb support is lessened by lateral and anterior tilt of the pelvis combined with stance limb ankle plantar flexion and knee flexion. Lowering of the body center by double limb support is reduced by terminal stance heel rise, initial heel contact combined with full knee extension, and horizontal rotation of the pelvis. Lateral displacement is similarly minimized by the pelvic rotations, medial femoral angulation, and the substitution of inertia for complete coronal balance. As a result, the body's center of gravity follows a smooth three-dimensional sinusoidal path that intermingles vertical and horizontal deviations.

Selective Control. By substituting passive posturing and available momentum

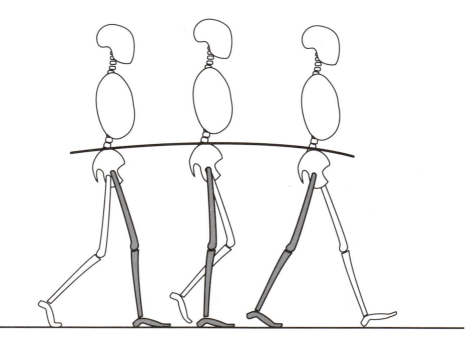

Figure 3.37 The addition of serial knee flexion and extension to the changes in ankle position reduces the relative lengthening of the limb and C/G displacement.

for muscle action whenever possible, less energy is expended as the desired progression and the necessary joint stability are accomplished. Both the timing and intensity of muscular activity are selectively modulated.

Throughout stance the muscles contract only when body alignment creates a torque antagonistic to weight-bearing stability of the limb and trunk. That is, the body vector is aligned to create instability. The demand torques that must be controlled in the sagittal plane are those that induce hip flexion, knee flexion and ankle dorsiflexion (Figure 3.38). In the coronal plane, the threatening alignments are hip adduction and abduction and subtalar joint inversion and eversion. There also are transverse rotational demands at each joint that must be controlled. The intensity of the muscular responses is proportional to the magnitude of the demand torque that must be restrained. As soon as an alternate means of joint control is available, the muscles relax. Hence, there is a continual exchange between the demand torque and the controlling mechanisms of muscle action, momentum, and passive tension of the ligaments or fascia.

The hip extensors contract only at the onset of limb loading (Figure 3.39a).[11] They then relax and allow momentum from the heel rocker and quadriceps action at the knee to extend the hip passively as the femur is advanced faster than the pelvis. At the knee, peak quadriceps action occurs only during loading

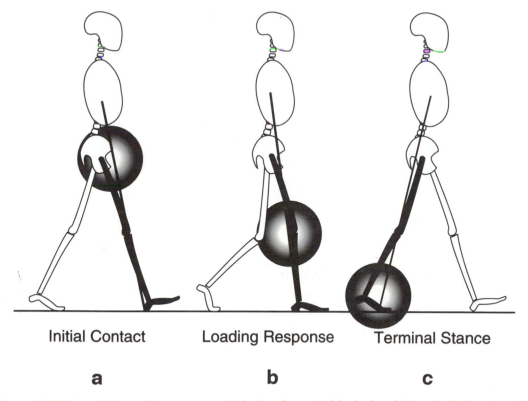

Initial Contact   Loading Response   Terminal Stance

a   **b**   **c**

Figure 3.38 The serial demand torques presented by the alignment of the body weight vector during stance. Dark line indicates the body vector. The circles identify the major site of passive instability created by vector alignment. (a) Initial contact hip flexion torque, vector anterior. (b) Loading response knee flexion torque, vector posterior. (c) Terminal stance ankle dorsiflexion torque, vector anterior.

response and the onset of mid stance when the vector is behind the joint axis (Figure 3.39b). As the vector moves forward of the knee axis, this muscle group relaxes, even though the knee has not reached full extension. Momentum completes the extensor motion.

Ankle control is the only area that requires persistent muscle action from loading response to early pre-swing. Energy is conserved by minimizing the extent of cocontraction by antagonists. Modulating the intensity of plantar flexor muscle activity during the individual gait phases is a second means of reducing the energy cost. The intensity is low during mid stance when the limb is rolling forward over a stationary foot and then high in terminal stance when body weight must be supported on the forefoot (Figure 3.39c).

Limb advancement in swing is a similar mixture of momentum, gravity and direct muscle control. The initiating action in pre-swing relies on residual force from the deactivated ankle plantar flexors combined with an unstable base of support. Hip flexion is a by-product of the adductor longus muscle action to restrain contralateral fall of the body. The result is 35° of knee flexion gained without any direct muscle action. In initial swing the combination of hip flexion and tibial inertia provides 60° of knee flexion with minimal use of the knee muscles. In mid swing the knee is extended passively. Even the ankle dorsiflexor muscles often relax for a brief time in late mid swing once the foot has passed the peak toe drag threat. Only in terminal swing is there vigorous

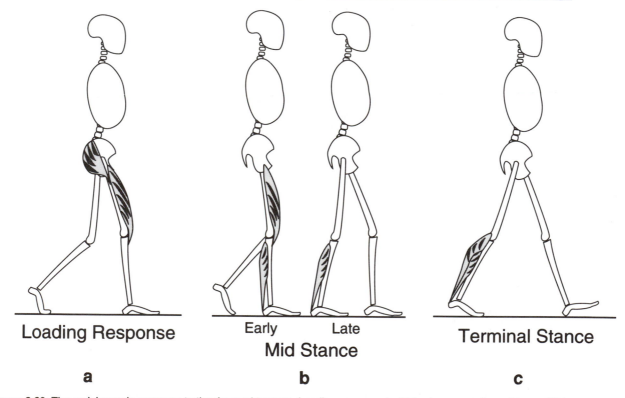

Loading Response

Early   Late
Mid Stance

Terminal Stance

a   **b**   **c**

Figure 3.39 The serial muscle response to the demand torques. Loading response by hip extensors and quadriceps. Mid stance (early) uses knee extensors and ankle plantar flexors. Terminal stance requires only ankle plantar flexors.

activity of the hip extensors, knee extensors and ankle dorsiflexors to prepare the limb quickly and assuredly for weight acceptance.

References

1. Adams JM, Baker LL, Perry J, et al.: *Quantitative assessment of static and dynamic postural stability in normal adults.* Master's paper, USC, Department of Physical Therapy, 1987.
2. Asmussen E: The weight-carrying function of the human spine. *Acta Orthop Scand.* 29:276-280, 1960.
3. Asmussen E, Klausen K: Form and function of the erect human spine. *Clin Orthop* 25:55-63, 1962.
4. Astrand PO, Rodahl K: *Textbook of Work Physiology.* 2nd edition, New York, McGraw-Hill Book Co., 1986, p. 513.
5. Beasley WC: Quantitative muscle testing: Principles and applications to research and clinical services. *Arch Phys Med Rehabil* 42:398-425, 1961.
6. Dempster WT: Space requirements of the seated operator. *WADC Technical Report.* Dayton, Ohio, Wright-Patterson Air Force Base, pp. 55-159, 1955.
7. Elftman H: The functional structure of the lower limb. In Klopsteg PE, Wilson PD (Eds): *Human Limbs and Their Substitutes.* New York, McGraw-Hill Book Co., 1954, pp. 411-436.
8. Hellebrandt FA, Fries EC: The eccentricity of the mean vertical projection of the center of gravity during standing. *Physiotherapy Review* 4:186-192, 1942.
9. Inman VT, Ralston HJ, Todd F: *Human Walking.* Baltimore, MD, Williams and Wilkins Comopany, 1981.
10. LeVeau BF: *Williams and Lissner Biomechanics of Human Motion.* 2nd edition, Philadelphia, W. B. Saunders Company, 1977, p. 207.
11. Lyons K, Perry J, Gronley JK, Barnes L, Antonelli D: Timing and relative intensity of hip extensor and abductor muscle action during level and stair ambulation: an EMG study. *Phys Ther* 63:1597-1605, 1983.
12. Mann RA, Hagy JL, White V, Liddell D: The initiation of gait. *J Bone Joint Surg* 63:1597-1605, 1983.
13. Mansour JM, et al.: A three-dimensional multi-segmental analysis of the energetics of normal and pathological human gait. *J Biomech* 15(1):51-59, 1982.
14. Mena D, Mansour JM, Simon SR: Analysis and synthesis of human swing leg motion during gait and its clinical applications. *J Biomech* 14(12):823-832, 1981.
15. Murray MP, Drought AB, Kory RC: Walking patterns of normal men. *J Bone Joint Surg* 46A(2):335-360, 1964.
16. Murray MP, Peterson RM: Weight distribution and weight-shifting activity during normal standing posture. *Phys Ther* 53(7):741-748, 1973.
17. Murray MP, Seireg AA, Sepic SB: Normal postural stability and steadiness: quantitative assessment. *J Bone Joint Surg* 57A(4):510-516, 1975.
18. Perry J, Ireland ML, Gronley J, Hoffer MM: Predictive value of manual muscle testing and gait analysis in normal ankles by dynamic electromyography. *Foot and Ankle* 6(5):254-259, 1986.
19. Ralston HJ: Effect of immobilization of various body segments on the energy cost of human locomotion. Proc. 2nd I.E.A. Conf., Dortmund. *Ergonomics* 53, 1965.
20. Saunders JBdeCM, Inman VT, Eberhart HD: The major determinants in normal and pathological gait. *J Bone Joint Surg* 35A(3):543-557, 1953.
21. Waters R, Hislop H, Perry J, Antonelli D: Energetics: Application to the study and management of locomotor disabilities. *Orthop Clin North Am* 9:351-377, 1978.

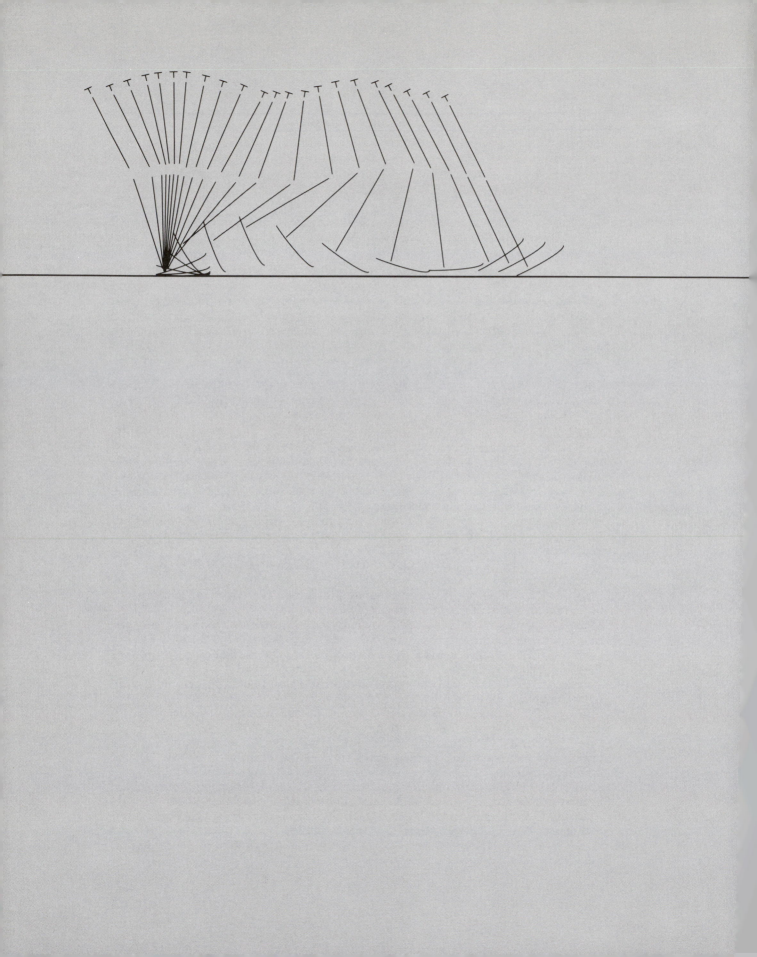

Section Two

Normal Gait

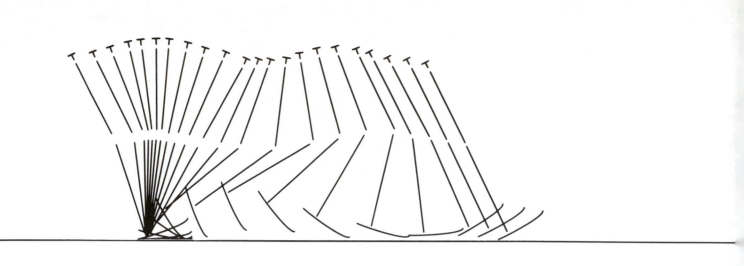

Chapter 4

Ankle Foot Complex

The junction between the leg (tibia) and foot presents a unique situation. At this anatomical area vertical weight-bearing forces are transmitted to a horizontal support system. Customarily, the ankle is considered to be the site of all leg-foot interactions. A more accurate interpretation includes the subtalar joint. The talus lies in the vertical weight-bearing axis of the leg, between the tibia and calcaneus, while the foot extends from the calcaneus to the toes. The talus is not an essential element of the horizontal, floor-contacting, foot support structure. Instead it serves as a weight-bearing link between the leg (tibia) and foot (calcaneus) that allows two single axis joints to provide three-dimensional mobility.

Inman emphasized the interplay between the subtalar and tibiotalar articulations under the term *joints of the ankle*.[26] This concept is correct, but redefining a commonly used term has proven futile in other endeavors and will not be attempted here. The original usage is too well preserved in prior writing and customs. The term *ankle* will relate to the junction between the tibia and the talus (tibiotalar joint), and the inferior joint will continue to be called *subtalar.* The actions of the other major joints within the foot (midtarsal and metatarsophalangeal, particularly) also influence ankle function. Thus, all these articulations will be treated as a functional complex.

Ankle

Motion

Terminology. For simplicity, ankle motion is commonly called flexion and extension.[1] Definition of these terms, however, has varied. Some authorities treat the ankle in the same manner as joint motion elsewhere in the body and apply the term *flexion* to motions that decrease the angle between the two bones (i.e., upward motion of the foot toward the tibia). Similarly, *extension* indicates straightening of the limb (foot moving away from the leg). Others consider upward motion of the foot (toward the anterior tibia) to be extension, because that is the term used for toe motion in the same direction. Following the same logic, downward motion of the foot is called flexion.

Neurologically, the first terminology is correct. Upward movement of the foot is part of the primitive flexor synergy, that is, it accompanies hip and knee flexion. Likewise, downward motion of the foot is part of the limb's extensor synergy. Due to such confusion, the only recourse is to use the term *dorsiflexion* to signify upward travel of the foot and *plantar flexion* for the ankle's downward motion. This will be the policy in this text.

Arcs of Motion

While the arcs of ankle motion are not large, they are critical for progression and shock absorption during stance (Figure 4.1). In swing, ankle motion contributes to limb advancement.

During each gait cycle the ankle travels through four arcs of motion. Most investigators[16,32,51] have differed little from Murray's data recorded on 60 normal adults (ages 20-60 years).[35] This, in turn, merely refined with a larger number of subjects the values reported earlier by Close and Inman.[11] Recent developments of three-dimensional motion analysis (3-D) have resulted in some reduction of the arcs of motion recorded.[30] The Rancho motion values cited in this text also recorded with a 3-D system, present a compromise between the two extremes.

Twice during each gait cycle the ankle alternately plantar flexes (PF) and then dorsiflexes (DF).[11,30,35,48,52] The first three arcs of motion occur in stance (PF, DF, PF). During swing the ankle only dorsiflexes. The sequence and timing of ankle motion arcs following initial floor contact with the heel are presented in Table 4.1.

The entire range of ankle motion used during walking averages 30° (20° to 40°).[9,30,35] Each arc of ankle motion relates closely to the foot's support pattern. Initial contact by the heel occurs with the ankle at neutral (or plantar flexed

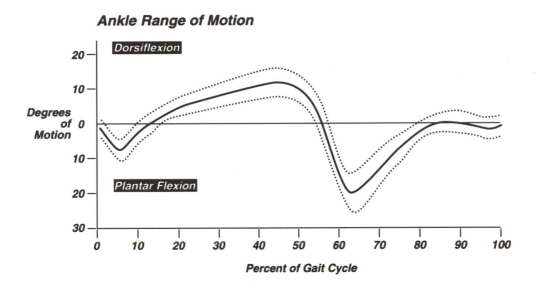

Figure 4.1 Ankle motion: Normal range during a stride. Black line = the mean, dotted line = 1 standard deviation.

3°-5°). This is followed by the first plantar flexion arc during the loading response (0-10% GC). With the onset of forefoot contact (foot flat) the ankle changes its direction toward dorsiflexion. Now the foot is stationary, and the tibia becomes the moving segment. Neutral alignment is reached at the 20% point in the gait cycle. Dorsiflexion continues through mid stance and the first half of terminal stance, reaching the maximum 10° angle by 48% GC. This position is held until the end of the single support period. Following the onset of terminal double support, there is rapid ankle plantar flexion, reaching the maximum 30° angle at the end of stance. Toe-off initiates the final dorsiflexion action. A neutral position (0°) is reached by mid swing and maintained during the rest of the phase. Often there is a drop into 3°-5° PF during terminal swing.

Table 4.1

Ankle Motion During A Stride

Plantar flexion to 7°	(0-12%gc)
Dorsiflexion to 10°	(12-48%gc) (in shoes it is 5°)
Plantar flexion 20°	(48-62%gc)
Dorsiflexion to neutral	(62-100%gc)

Body Vector

The functional demands placed on the ankle joint during the three arcs of motion occurring during the stance phase follow the load imposed on the limb and the alignment of the body weight vector. In swing, only the weight of the foot and speed of motion influence ankle motion.

Throughout stance the base of the body vector (center of pressure) advances along the length of the foot from the heel to the MP joint and proximal phalanges.[31,33] This creates two alignments of the body vector in relation to the ankle joint axis. At the onset of the loading response the body vector is posterior to the ankle axis. By the 5% point in the gait cycle the vector passes anterior to the ankle axis. This alignment continues throughout the rest of stance (Figure 4.2).

At initial contact the weight line is centered in the heel. This places the vector behind the ankle, and a plantar flexion torque is generated. While the rate of limb loading is rapid, the short heel level results in a small maximum, yet functionally significant, loading response torque (1.5 body weight leg length units [BWLL]) which occurs early in the phase (2% GC). From this point the plantar flexion torque progressively diminishes, due to the rapid advancement of the center of pressure from the point of heel contact to the

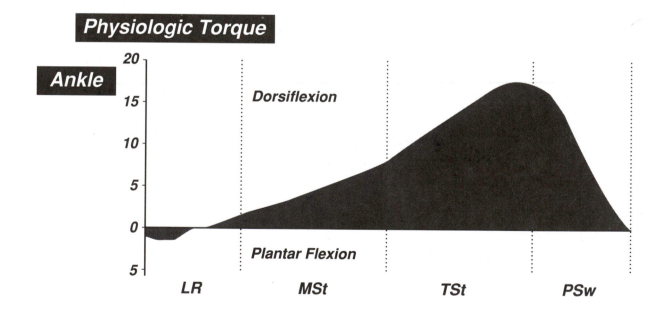

Figure 4.2 Ankle torques: Normal weight-bearing pattern generated by the sagittal vector during walking. The brief plantar flexion torque at the onset of stance is followed by progressive dorsiflexion into terminal stance and then decreases to 0 at toe-off (end of pre-swing). Deviation of the shadow from 0 indicates the magnitude of the torque in physiological units (BW×LL). LR = loading response, MSt = mid stance, TSt = terminal stance, PSw = pre-swing.

ankle joint. The plantar flexion torque is reduced to zero by the midpoint of the loading response phase (5% GC). Beyond this point, a dorsiflexion torque develops and increases in magnitude as the center of pressure (C/P) progressively moves ahead of the ankle joint. This continues at virtually the same rate until just before the other foot strikes the floor (48% GC). Peak dorsiflexion torque (17 BWLL) occurs in late terminal stance. The center of pressure is at the metatarsophalangeal joints, and the effect of body weight is accentuated by the acceleration of the downward fall.

Muscle Control

As the ankle joint moves in a single plane, all the controlling muscles function either as dorsiflexors or plantar flexors. Timing of ankle muscle action is very phasic. The plantar flexors consistently are active in stance. Conversely, the dorsiflexors are swing phase muscles. An exception to this rule occurs as the dorsiflexor muscles participate during the loading response phase of stance to control the rate of ankle plantar flexion.

The phasic clarity of the ankle muscles varies with the type of electromyographic electrodes used to record muscle action. Surface electrodes display a low level of continuous action in between the peaks. This continuity is absent when the recording is made within the muscle by wire electrodes.

The functional potential (torque) of the ankle muscles is proportional to their size (physiological cross section) and leverage. Both of these values have been well defined in the literature.[28,50] Knowing each muscle's potential is an important factor in understanding the pattern of ankle control that occurs during gait. While muscle leverage is modified by joint position, a useful relative scale can be gained by comparing the torques available with the ankle at neutral. The soleus, as the largest ankle muscle, has been selected as the reference model to which others are related (Tables 4.2 and 4.3).

Dorsiflexors

Three major muscles lie anterior to the ankle joint: tibialis anterior, extensor digitorum longus, and extensor hallucis longus (Figure 4.3). The peroneus tertius is an inconstant accessory to the extensor digitorum longus and anatomically they are difficult to separate. EMG differentiation of peroneus tertius and the extensor digitorum longus is lacking. As the two muscle bellies blend into each other and share the lateral tendon, the action of the peroneus tertius will be assumed to be equivalent to that of the extensor digitorum longus.

All of the potential dorsiflexors have lever arms of similar length, but their size varies markedly. The tibialis anterior (TA) has the largest cross section. Both toe extensors are markedly smaller. The combined extensor digitorum longus and peroneus tertius mass is 40% of the TA, and the very visible extensor

Table 4.2

Ankle Vectors

	Peak	Duration
Posterior	1.5 BWLL (2% GC)	5% GC
Anterior	17.4 BWLL (45% GC)	48% GC

hallucis longus is less than 20%. Their dorsiflexion capabilities (torques) therefore are much less.

The onset of dorsiflexor muscle activity starts in pre-swing. First to contract is the extensor hallucis longus, which is active throughout pre-swing. Its peak effort is about 8% manual muscle test (MMT). Activity of the tibialis anterior and extensor digitorum longus quickly follows in mid-swing. Tibialis anterior intensity promptly rises throughout initial swing, reaching 35% MMT by the end of the phase. During mid swing muscle action becomes minimal (10% MMT). In terminal swing the intensity gradually rises again to position the foot for stance. Action of the extensor digitorum longus (and presumably the peroneus tertius) parallels that of the tibialis anterior but at a slightly lower amplitude.

At initial contact all the pretibial muscles are significantly active. The intensity of the tibialis anterior promptly rises to 45% MMT, and the extensor hallucis reaches 35%. Action of extensor digitorum longus remains at 25% MMT. All three dorsiflexors terminate their action by the end of loading response. Thus, the typical pattern of dorsiflexor muscle action is biphasic, with initial swing and the loading response phases being the intervals of peak intensity.

Table 4.3

Relative Dorsiflexor Torque

	(% Soleus)
Tibialis Anterior	6.9%
Extensor Digitorum Longus	2.7%
Extensor Hallucis Longus	1.1%

Ankle Dorsiflexor Muscles

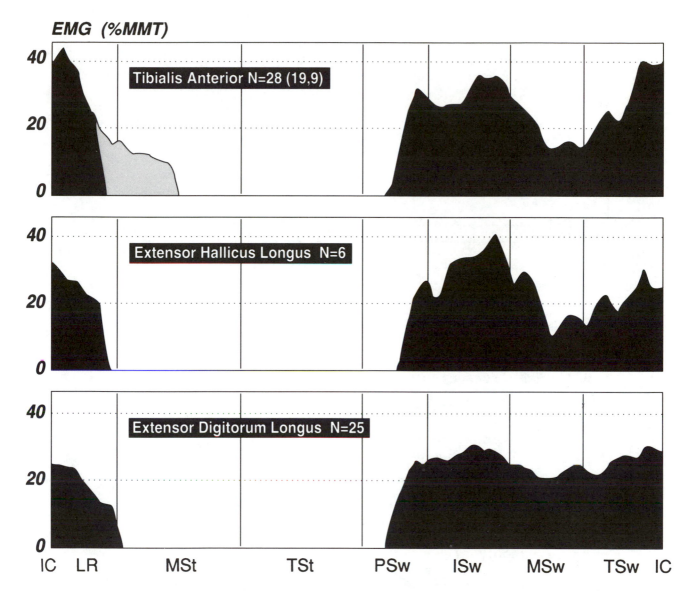

Figure 4.3 Ankle dorsiflexor muscles. Normal mean intensity and timing during free walking (quantified electromyogram Intensity as a percent of maximum manual muscle test value (% MMT) indicated by height of gray area. Vertical bar designate the gait phases.

Plantar Flexors

Seven muscles pass posterior to the ankle and thus can serve as plantar flexors (Figure 4.4). Their actual capacity, however, varies markedly. The soleus and gastrocnemius account for 93% of the theoretical plantar flexor torque, while the five perimalleolar muscles provide 7%.[21] This means there are two distinct functional groups of plantar flexors: the triceps surae and the perimallolar muscles. The soleus and medial and lateral heads of the gastrocnemius have the advantage of large size and a full calcaneal lever. In contrast, the perimalleolar muscles are relatively small and wrap closely around the medial and lateral malleoli as their tendons turn from a vertical alignment along the leg to a horizontal path for action on the foot. Among the perimalleolar muscles, the flexor hallucis longus (FHL) generates the greatest plantar flexor torque. While similar in size to the posterior tibialis or peroneus longus, the flexor hallucis longus has the advantage of a longer lever from the ankle axis, as it tendon passes behind the posterior margin of the tibia rather than the more anterior malleoli (Table 4.4).

Table 4.4

Ankle Plantar Flexor Torques

	(% Soleus)
Soleus	100.0%
Gastrocnemius	68.0%
Tibialis Posterior	1.8%
Flexor Hallucis Longus	6.1%
Flexor Digitorum Longus	1.8%
Peroneus Longus	2.4%
Peroneus Brevis	1.0%

Triceps Surae. Soleus muscle action begins near the end of the loading response phase, rises quickly to 25% MMT and continues at this level of effort throughout mid stance (Figure 4.4). With the onset of terminal stance (30% GC) there is a rapid and marked rise in amplitude to 75% MMT by the 45% point in the gait cycle. Then the intensity of soleus action declines with similar speed, dropping to zero by the onset of double stance (pre-swing).

The medial head of the gastrocnemius parallels the soleus while the onset of the lateral head may be delayed until midstance.[49] The onset of gastrocnemius action quickly follows the soleus (12% versus 8% GC). Its rise in mid stance is slower and less intense (25% MMT) than that of the soleus. With the onset of terminal stance there is a rapid increase in intensity to a peak of 60% MMT at the 40% GC point. This is followed by an equally rapid decline and then cessation shortly after the onset of pre-swing. A brief contraction of the gastrocnemius in mid swing is a common finding, but the reason is not clear.

Authors have differed in the relative onset times of the two muscles.

Ankle Plantar Flexor Muscles

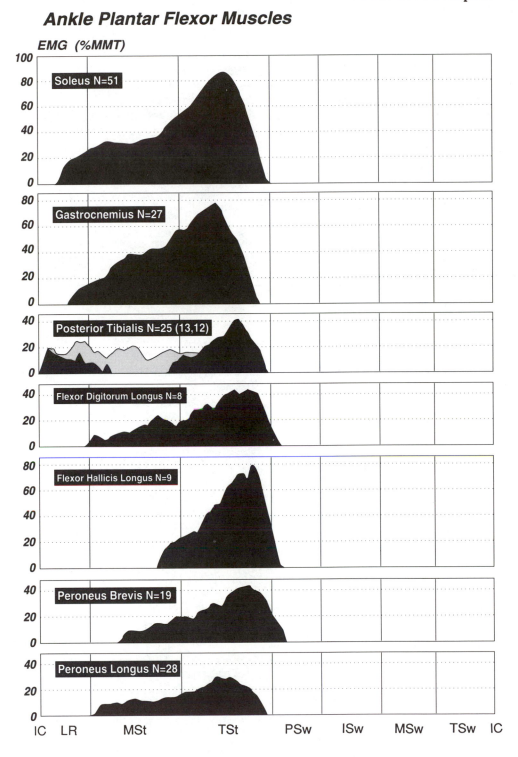

Figure 4.4 Ankle plantar flexor muscles. Normal mean intensity and timing during free walking (quantified electromyogram). Intensity as a percent of maximum manual muscle test value (% MMT) indicted by height of gray area. Vertical bars designate the gait phases.

Sutherland found a 10% GC delay by the gastrocnemius action compared to that of the soleus, while Carino reported only a 2% difference.[7,48] Our current data are midway between the earlier reports.[39] Both muscles markedly reduce their action by the end of terminal stance, (i.e., as the other foot contacts the ground), with only minimal action persisting into pre-swing.

Other gait characteristics that increase calf muscle action are a lengthened stride[22] and speed.[5] Both qualities were studied during treadmill walking. Hof found a linear relationship between stride length and peak calf muscle action by surface electromyography (EMG). In Hof's study, gait velocity was not a statistically significant factor, though there was a strong trend. When step rate was the means of increasing gait velocity, no relationship between calf muscle action and speed of walking was found.[22]

Perimalleolar Muscles. The other five muscles crossing the ankle posteriorly have low plantar flexor capability, because they are aligned for a different primary role during walking, that is, to control the subtalar joint and other articulations within the foot. In the process of providing their basic functions, these muscles also create a force at the ankle that should be considered.

The tibialis posterior becomes active at the time of initial contact (0% GC) and continues through single stance.[48] This is promptly followed by the flexor digitorum longus (10% GC) and, finally, the flexor hallucis longus (25% GC). Contralateral foot contact (50% GC) is the signal for the tibialis posterior and flexor digitorum longus to relax, while the toe flexors (FDL, FHL) continue briefly into pre-swing (52% GC). Sutherland found that both toe flexor muscles may show much earlier action, and there may be prolonged action of the FHL and TP.[48]

Peroneal muscle action starts early in the gait cycle.[10,18,48] The timing and relative intensity of the peroneus brevis and peroneus longus are very similar.[23,24,29,36,37] Both muscles tend to relax in mid pre-swing (55-58% GC). In some individuals the peroneus longus displays earlier and more prolonged action.

Functional Interpretation of the Ankle

The significance of relative weight imposed on the limb and the location of the vector on the intensity of muscle action are particularly evident during the double support intervals. Similar arcs of motion stimulated by different circumstances within the stride serve very dissimilar functions.

Both arcs of plantar flexion are found during periods of double support, but neither their weight bearing nor muscle control requirements are the same. The initial plantar flexion interval, occurring in loading response, presents a high demand on the pretibial muscle group. Within a short interval (5% GC) 60% of body weight is dropped onto the heel, and the pretibial muscles must respond to decelerate the rate of ankle plantar flexion.[14,27] Conversely, the second PF arc, displayed in pre-swing, is a period of low demand, even though the range is greater. The muscles of concern are the ankle plantar flexors. Because weight is being quickly transferred to the other foot, there is a 60-80% decrease in the muscle's load within the first half of pre-swing (5% GC). This, correspondingly, lessens the demand on the major plantar flexor muscles (soleus and gastrocnemius). Final floor contact in late pre-swing, presumably to assist balance, is maintained by just the long toe flexors and peroneals. Hence, this is a period of minimal muscle action.

A similar relationship exists between the two periods of dorsiflexion. The first dorsiflexion arc, occurring during single limb support, is an interval of high demand as the soleus and gastrocnemius decelerate the rate of tibial advancement over the foot against the body's progressional forces.[27] In contrast the second dorsiflexion action occurs during swing, when only the weight of the foot must be controlled by the tibialis anterior and long toe extensors.

Ankle Function by Gait Phase

The complexities of ankle function are best visualized by correlating motion, demand vectors and muscle action according to the gait cycle phases. The balance between functional demand and response becomes evident.

Initial Contact.

Posture: Ankle at 90° to initiate a heel rocker

Floor contact by the heel places the body vector posterior to the ankle. This prepares the limb for the loading response actions needed to preserve progression and provide shock absorption (Figure 4.5).

To provide a significant period of heel-only support, the ankle is positioned at 90° (neutral) so there is an optimum upward tilt of the forefoot. Support of the foot is provided by the dorsiflexion pull of the pretibial muscles. Less precise control will allow the ankle to drop into 3° or 5° of plantar flexion and reduce the potential heel rocker accordingly.

Loading Response.

Motion: First arc of ankle plantar flexion
Function: Heel rocker

At the onset of the loading response, the initial impact vector is vertical, that is, the forces are directed into the floor. This provides for limb stability but not progression. To keep the body moving forward without interruption, a *heel rocker* is used (Figure 4.6).

With the body vector posterior to the ankle, rapid loading of the limb (60% BW by 2% of the gait cycle) immediately generates a plantar flexion torque that drives the foot toward the floor. Brisk response of the pretibial muscles (tibialis anterior and long toe extensors) decelerates the rate of ankle plantar flexion. Two purposes are served by this dynamic response. The heel support period is extended, and the tibia is drawn forward as the foot drops. Both actions contribute to limb progression. The combined effects of the passive foot drop and active tibial advancement roll the body weight forward on the heel. Hence, the term *heel rocker.*

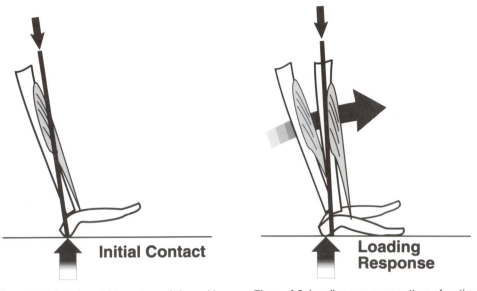

Figure 4.5 Initial contact posture of the ankle and alignment of the vector. The vector is within the heel, controlled by the tibialis anterior.

Figure 4.6 Loading response pattern of motion, muscle control and vector alignment at the ankle. The pretibial muscles restrain the rate of passive ankle plantar flexion created by the vector within the heel and advance the tibia. Arrow indicates the direction of motion.

The 10° of plantar flexion motion that occurs during the loading response actually reduces (rather than contributing to) the heel rocker effect so the tibia will not advance too fast. If the ankle had remained in a 90° position, the tibia would follow the foot through its 25° to 30° arc as it dropped to the floor from its tilted position at initial contact.

Shock absorption is the second advantage of restrained ankle plantar flexion during the loading response. This too is facilitated by the pretibial muscle action. As greater force is required to restrain the plantar flexion torque than was used to support the foot in swing, there is a lag in muscle effectiveness. The result is an initial arc of rapid ankle plantar flexion.[34] This serves as a brief "free fall" period for body weight (BW). The vertical height of the ankle is lowered by the rapid drop of the foot as it rolls freely on the rounded undersurface of the calcaneus (heel). Once the pretibial muscle force becomes sufficient, the downward motion of the foot is slowed, making forefoot contact a quiet event. In this way the heel rocker redirects some of the body's downward force to the pretibial muscles as they restrain ankle motion. These actions absorb some of the shock that accompanies rapid limb loading.

Throughout the initial arc of ankle plantar flexion the foot has been the moving segment and the leg relatively stationary. Once the forefoot contacts the floor the site of motion changes from the foot to the leg (shank). At the same time ankle motion is reversed toward dorsiflexion. This begins at the end of the loading response phase. Exact timing varies with the person's gait

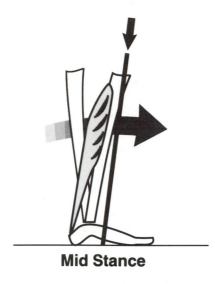

Mid Stance

Figure 4.7 Mid stance pattern of motion, muscle control and vector alignment at the ankle. Passive dorsiflexion is restrained by the soleus and gastrocnemius muscle action. Arrow indicates the direction of motion.

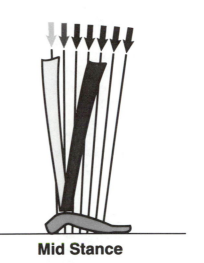

Mid Stance

Figure 4.8 Mid stance advancement of the vector over the foot as the ankle dorsiflexes. Each vertical line represents one vector sample. The arrows indicate body weight.

velocity. Fast walkers experience forefoot contact with the onset of single stance.

Mid Stance.

Motion: First arc of ankle dorsiflexion

Function: Ankle rocker for progression

Ankle motion during mid stance serves as an *ankle rocker* to continue progression. At the same time the soleus acts to maintain stance stability of the limb (Figure 4.7).

Throughout mid stance the body vector advances across the foot in response to momentum from the swing limb and forward fall of body weight (Figure 4.8). This creates an ever-increasing dorsiflexion torque that rolls the tibia forward from an initial 8° plantar flexed position to 5° dorsiflexion (i.e., anterior to the vertical axis), while the heel and forefoot remain in contact with the floor.

The soleus muscle (soon assisted by the gastrocnemius) reacts quickly to restrain the initial rapid rate of ankle dorsiflexion that follows forefoot floor contact. Starting with the onset of mid stance (10% GC), the soleus reaches its ankle rocker peak of 25% MMT at the 20% GC point. This activity slows the rate of tibial advancement to half of its former speed. Soleus activity continues at the same level of intensity until the end of mid stance (30% GC), while the ankle continues to dorsiflex at the slower rate. Thus, the soleus contributes modulated control of the ankle for simultaneous progression and stability (eccentric muscle action).

Soleus activity is the dominant decelerating force (compared to the gastrocnemius) because it provides a direct tie between the tibia and calcaneus. Also, the soleus is the largest plantar flexor muscle. In contrast, the gastrocnemius has no direct tie to the tibia because it arises from the distal femur. Consequently, until body weight is anterior to the knee joint axis (late mid stance), the gastrocnemius also acts as a knee flexor, as it lies posterior to the knee joint axis. This increases the demand on the quadriceps, but that is not a problem for persons with normal strength or control. Sutherland's data demonstrate a distinct delay in the onset of gastrocnemius activity.[48] The Rancho data also show a slight delay in gastrocnemius onset compared to that of the soleus. In addition, there is a slower rise in the intensity of action by the gastrocnemius. Both data indicate a sensitivity to the functional difference between the mechanics of the two plantar flexor muscles. Progression and stability are both served by the normal balance between mobility and muscular control.

While the posterior tibialis and peroneal muscles also are active in mid stance, their short plantar flexor leverage as they pass closely behind the malleoli offers no significant tibial control. Their actions are on the foot.

Terminal Stance.
Motion: Heel rise with continued ankle dorsiflexion.
Function: Forefoot rocker for progression.
By the end of mid stance the base of the body vector lies in the forefoot. With the ankle virtually locked by the soleus and gastrocnemius, the heel rises as the tibia continues to advance.[35] This makes the forefoot the sole source of foot support. The rounded contours of the metatarsal heads and the adjacent bases of the proximal phalanges provide a forefoot rocker that allows the vector to roll forward for continued progression (Figure 4.9).

With the body vector based in the area of the metatarsal heads the dorsiflexion lever (moment arm) is the full length of the forefoot (Figure 4.10). This combined with falling body weight generates a maximal dorsiflexion torque at the ankle. The heel rise posture means body weight must be supported as well. Consequently there is a demand for strong soleus and gastrocnemius action (80% MMT), which is approximately three times that needed during mid stance. Active gastrosoleus deceleration of the dorsiflexion torque results in minimal ankle motion, being limited to a mere 5° increase in dorsiflexion (to 10°) as the tibia follows the forward moving body vector.[17,35]

The high intensity reported for terminal stance plantar flexor muscle action must be put in perspective with the available clinical test. Manual resistance (as done elsewhere in the body) challenges less than 30% of the muscular activity occurring in a single heel rise. Dynamometer torque testing is not routine, because it a very time-consuming process. Consequently, the clinically expedient normalizing test (MMT) represents a single heel rise to maximum range. The plantar flexors of normal, active persons accomplish 20 maximum heel rises before exhaustion.

The combination of ankle dorsiflexion and heel rise in terminal stance places the body's center of gravity anterior to the source of foot support. As the center of pressure moves more anterior to the metatarsal head axis, the foot rolls with

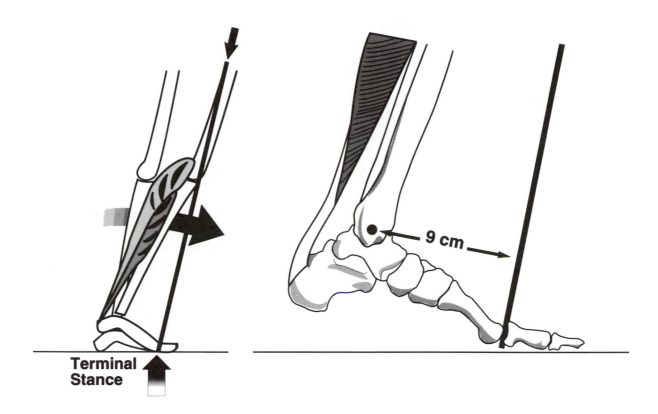

Figure 4.9 Terminal stance pattern of motion, muscle control and vector alignment at the ankle. The vector at the metatarsal head initiates progression over the forefoot rocker (arrow). Strong soleus and gastrocnemius muscle action stabilizes the dorsiflexing ankle and allows heel rise.

Figure 4.10 Terminal stance dorsiflexion lever arm of the body vector. The adult length is approximately 9cm between the base of the vector and the center of the ankle joint.

the body, leading to greater heel rise. The effect is an ever-increasing dorsiflexion torque. This creates a free forward fall situation that passively generates the major progression force used in walking. As forward roll and downward fall are combined, a force is created against the floor that is greater than body weight. The actual magnitude of the floor reaction force varies with the gait velocity.

By the end of terminal stance, advancement of the base of the body vector to the metatarsal joints and the forward fall has progressed to a state where there is no available restraint. Also, there is no stabilizing force within the foot, so it is free to plantar flex in response to gastrosoleus muscle action. Terminal stance is ended by the other foot contacting the floor to reestablish stability.

Push-off commonly is considered to be the primary function of the gastrosoleus muscle group. The peak triceps surae muscle action at this time, in combination with a high ground reaction force and the large arc of ankle plantar flexion which follows in pre-swing, has fostered this concept of there being a push-off force for body progression. This interpretation overlooks three very pertinent facts. The ankle remains in dorsiflexion until the other foot contacts the ground (terminal double support). At the time of contralateral foot floor contact, rapid transfer of body weight begins. The reduction in soleus and gastrocnemius action parallels the rapid decline in the force plate pattern. The peak intensities of both the soleus and gastrocnemius just support a heel rise in an eccentric mode (Figure 4.9). No added force has been provided to thrust the body forward. Also, biomechanical studies identify deceleration rather than increasing tibial advancement.[17,43]

A careful study relating the pattern of body advancement to the external vector demonstrated that the plantar flexor muscles restrain the body's momentum rather than propelling it forward.[43] Direct shank accelerometry found a deceleration force in terminal stance about equal to that occurring in loading response.[17] These findings contradict Hof's conception of an elastic after force catapulting the body forward.[22] In reality the muscles provide critical ankle stabilization that allows both the foot and tibia to roll forward on the forefoot rocker. There are two significant effects: a reduction in the amount of fall by the body's center of gravity and enhancement of progression.[43] Both relate to the increase in relative limb length from using the forefoot rather than the ankle as the fulcrum. Hence, *roll-off* (the forefoot rocker) is a more appropriate term than *push-off.*

The signs of effective ankle function during terminal stance are heel rise, minimal joint motion and a nearly neutral ankle position.

Pre-Swing.

Motion: Second arc of ankle plantar flexion

Function: Initiate knee flexion for swing

This is a very complex phase of gait. The actions at the ankle are related to events other than the weight-bearing capability of the limb. Continued floor contact assists body balance as body weight is transferred to the other limb, while the synergy of muscle action and ankle motion are the primary factors in initiating swing.

Following the onset of double limb support (opposite foot contact), body weight is rapidly transferred to the other limb. The need for forceful stabilization of the ankle and foot is past. As a result, the soleus and gastrocnemius promptly reduce the intensity of their action. This also is true for the perimalleolar muscles. At the same time the ankle rapidly plantar flexes 20°. While the activity of the gastrocnemius and soleus decreases too rapidly to lift the body, it is sufficient to accelerate advancement of the unloaded limb. This is an important contribution to swing. The foot is free to plantar flex because the body vector is based at the MP joint. The residual plantar flexor muscle action nudges the tibia forward as the toe is stabilized by floor contact. The effect is rapid knee flexion in preparation for swing (Figure 4.11).

The onset of tibialis anterior and toe extensor muscle action at the end of pre-swing decelerates the rate of foot fall. This also prepares the muscles controlling the ankle for the demands of initial swing. Throughout most of the pre-swing phase the foot is not bearing significant weight. Hence, the terminal double support period indicates bilateral floor contact but not equal load sharing.

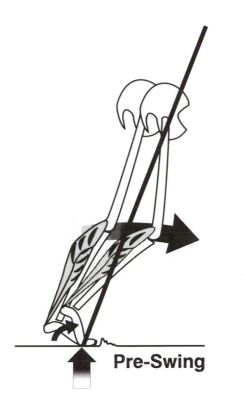

Pre-Swing

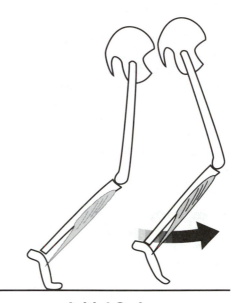

Initial Swing

Figure 4.11 Pre-swing pattern of motion, muscle control and vector alignment at the ankle. The vector is at MP joint, which frees the foot to roll forward in response to the dorsiflexion torque. Calf muscle action is markedly reduced as the limb is rapidly unloaded. Advancement of the tibia places the vector behind the knee, creating a flexion torque.

Figure 4.12 Initial swing pattern of motion, muscle control and vector alignment at the ankle. Limb advancement (arrow) creates a plantar flexion drag at the ankle that requires tibialis anterior control.

Initial Swing.

Motion: Initiation of the second arc of dorsiflexion

Function: Floor clearance for limb advancement

The actions occurring during initial swing are designed to facilitate progression. At the ankle this involves lifting the foot to aid limb advancement (Figure 4.12).

At the moment of toe-off, which signifies the onset of the swing phase, the ankle is in 20° plantar flexion. This position does not immediately obstruct advancement of the limb, because of its trailing posture. That is, having the tibia behind the body places the foot into a toe down posture (i.e., natural equinus). Now it is necessary to reverse ankle motion into dorsiflexion for subsequent floor clearance by the toes in mid swing. The pretibial muscles quickly increase their intensity, reaching 25% MMT within the first 5% gait cycle interval in initial swing. This almost lifts the foot to neutral (5° PF) by the time the swing foot is opposite the stance limb. As the toe extensor muscles are as active as the tibialis anterior, there also is visible dorsiflexion of the toes.

Mid Swing.

Motion: Continued ankle dorsiflexion

Function: Floor clearance

As the tibia becomes vertical, foot weight creates a stronger downward torque. The tibialis anterior and extensor hallucis longus respond by increasing their action to a peak of 40% MMT. Ankle dorsiflexion to neutral or a couple of degrees above is accomplished but not totally maintained (Figure 4.13). Failure of the extensor digitorum longus to increase its activity may relate to the medial side of the foot being the heavier mass.

This muscular reaction occurs during the early part of mid swing. The following decline in muscular action implies that supporting the foot at neutral (an isometric action) is less demanding than the concentric muscle action required to meet the demands of completing foot lift against a more challenging limb posture.

Terminal Swing.

Motion: Support of the ankle at neutral

Function: Prepare for initial contact

The increase in pretibial muscle action during terminal swing assures the ankle will be at neutral for optimum heel contact in stance (Figure 4.14), though commonly there is a 3° to 5° drop into plantar flexion, suggesting the response is not precise. Inertia of the foot while the tibia is being actively advanced is the

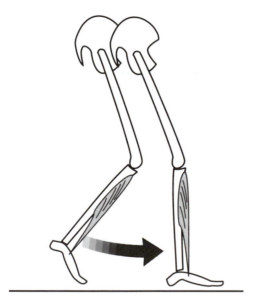

Mid Swing

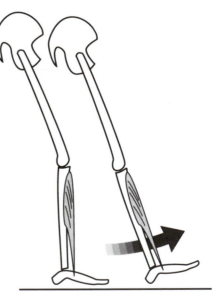

Terminal Swing

Figure 4.13 Mid swing limb advancement (arrow) continues the demand on the tibialis anterior.

Figure 4.14 Terminal swing advancement (arrow) of the tibia also presents a demand for tibialis anterior support of the foot against the plantar flexion force of gravity.

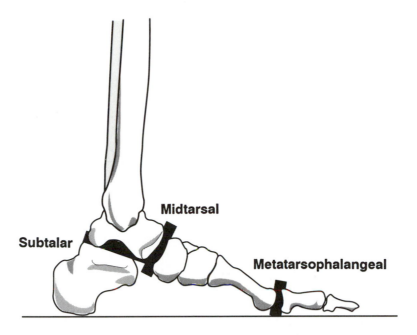

Figure 4.15 The joints in the foot with major functional significance during walking (black areas): subtalar, midtarsal, metatarsophalangeal.

probable stimulus for the added muscular effort. The greater action by the largest muscle (tibialis anterior) supports this interpretation. Terminal swing muscle activity also prepares the pretibial muscles for the higher demand they will experience during limb loading.

Conclusion

The conspicuous events during a gait cycle are ankle plantar flexion during the loading response and pre-swing phases of gait. Most critical, however, is the gradual dorsiflexion that progresses through mid and terminal stance. This is the main determinant of progression. Another critical event is heel rise at the onset of terminal stance. This signifies adequate triceps surae stabilization of the ankle. During swing, recovery of dorsiflexion to neutral is the only obligation of the ankle and its controlling muscles.

The Foot

There are three major articulations within the foot that relate to the mechanics of walking. These are the subtalar (ST), midtarsal (MT) and metatarsophalangeal (MP) joints (Figure 4.15).

The subtalar joint is the junction between the talus and calcaneus. This places it within the vertical weight-bearing column between the heel and tibia. Subtalar action adds coronal and transverse plane mobility to the sagittal plane function available at the ankle. In addition, subtalar motion modifies the mobility of the other joints within the foot.

The midtarsal (or transverse tarsal) joint is the junction of the hind and forefoot. It is formed by two articulations, talonavicular and calcaneocuboid. Midtarsal motion contributes to the shock absorption of forefoot contact.

The MP joint is the *toe break*, which allows the foot to roll over the metatarsal heads rather than the tips of the toes. The five metatarsal heads provide a broad area of support across the forefoot. In addition, the proximal phalanges allow an adjustable lengthening of the forefoot for progressional stability as needed.

Motion

Subtalar Joint. The subtalar joint has a single, obliquely oriented axis that allows the foot to tilt medially (inversion) and laterally (eversion). These actions occur in both stance and swing, but the stance phase motions are more significant as they influence the weight-bearing alignment of the whole limb.

Eversion begins as part of the loading response immediately after the heel contacts the floor. Peak eversion is reached by early mid stance (14% GC). The arc is small though rapid, averaging 4°-6° (Figure 4.16).[6,12,52] These represent both shod and barefoot measurements. Subtalar motion then slowly reverses toward inversion throughout terminal stance. Peak inversion is attained at the onset of pre-swing (52% GC). In swing the foot drifts back to neutral, followed by terminal inversion during the last 20% of the cycle.[52]

Midtarsal Joint. Midtarsal mobility has been observed but not measured. The signs of action are flattening and recovery of the arch. Flattening quickly follows forefoot contact. The motion is dorsiflexion. This occurs during the

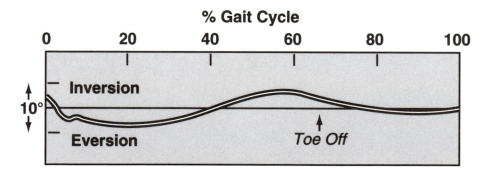

Figure 4.16 Normal subtalar joint motion during free walking. (Adapted from Wright DG, Desai SM, Henderson WH. Action of the subtalar and ankle-joint complex during the stance phase of walking. *J Bone Joint Surg.* 46A:361-382, 1964.)

early mid stance phase of single limb support. With heel rise, restoration of the arch is observed, implying the midtarsal dorsiflexion has been reversed.

Metatarsophalangeal Joint. At initial contact the MP joints are in 25° dorsiflexion with the toes up. Following forefoot contact at the end of loading response, the toes drop towards neutral alignment and maintain this position throughout mid stance. With heel rise in terminal stance, the MP joints dorsiflex (extend) 21°.[4] During this motion the toes remain in contact with the floor, and the metatarsal shafts angle upward as the hind foot is lifted. This motion continually increases throughout pre-swing to a final position of 55° extension (Figure 4.17).

Lifting the foot for swing allows the toes to drop toward the line of the metatarsal shafts. In mid swing slight dorsiflexion is maintained. Then the MP joints increase their dorsiflexion (toes up) in preparation for initial contact.

Muscle Control

The sequence of muscular control within the foot progresses from the hind foot to the forefoot and then the toes. Ten muscles are involved. As subtalar control is dominant, the muscles generally are grouped according to their relationship to the subtalar joint axis (i.e., as the long invertors, long evertors and plantar intrinsics). Most of the muscles have another primary function, and thus their effectiveness at the subtalar joint varies markedly (Table 4.5).

Invertor Muscles. Five muscles cross the subtalar joint medially. In the order of their inverting leverage, these are the tibialis posterior, tibialis anterior, flexor digitorum longus, flexor hallucis longus, and soleus. All but the tibialis anterior also lie posterior to the ankle. Their onset of activity during stance occurs in a serial fashion and continues relative to their need by more distal joints.

Tibialis anterior action markedly increases its intensity during loading

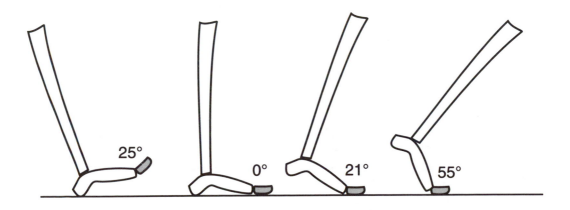

Figure 4.17 Metatarsophalangeal joint motion during stance. Shaded toe indicates area of motion.

Table 4.5

Relative Muscle Leverage at the Subtalar Joint
(Tibialis Posterior, the reference base)

Inversion

Tibialis Posterior	1.00
Tibialis Anterior	0.63
Flexor Hallucis Longus	0.51
Soleus	0.43

Eversion

Peroneus Longus	1.08
Peroneus Brevis	1.00
Extensor Digitorum Longus	0.92
Extensor Hallucis Longus	0.23

---

response from the level in swing to 45% MMT. Then there is a rapid decline and relaxation in early mid stance (15% GC) (Figure 4.3).[38]

Tibialis posterior action is more variable. Close and Sutherland[13,48] reported good TP activity, but not Gray and Basmajian.[3,18] The Rancho data showed considerable variability, but the dominant pattern was early subtalar control. Following the onset of action in early loading response (5% GC),[48] there are two periods of peak intensity. The first is a 20% MMT effort at the end of loading response (10% GC). The middle of terminal stance (40% GC) is the time of the second tibialis posterior rises (30% MMT), which persists into early pre-swing (Figure 4.4).

Soleus muscle activity showed two levels of control. During mid stance there was a 25% effort. This was followed by a progressive rise in terminal stance to 80% MMT. In pre-swing, soleus muscle action promptly declines.

Both of the long toe flexors (FDL and FHL) begin their action in mid stance (15% and 25% GC respectively) and progressively increase their intensity through terminal stance. Then there is a rapid decline in pre-swing (Figure 4.4).[48]

Evertor Muscles. Five muscles lie on the lateral side of the subtalar joint axis. Two are anterior, the extensor digitorum longus and peroneus tertius. Posteriorly there are the gastrocnemius, peroneus longus and peroneus brevis.

Extensor digitorum longus action in stance occurs during loading response at about 25% MMT and terminates with the onset of mid stance. Clinically, the peroneus tertius displays similar timing, but it has not been documented by EMG.

Gastrocnemius action progressively increases after its onset in early mid stance (10% GC). Peak action (75% MMT) is reached at the end of terminal stance (50% GC). During pre-swing, gastrocnemius action rapidly declines.

The two posterior peroneal muscles begin their action with the onset of forefoot loading (15% GC) and reach a peak of intensity by the end of the phase.[13,18,48] The timing and relative intensity of the peroneus brevis and peroneus longus are very similar (Figure 4.4).[23,24,29,36,37] In many individuals the peroneus longus displays an earlier onset and more prolonged action. Both muscles tend to relax in mid pre-swing (55-58% GC).

Intrinsics. The intrinsic muscles of the foot constitute one on the dorsum (extensor digitorum brevis) and five on plantar surface of the foot. Intrinsic muscle action follows two patterns (Figure 4.18). Three begin their activity in early mid stance (20% GC). These are the abductor digiti quinti in Figure 4.18, flexor hallucis brevis and extensor digitorum brevis. The other three muscle groups, abductor hallucis, flexor digitorum brevis and interossei, become active in terminal stance (40% GC).

The plantar fascia offers passive support to the mid foot and MP joints. Extending from the calcaneus to the toes, it becomes tense with heel rise. MP joint dorsiflexion serves as a windlass to tighten the fascia (Figure 4.19). A force plate study showed that in maximum dorsiflexion the toe flexor force was twice that available by maximum voluntary contraction of the flexor muscles.

Functional Interpretation of the Foot

Foot motion and muscular control relate to three events: shock absorption, weight-bearing stability and progression. These tasks occur sequentially as floor contact proceeds from initial heel contact to total forefoot support.

Shock Absorption. Lessening the impact of body weight dropping onto the supporting foot is a major function of tarsal mobility. The shock absorbing mechanisms are subtalar eversion and midtarsal dorsiflexion. These actions begin with initial contact and continue until the forefoot is sharing the weight-bearing load. Loading response and early mid stance are the gait phases involved.

Initiating floor contact with the heel introduces subtalar joint eversion as a normal, passive event during limb loading. This occurs because the body of the calcaneus is lateral to the longitudinal axis of the tibia (Figure 4.20).[38] Hence, the load imposed on the talus causes eversion at the subtalar joint (Figure 4.21a). As the foot moves laterally, calcaneal support for the talus is reduced and the bone falls into inversion. Due to the tightly fitted rectangular shape of the ankle joint (Figure 4.21b), the tibia also rotates inward (Figure 4.21c).[33]

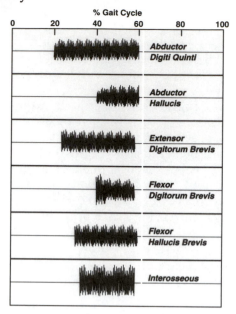

Figure 4.18 Intrinsic foot muscle action during stance. (Adapted from Mann R, Inman VT. *J Bone Joint Surg* 46A:469-481, 1964.)

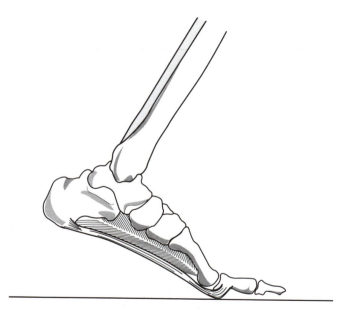

Figure 4.19 Plantar fascia of the foot (superficial to the intrinsic foot muscles in the arch). Fascia tensed by MtP joint dorsiflexion.

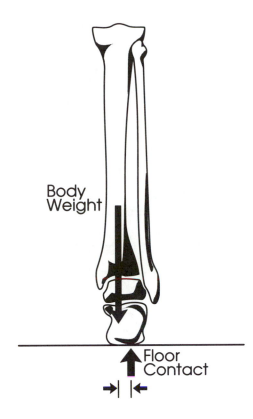

Body
Weight

Floor
Contact

Figure 4.20 Lateral alignment of heel contact (fat arrow) and weight-bearing axis in tibia and talus (long arrow). Offset indicated by interval between the small horizontal arrows.

Response by the inverting muscles absorbs some of the shock of floor impact as subtalar eversion is decelerated. Tibialis anterior action restrains the subtalar joint during the heel rocker period. This is assisted by the early onset of the tibialis posterior in loading response (5% GC). By the time of peak eversion (14% GC) the tibialis anterior has relaxed as its primary function, since a dorsiflexor no longer is needed. At the same time the soleus has reached its moderate level of action. The dominant functions of the tibialis anterior and soleus relate to ankle control, but both muscles also have considerable inversion leverage (Table 4.5). The much larger size of the soleus compared to the tibialis posterior (5X) makes it a significant invertor, even though the tibialis posterior has twice as long an inversion lever arm (Figure 4.22). The variability in posterior tibialis activity suggests it is a reserve force ready to supplement insufficient varus control by the ankle muscles.

Midtarsal joint dorsiflexion also contributes to shock absorption. The motion, stimulated by forefoot contact at the onset of mid stance, follows the subtalar eversion that occurred during loading response.

Dynamic support of the midtarsal joints is provided by several muscles. The tibialis posterior muscle appears to be the major muscle supporting the midtarsal joint. However, the onset of the flexor digitorum longus (15% GC) and lateral plantar intrinsic (20% GC) muscle action before any change in toe position implies these toe muscles also contribute to support of the midtarsal

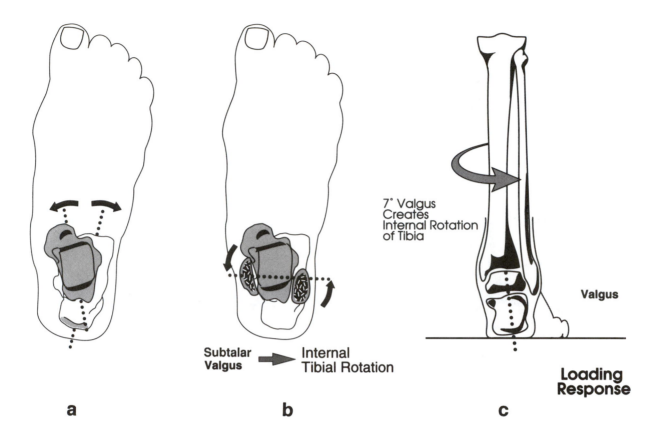

Figure 4.21 Loading response subtalar action. (a) Foot everts, and the unsupported talus rotates inward. (b) Ankle axis (dotted line) rotates medially (arrows) as talus reacts to everted foot. (c) Tibia follows internal rotation of talus.

joint. Subsequent action by the flexor hallucis longus (25% GC) and finally the medial intrinsics (40% GC) is consistent with the lateral side of the forefoot (MT 5) contacting the floor prior to the medial metatarsals (MT 1).

Stability. Advancement of the body vector across the foot directs an increasing percentage of the load onto the forefoot. This necessitates good intertarsal stability, for the weight-bearing column extends from the talus to metatarsal heads. The demand is greatest with heel rise when there is total forefoot support.

To meet this demand for mid foot stability, the subtalar joint reverses its everted position to one of inversion (Figure 4.23). This action also locks the midtarsal joint.

Dynamic locking of the midtarsal joints through subtalar inversion occurs incidental to soleus muscle action at the ankle. There also is continued action of the tibialis posterior and increasing toe flexor involvement. In terminal stance all four inverting muscles (soleus, tibialis posterior, flexor digitorum longus and flexor hallucis longus) markedly increase their intensity to provide the added

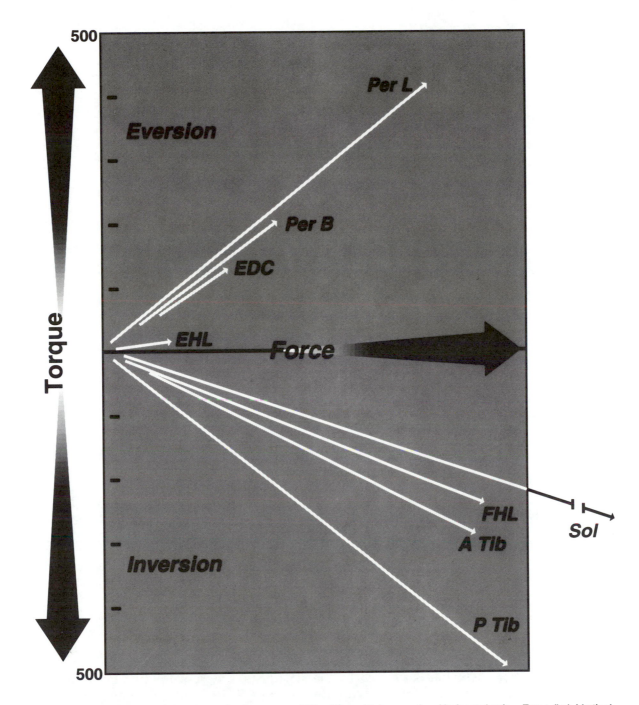

Figure 4.22 Relative inversion and eversion torque capability of the subtalar muscles. Horizontal axis = Force (kg). Vertical = lever arm as well as torque as the end point is the diagonal line length. Torque = the diagonal line length. (Adapted from Perry J. Anatomy and biomechanics of the hind foot. *Clin Ortho* 177:9-16, 1983.)

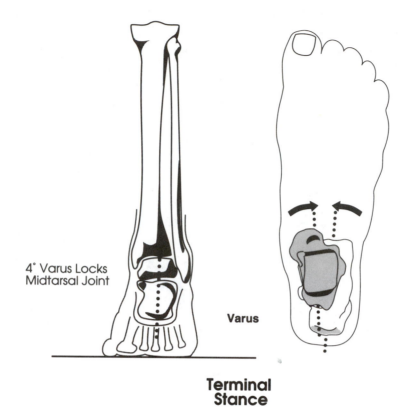

4° Varus Locks
Midtarsal Joint

Varus

**Terminal
Stance**

Figure 4.23 Terminal stance subtalar action. Inversion moves the calcaneus under the talus, externally rotates tibia.

stability needed for isolated forefoot support. The deep intrinsic muscle layer has the advantage of proximity, but the other muscle groups provide greater force due to their larger mass.

The plantar fascia also offers passive stability in terminal stance and pre-swing. Extending from the calcaneus to the fascia about the base of the toes (proximal phalanges), this fascial band is tightened by metatarsophalangeal (MP) dorsiflexion. Effectiveness of tightening of the plantar fascia during routine walking, however, is limited, as 50% shortening of the aponeurosis requires 30° of MP dorsiflexion. Only two-thirds of this range of dorsiflexion is reached by the end of terminal stance when maximum stability is needed.[4] Plantar fascial stability, however, would be of significance in more vigorous activities.

Excessive inversion is avoided by the synergistic action of the two peroneal muscles. Their activity begins with heel rise (30% GC) and continues into pre-swing.

Ankle/subtalar synergy. Subtalar motion lessens the potential strain on the ankle during walking. Throughout stance the body moves from behind to ahead of the supporting limb, which creates a rotatory torque on the supporting joints. The externally rotated alignment of the ankle axis (20°) is not compatible with the path of the body's motion in loading response. The potential medial joint strain this presents is avoided by simultaneous subtalar motion. As the foot everts during the loading response, support for the head of the talus is reduced (Figure 4.21a). This causes the whole talus to internally rotate, carrying the ankle joint mortise with it. The resulting transverse rotation improves the ankle joint's progressional alignment, and medial joint impingement is avoided (Figure 4.21c).

Then, as the body moves ahead of the ankle during mid and terminal stance, subtalar action is reversed to inversion (Figure 4.23). This lifts the head of the talus and restores the externally rotated alignment of the ankle axis. Again, strain from body weight torque is avoided at the snugly contoured, single axis ankle joint. Rotatory moments measured at the floor are small but functionally significant, as intrarticular shear is poorly tolerated.

Subtalar/midtarsal synergy. The subtalar joint controls midtarsal mobility by altering the relative alignment of the talonavicular (TN) and calcaneocuboid (CC) joints. With subtalar joint eversion the axes of the TN and CC joints are parallel, and the midtarsal joint is free to move and serve as a shock-absorbing mechanism during the loading response (Figure 4.24).

The subtalar inversion that occurs in late mid stance and terminal stance causes the axes of the TN and CC joints to diverge. This locks the midtarsal joint into relative plantar flexion (high arch). The tarsometatarsal joints also are locked by this mechanism. Now the foot has the intertarsal stability to support all of body weight on the forefoot.

Progression. Controlled mobility of the MP joint is essential for optimum forward roll across the forefoot. During mid stance foot flat contact, body weight is shared by the heel and forefoot. The metatarsal joints lie in neutral (Figure 4.25). In terminal stance, as the heel rises with continued forward progression body weight is transferred fully onto the forefoot, and dorsiflexion is induced at the MP joints (Figure 4.26).

Deceleration by toe flexors assures a broad, stable area of support. The total area can be expanded by inclusion of the toes. This allows a greater forward roll if the MP joint yields appropriately. Stance phase action of the toe flexors controls the shape and stability of the forefoot rocker. Floor contact by the distal phalanges is the obvious action. The more significant, but subtle, function is the muscles' compressive force across the MP joints. This expands the forefoot contact area by adding the base of the proximal phalanx to that of the metatarsal heads. As a result, the weight-bearing pressure (force per unit area) is reduced. Supplementing the muscles is the passive compression by the plantar fascia, which has been tightened by MP dorsiflexion.

A further stabilizing force that improves the forefoot support area is the action of the peroneus longus on the first metatarsal. By plantar flexing the first ray, the weight-bearing capacity of the medial side of the forefoot (i.e., hallux) is improved. This is particularly significant as body weight rolls toward the first ray in preparation for weight acceptance by the other limb. As a result the terminal location of the body vector is between the first and second MP joints.

Freedom for the foot to roll across the rounded metatarsal surfaces

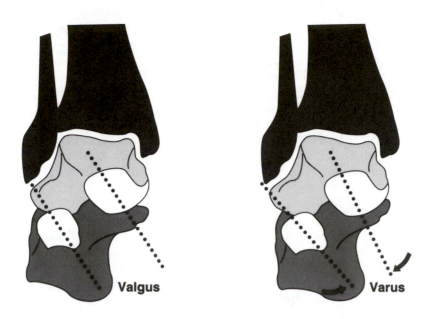

Figure 4.24 Midtarsal joint reactions. Talonavicular and calcaneal cuboid joint axes (dotted lines) parallel with subtalar valgus. The joint axes converge with subtalar varus (arrows). (Adapted from Mann RA. Biomechanics of the foot in American Academy Orthopaedic Surgeons (ed) Atlas of Orthotics: Biomechanical Principles & Application, 1975.)

depends on there being adequate passive mobility of the MP joint and yielding control by the flexor muscles. The small flexor leverage available to the long toe flexor muscles allows them to maintain the desired compressive force for MP joint stability and still permit progressive dorsiflexion. This enables the center of pressure to move beyond the end of the metatarsal head, thereby adding to the length of the stride.

Floor Contact

Foot Support Patterns

Differences in timing of heel and forefoot contact with the floor create three foot-support patterns. These normally occur in the following sequence: heel, foot flat (heel and forefoot) and forefoot (Figure 4.27). The last area of the forefoot in contact with the ground is the first metatarsal as body weight rolls onto the other foot (Figure 4.27). Timing of toe contact varies. There also are differences in the mode of forefoot loading during the foot flat period. Equivalent Latin terminology is calcaneograde (heel only), plantigrade (flat), digigrade (forefoot), and unguligrade (toe tips).[4]

Heel Support (Calcaneograde). The stance period normally is initiated by just the heel contacting the floor. Rapidity of this action has led to the term

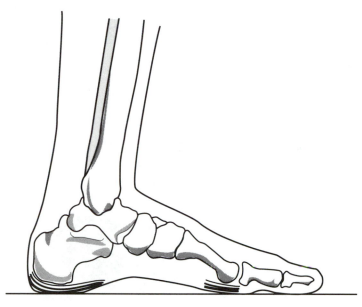

Figure 4.25 Foot flat weight-bearing on heel and forefoot, metatarsal joint neutral.

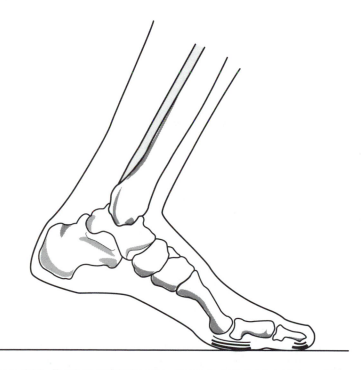

Figure 4.26 Forefoot weight-bearing. Support area increased by addition of proximal phalangeal base to metatarsal head. Toe tip contact is the visible sign of toe flexor action.

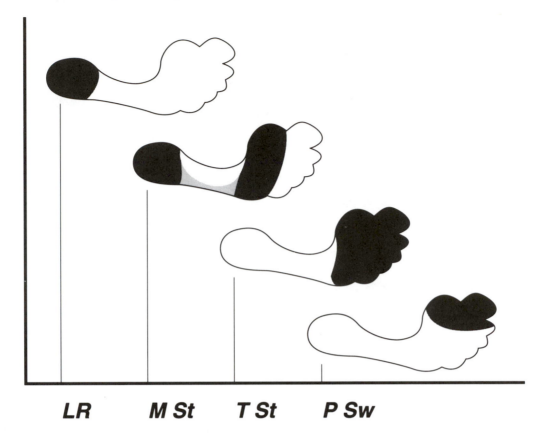

LR   **M St**   **T St**   **P Sw**

Figure 4.27 Sequence of foot support areas during stance. Heel only in loading response (LR). Foot flat in mid stance (MSt). Forefoot and toes in terminal stance (TSt). Medial forefoot in pre-swing (PSw). (Adapted from Barnett CH. The phases of human gait. *Lancet* 82(9/22):617-621, 1956.)

heel strike. After contacting the floor, the heel continues as the sole source of support for the first 6% to 10% of the gait cycle.[4,20,25,38,40,41] Consistency among studies has followed the development of more responsive equipment. In contrast, the early pedographs indicated a heel support time to be 15% GC.[2] Timing also is influenced by the size and location of sensor used, as contact is first made by the posterior margin and followed by a quick roll onto the center of the heel.[2,33,45]

Foot Flat Support (Plantigrade). Forefoot contact terminates the heel only support period and introduces a plantigrade or foot flat posture. This persists for approximately 20% of the gait cycle. The manner of forefoot contact varies among individuals. Most commonly (71%) the fifth metatarsal head is the first to touch the floor, resulting in at least a 0.1 second interval of H-5 support. The average is 10% GC.[25,38] A moderate number (22%) make contact with the total forefoot (H-5-1) and 8% of the subjects initiate forefoot support with the first metatarsal (H-1). Regardless of the means of starting forefoot contact, all segments from fifth to first soon are involved (H-5-1).

Recent studies with a segmented force plate show quick progression from the the lateral side of the foot (fifth and fourth metatarsal heads) to the medial side.[25] Less than 1% omit the foot flat interval.

Forefoot Support (Digigrade). Heel rise (5-1) changes the mode of foot support from flat to forefoot. This occurs at the 30% point in the gait cycle and persists until the end of stance. All the metatarsal heads are involved, though the simplified foot switch indicates only the 5-1 metatarsals.

Toe contact with the floor is quite variable. Scranton identified very early onset, while Barnett found the onset of toe involvement followed isolated forefoot support by 10% of the stance period.[2,42] Having the toe the last segment

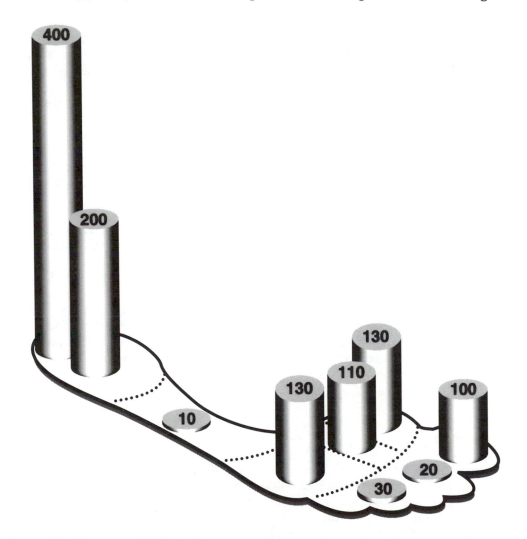

Figure 4.28 Sequence of weight-bearing pressure (KPa) from initial impact at the heel to toe roll off. (Adapted from Cavanagh PR, Michiyoshi AC. A technique for the display of pressure distributions beneath the foot. *J Biomech* 13:69-75, 1980.)

to lift from the floor at the end of stance is common.[4,38] Bojsen calls this the *unguligrade* phase of gait.[4] Simultaneous first metatarsal and toe departure also is a normal finding.

Foot Pressures

As body weight is dropped onto the supporting foot, pressure is imposed on the plantar tissues. The magnitude of the compression is a balance between the intensity of the loading force and the area of the foot in contact with the floor.

Heel pressure shows two patterns. Initial loading occurs on a small posterior lateral area, and body weight is dropped rapidly. This results in the largest pressure experienced by the foot (Figure 4.28).[2,15,25,45,47] A total force, ranging between 70% and 100% of body weight, occurs within 0.05 seconds.[25,46] Cavanagh identifed this pressure as 1018 kPa during a slow walk.[8] For comparison with other areas, this peak high pressure will be called 100%.

Advancement of body weight onto the center of the heel reduces the pressures to a third (33%).[8] When the sensors are placed only in the middle of the heel, this becomes the only identified heel pressure. Then maximum pressure is identified in another area of the foot.[19,20]

Lateral mid foot contact with the floor is moderately common but of low intensity. The pressure in this area averages 10% of body weight,[25] or it also has been expressed as 10% of heel maximum.[45]

Metatarsal head pressure differs among the individual bones. Generally the highest pressures are registered under the second and third metatarsal heads.[15,19,45] Whether the forces are equal or one is slightly greater than the other is highly variable among individuals. Compared to the posterior heel value, the metatarsal head pressures varied between 60% and 100%. One author found a low of 30%.[25]

Toe pressures differ markedly. The hallux has the greatest pressure. It ranged between 30% and 55% of that at the heel.[15,19,25,45,47] The fifth metatarsal head always registered the least pressure within the forefoot. The range was 5%, 20% and 45% of heel maximum or half that experience by the central (third) ray.[15,19] Only one investigator found fifth metatarsal pressures similar to that on the other heads.[45]

Conclusion

The ankle moves through four arcs of motion during each stride. Each has a specific function. The restrained dorsiflexion during mid and terminal stance is least apparent, yet the most significant. It combines progression and stability during the single limb support interval.

Subtalar motion provides shock absorption during limb loading and foot stability in terminal stance. Motion at the subtalar joint reduces the rotatory strain at the ankle and controls the mobility of the midtarsal joint.

Midtarsal mobility contributes to shock absorption. Rigidity of this area is needed for body weight transfer to the forefoot.

Controlled metatarsophalangeal joint motion uses the toes to lengthen the forefoot support area without obstructing the rocker effect. Progression is enhanced by this action.

References

1. American Academy of Orthopaedic Surgeons: *Joint Motion—Method of Measuring and Recording*. American Academy of Orthopaedic Surgeons, 1965.
2. Barnett CH: The phases of human gait. *Lancet* 2:617-621, 1956.
3. Basmajian JV, Stecko G: The role of muscles in arch support of the foot. *J Bone Joint Surg* 45A(6):1184-1190, 1963.
4. Bojsen-Moller F, Lamoreux L: Significance of dorsiflexion of the toes in walking. *Acta Orthop Scand* 50:471-479, 1979.
5. Brandell BR: Functional roles of the calf and vastus muscles in locomotion. *Am J of Phys Med* 56(2):59-74, 1977.
6. Buchthal F, Guld C, Rosenfalck P: Multielectrode study of the territory of a motor unit. *Acta Physiol Scand* 39:83-103, 1957.
7. Carino JM: Force and gait evaluation in normal individuals. *Orthopedic Seminars, RLAMC* 4:63-71, 1971.
8. Cavanagh PR, Michiyoshi AC: A technique for the display of pressure distributions beneath the foot. *J Biomech* 13:69-75, 1980.
9. Cerny K, Perry J, Walker JM: Effect of an unrestricted knee-ankle-foot orthosis on the stance phase of gait in healthy persons. *Orthopedics* 13(10):1121-1127, 1990.
10. Close JR: *Functional Anatomy of the Extremities*. Springfield, Charles C. Thomas, 1973.
11. Close JR, Inman VT: The Action of the Ankle Joint. *Prosthetic Devices Research Project, Institute of Engineering Research, University of California, Berkeley*, Series 11, Issue 22. Berkeley, The Project, 1952.
12. Close JR, Inman VT, Poor PM, Todd FN: The function of the subtalar joint. *Clin Orthop* 50(1-2):159-179, 1967.
13. Close JR, Todd FN: The phasic activity of the muscles of the lower extremity and the effect of tendon transfer. *J Bone Joint Surg* 41A(2):189-208, 1959.
14. Cochran GVB: *A Primer of Orthopaedic Biomechanics*. New York, Churchill Livingstone, 1982, pp. 268-293.
15. Collis WJ, Jayson MI: Measurement of pedal pressures. *Ann Rheum Dis* 31:215-217, 1972.
16. Eberhart HD, Inman VT, Bressler B: The principle elements in human locomotion. In Klopsteg PE, Wilson PD (Eds): *Human Limbs and their Substitutes*. New York, Hafner Publishing Company, 1968, pp. 437-471.
17. Gilbert JA, Maxwell GM, McElhaney JH, Clippinger FW: A system to measure the forces and moments at the knee and hip during level walking. *J Orthop Res* 2:281-288, 1984.
18. Gray EG, Basmajian JV: Electromyography and cinematography of leg and foot ("normal" and flat) during walking. *Anat Rec* 161:1-16, 1968.
19. Grieve DW, Rashid T: Pressure under normal feet in standing and walking as measured by foil pedobarography. *Ann Rheum Dis* 43:816-818, 1984.
20. Grundy M, Tosh PA, McLeish RD, Smidt L: An investigation of the centers of pressure under the foot while walking. *J Bone Joint Surg* 57B(1):98-103, 1975.
21. Haxton HA: Absolute muscle force in the ankle flexors of man. *J Physiol* 103:267-273, 1944.
22. Hof AL, Geelen BA, Van den Berg J: Calf muscle moment, work and efficiency in

level walking; role of series elasticity. *J Biomech* 16(7):523-537, 1983.

23. Houtz JH, Fischer FJ: Function of leg muscles acting on foot as modified by body movements. *J Appl Physiol* 16:597-605, 1961.

24. Houtz SJ, Walsh FP: Electromyographic analysis of the function of the muscles acting on the ankle during weight bearing with special reference to the triceps surae. *J Bone Joint Surg* 41A:1469-1481, 1959.

25. Hutton WC, Dhanendran M: A study of the distribution of load under the normal foot during walking. *Int Orthop* 3:153-157, 1979.

26. Inman VT: *The Joints of the Ankle*. Baltimore, MD, Williams and Wilkins Company. 1976, pp. 26-29.

27. Inman VT, Ralston HJ, Todd F: *Human Walking*. Baltimore, MD, Williams and Wilkins Company, 1981.

28. Jergesen F: *A Study of Various Factors Influencing Internal Fixation as a Method of Treatment of Fractures of the Long Bones*. Washington, D.C., National Research Council, Committee on Veterans Medical Problems Report, 1945.

29. Jonsson B, Rundgren A: The peroneus longus and brevis muscles. A roentgenologic and electromyographic study. *Electromyogr Clin Neurophysiol* 11(1):93-103, 1971.

30. Kadaba MP, Ramakaishnan HK, Wootten ME, Gainey J, Gorton G, Cochran GVB: Repeatability of kinematic, kinetic and electromyographic data in normal adult gait. *J Orthop Res* 7:849-860, 1989.

31. Katoh Y, Chao EYS, Laughman RK, Schneider E, Morrey BF: Biomechanical analysis of foot function during gait and clinical applications. *Clin Orthop* 177:23-33, 1983.

32. Locke M, Perry J, Campbell J, Thomas L: Ankle and subtalar motion during gait in arthritic patients. *Phys Ther* 64(4):504-509, 1984.

33. Mann RA, Baxter DE, Lutter LD: Running symposium. *Foot Ankle* 1(4):190-224, 1981.

34. Murray MP, Clarkson BH: The vertical pathways of the foot during level walking. I. Range of variability in normal men. *Phys Ther* 46(6):585-589, 1966.

35. Murray MP, Drought AB, Kory RC: Walking patterns of normal men. *J Bone Joint Surg* 46A(2):335-360, 1964.

36. O'Connell AL: Electromyographic study of certain leg muscles during movements of the free foot and during standing. *Am J Phys Med* 37:289-301, 1958.

37. O'Connell AL, Mortensen OA: An electromyographic study of leg musculature during movements of the free foot and during standing. *Anat Rec* 127:342, 1957.

38. Perry J: Anatomy and biomechanics of the hindfoot. *Clin Orthop* 177:9-16, 1983.

39. Perry J, Ireland ML, Gronley J, Hoffer MM: Predictive value of manual muscle testing and gait analysis in normal ankles by dynamic electromyography. *Foot and Ankle* 6(5):254-259, 1986.

40. Schwartz RP, Heath AL: The feet in relation to the mechanics of human locomotion. *Phys Ther Review* 16:46-49, 1936.

41. Schwartz RP, Heath AL: The definition of human locomotion on the basis of measurement with description of oscillographic method. *J Bone Joint Surg* 29A:203-213, 1947.

42. Scranton PE, McMaster JH: Momentary distribution of forces under the foot. *J Biomech* 9:45-48, 1976.

43. Simon SR, Mann RA, Hagy JL, Larsen LJ: Role of the posterior calf muscles in normal gait. *J Bone Joint Surg* 60A:465-472, 1978.

44. Skinner SR, Antonelli D, Perry J, Lester DK: Functional demands on the stance limb in walking. *Orthopedics* 8(3):355-361, 1985.

45. Soames RW: Foot pressure patterns during gait. *J Biomed Eng* 7(2):120-126, 1985.

46. Stokes IAF, Stott JRR, Hutton WC: Force distributions under the foot—a dynamic measuring system. *Biomed Eng* 9(4):140-143, 1974.

47. Stott JR, Hutton WC, Stokes IA: Forces under the foot. *J Bone Joint Surg* 55B(2):335-344, 1973.
48. Sutherland D: An electromyographic study of the plantar flexors of the ankle in normal walking on the level. *J Bone Joint Surg* 48A:66-71, 1966.
49. Sutherland DH, Cooper L, Daniel D: The role of the ankle plantar flexors in normal walking. *J Bone Joint Surg* 62A:354-363, 1980.
50. Weber EF: *Ueber die Langenverhaltnisse der Fkeuscgfaserb der Muskeln im Allgemeinen.* Math-phys Cl, Ber. Verh. K. Sachs. Ges. Wissensch, 1851.
51. Winter DA, Quanbury AO, Hobson DA, Sidwall HG, Reimer G, Trenholm BG, Steinkle T, Shlosser H: Kinematics of normal locomotion—a statistical study based on T.V. data. *J Biomech* 7(6):479-486, 1974.
52. Wright DG, Desai SM, Henderson WH: Action of the subtalar and ankle-joint complex during the stance phase of walking. *J Bone Joint Surg* 46A(2):361-382, 1964.

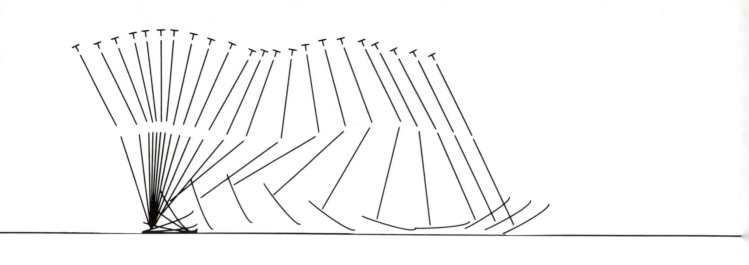

Chapter 5

Knee

The knee is the junction of the two long bones (femur and tibia) that constitute the major segments of the lower limb. Small arcs of motion result in significant changes in either foot or body location. Consequently, knee mobility and stability are major factors in the normal pattern of walking. During stance the knee is the basic determinant of limb stability. In swing, knee flexibility is the primary factor in the limb's freedom to advance. The number of two joint muscles involved in knee control also indicates close functional coordination with the hip and the ankle.

Motion

The knee is a very complex joint characterized by a large range of motion in the sagittal plane and small arcs of coronal and transverse mobility (Figure 5.1). Sagittal motion (flexion and extension) is used for progression in stance and limb advancement in swing. Motion in the coronal plane facilitates vertical balance over the limb, particularly

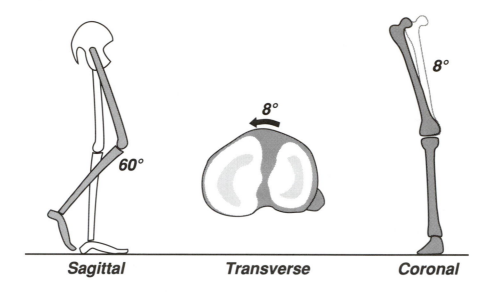

Figure 5.1 Three-dimensional knee motion and arcs used in free walking: Sagittal plane flexion (60°); Transverse plane rotation (8°); Coronal plane abduction (8°).

during single support. Transverse rotation accommodates the changes in alignment as the body swings from behind to ahead of the supporting limb. Unless joint mobility is exaggerated by pathology, visual analysis identifies only the sagittal motion. Instrumented measurement systems are needed to discern the other events.

Sagittal Motion

During each stride, the knee passes through four arcs of motion, with flexion and extension occurring in an alternating fashion (Figure 5.2).[5,7-9,11,14] Normal knee motion during walking represents greater and lesser degrees of flexion within the full range of 0° to 70°. The exact limits of each flexion or extension arc vary with the study reported. These differences are related to variations in walking speed, subject individuality and the landmarks selected to designate limb segment alignments. As not all studies identified the velocity of walking at the time knee motion was recorded, an exact relationship between these two factors can not be calculated.

The average magnitude, timing and sequence of knee motion during each stride is as follows (Table 5.1).

The type and extent of motion occurring at the knee is related to the functional demands of the individual gait phases. The numerical values quoted represent a consensus of the data reported in the literature. Not all functions have been assessed by all investigators.

At initial contact the knee is flexed about 5°. Subjects vary in their knee posture at initial contact between slight hyperextension (−2°) and flexion (5°).[9]

Knee Range of Motion

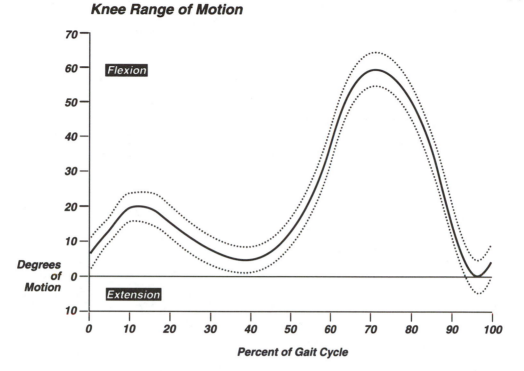

Figure 5.2 Knee motion. Normal range during a gait cycle for free walking.

Following the onset of stance, the knee rapidly flexes throughout the loading phase. The rate of flexion at this time (300°/sec) almost equals that occurring in swing. With the onset of single limb support (12% GC), the knee immediately completes its stance phase flexion (18° at 15% GC). This is the time when the flexed knee is under maximum weight-bearing load.

The differences in knee position at initial contact were unrelated to walking speed. There was a notable influence by walking speed, however, on the amount of flexion occurring during the loading response. Slowing the pace led to a greater change than going faster. Compared to the motion at 90m/min, walking at 60m/min reduced knee flexion by 67%, while increasing the gait speed to 120m/min led to 38% more knee flexion in loading.[9]

During the rest of mid stance, the knee gradually extends. Minimum stance phase flexion (averaging 3°) is reached about midway in terminal stance (40% GC) and persists for only a short time before the knee slowly begins to flex again. The rate of knee extension is approximately half that of flexion during limb loading.

The second wave of knee flexion begins during the end of terminal stance. Approximately 7° flexion is present at the time single limb support is completed by the other foot contacting the floor. With the onset of double limb support the knee flexes rapidly. A 40° position is reached by the end of pre-swing (62% GC). Knee flexion continues at the same fast rate throughout initial swing. The final position of 60° is the maximum knee angle occurring during the gait cycle.[10]

Table 5.1

Knee Motion	
Motion	Timing
Flexion to 18°	0-15% GC
Extension to 5°	15-40% GC
Flexion to 65°	40-70% GC
Extension to 2°	70-97% GC

Murray reported 70° flexion.[14] To reach this position in the time available (pre-swing and initial swing phases), the knee flexes at 350°/sec.

Following a momentary pause in mid swing, the knee begins to extend as rapidly as it flexed in the preceding phases.[3,16] Half of the recovery toward maximum extension occurs during mid swing. Knee extension continues in terminal swing until full extension (3° flexion) is gained. Actual knee position varies among individuals. Some attain slight hyperextension (3°). Others maintain a minor degree of flexion (5°). Peak knee extension is attained slightly before the end of the swing phase (97% GC). Then the knee tends to drop into a minor degree of flexion. The final knee posture at the end of terminal swing averages 5° flexion.

Transverse Rotation

From a position of maximum external rotation at the end of stance, the entire limb (pelvis, femur, tibia) begins internal rotation at toe-off and continues through swing and loading response. During the rest of stance these body segments externally rotate.

Skeletal pins in the femur and tibia demonstrated an average of 9° rotation within the knee.[12] Triaxial goniometric recordings identified a greater range of rotation (13°).[11]

The magnitude as well as the direction of rotation changes with the gait phases. At initial contact the femur is in slight external rotation relative to the tibia (i.e., the knee is locked). During the loading response, internal rotation of the tibia is markedly accelerated, and the femur follows but at a slightly slower rate. While the entire limb responds, the motion is greater at the knee: 7° with the pin markers.[12] Transfer of the subtalar inversion to the tibia has unlocked the knee. By the end of loading response (i.e., initial double support), the bone pin data indicated both the knee joint and the total limb have reached their peak of inward rotation. According to electrogoniometer data, internal rotation might persist.[11] As the knee fully extends in terminal stance, there also is external rotation and the knee is locked. With body weight shifted to the other foot in pre-swing, the knee internally rotates as it is flexed and adducted. This could relate to adductor longus action at the hip.

Initial swing continues internal rotation of the whole limb. Motion at the knee has been described differently by pin and electrogoniometer data. The bone pin data indicated an increase in tibial rotation that ceased with knee extension. Electrogoniometer recordings registered external rotation as the knee was extended in terminal swing. This would be a second knee locking episode.

Coronal Plane Motion

Within each gait cycle the knee moves into both abduction and adduction. During stance the motion is abduction. A third of the subjects studied by Kettlecamp had maximum knee abduction on initial contact.[11] Most of the people (64%), however, experienced an additional 3° of abduction in loading response. During swing the knee returned to a more neutral posture by adducting 8°.

Vector Pattern

During stance the relationship of the body weight vector to the knee creates four torque patterns.[15] The sequence is extension, flexion, extension, flexion as the limb moves through the gait phases (Figure 5.3).

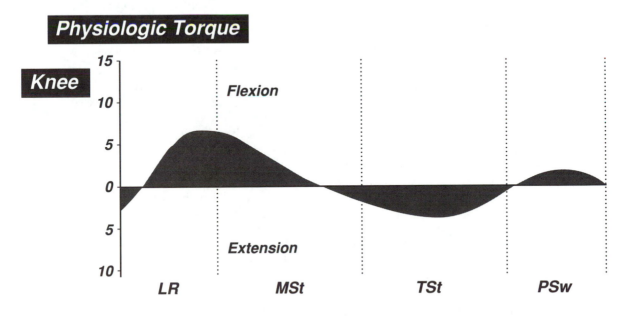

Figure 5.3 Knee joint torques: Normal weight-bearing pattern generated by the sagittal vector during walking. There are four peaks, two extensor torques each followed by a flexion torque interval of similar magnitudes (4 and 2 BW/LL).

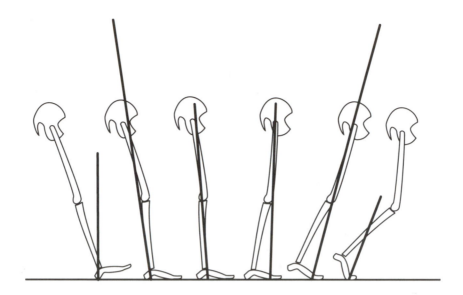

Figure 5.4 Sequence of visible vector relations to the knee from initial contact through pre-swing. The vertical lines represent the instantaneous body weight vectors.

The initial impulse of striking the ground creates a vertical vector. Since the point of floor contact is anterior to the knee so is the vector (Figure 5.4). This provides a momentary extensor torque during the initial 2% of the gait cycle. Its peak value is 2.6 BWLL in anatomical units (body weight × leg length) or a mean absolute value of 25 Nm.[4]

As body weight drops on to the limb during the loading response, the vector rapidly aligns itself with the source of the ground reaction force. This moves the weight line back toward the body center. By the 3% point in the gait cycle the vector reaches the knee joint center and then progressively becomes more posterior. A flexor moment of increasing magnitude is introduced. This results in a torque of 7.8 BWLL or 51 Nm[4] by the end of loading response.

With the onset of single limb support (early mid stance), the relationship between body mass and the supporting limb begins to change. This reverses the direction of the vector. The effect is a progressive decline in the knee flexion torque. By the middle of mid stance (20% GC), neutral alignment (zero torque) is reached. Further advancement of the body mass over the supporting foot moves the vector anterior to the knee. An extensor torque is generated that progressively increases until the middle of terminal stance (42% GC). A mean peak extensor torque of 3.8 BWLL (or 30 Nm)[4] is generated.

Once advancement of the extensor torque ceases, the body weight line moves closer to the knee, with neutral alignment occurring at the end of single limb support (50% GC). In pre-swing the vector again moves posterior to the knee, creating a flexion torque. This rapid reversal of vector alignment creates a peak torque of 1.5 BWLL (20 Nm) by the middle of the pre-swing phase (56% GC).

Muscle Control

The fourteen muscles contributing to knee control contract at selected intervals within the gait cycle. Their purpose is to provide the stability and mobility needed for walking. At the same time, they are quiescent whenever possible to conserve energy. During stance the extensors act to decelerate knee flexion. In swing both the flexors and extensors contribute to limb progression. Muscle action varies with the demands of the individual phases.

Among the multiple muscles acting on the knee, only six have no responsibility at another joint. These are the four vasti heads of the quadriceps that extend the knee and two knee flexors, popliteus and short head of the biceps femoris. All the other muscles (except one) also control hip motion (either flexion or extension). The final muscle acting on the knee is the gastrocnemius, which has its primary role as an ankle plantar flexor.

Knee Extension

The quadriceps is the dominant muscle group at the knee. Four heads cross only the knee joint (vastus intermedius, vastus lateralis, vastus medialis oblique, vastus medialis longus). The fifth head (rectus femoris) includes both the knee and hip.

Activity of the vasti muscles begins in terminal swing (90% GC) (Figure 5.5). Muscle intensity rapidly increases to a peak of 25% MMT early in loading response (5% GC). This level of effort is maintained throughout the remainder of the loading response period. With the onset of mid stance, the quadriceps rapidly reduces its effort and ceases by the 15% gait cycle point.

The timing and intensity of rectus femoris action is much different from that of the vasti (Figure 5.5). Activity of the rectus femoris, demonstrated with the selectivity of wire electrodes, has a short period of action between late pre swing (56% GC) and early initial swing (64% GC). During this interval, the intensity is under 20% MMT. Seldom does the muscle accompany the vasti in loading response (unless surface electrodes have been used and there is cross talk from the vasti).

One hip extensor muscle also contributes to knee extension in early stance. The upper gluteus maximus provides a knee extensor force through its iliotibial band insertion on the anteriorlateral rim of the tibia (Figure 5.6). Activity of this muscle begins in late terminal swing (95% GC) and terminates by the middle of mid stance (20% GC). Throughout most of this time period the upper gluteus maximus registers a significant effort level (30% and then 20% MMT).

Knee Flexion

Two single joint muscles, popliteus and the short head of the biceps femoris (BFSH), provide direct knee flexion. The BFSH is primarily active in initial and mid swing (65-85% GC). Less frequently, there may be activity in terminal stance (32-45% GC). EMG recordings of the popliteus show no

Knee Extensor Muscles (Vasti)

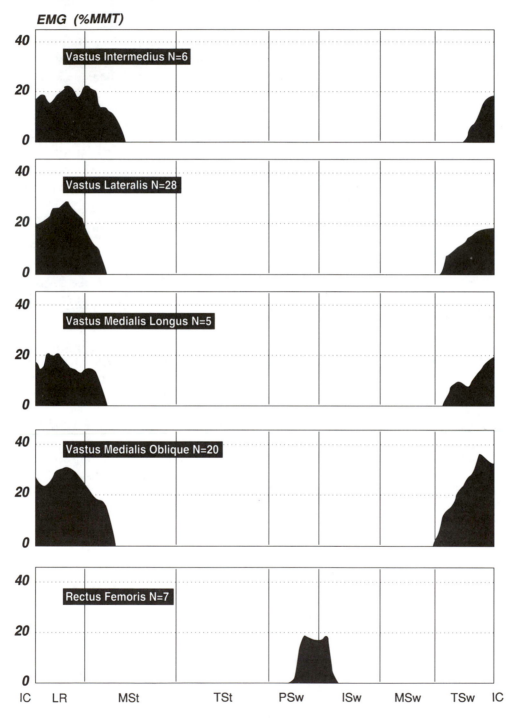

Figure 5.5 Knee extensor muscles: Normal mean intensity and timing during free walking (quantified electromyogram). Intensity as a percent of maximum manual muscle test value (%MMT) indicated by height of gray area. Vertical bars designate the gait phase divisions. N = samples included in data.

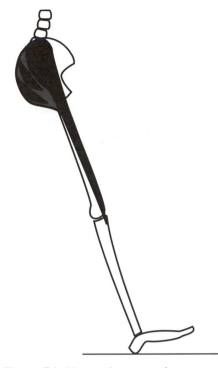

Figure 5.6 Upper gluteus maximus as a knee extensor through its insertion on the iliotibial band.

consistent pattern. While individuals are consistent in their use of the popliteus, its action occurs during all phases of the gait cycle except initial and mid swing (Figure 5.7). The muscle's greatest intensity generally begins in terminal swing and continues through the loading response. Another period of relatively high (25% MMT) effort is in pre-swing.

The three hamstring muscles (semimembranosis, biceps femoris long head, semitendinosis) are primary hip extensors, but these muscles are better known for their flexor role at the knee (Figure 5.8). Two patterns of action are seen. All three hamstrings have their most intense action in late mid- and terminal swing (onset 75% GC) and continue at a lesser level into the early loading phase (cessation 5% GC). The two medial hamstring muscles (semimembranosis and semitendinosis) often continue their activity throughout mid stance.

One additional stance phase muscle that relates to the knee is the gastrocnemius. While principally acting at the ankle, this muscle also is a knee flexor. The gastrocnemius progressively increases its intensity from the time of onset (15% GC) until the middle of terminal stance (75% MMT at 50% GC) (Figure 5.7). Then there is a rapid decline of action until it ceases with the onset of pre-swing.

Two hip flexor muscles also contribute to swing phase knee flexion. These are the gracilis and sartorius (Figure 5.9). Both muscles become active in initial swing and early mid swing (65% to 75% GC). The intensity of this action is moderate (20% MMT).

Knee Flexor Muscles

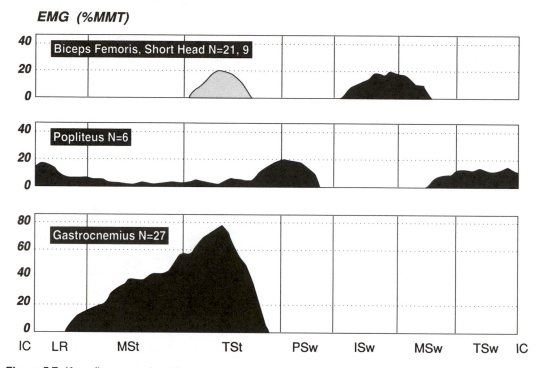

Figure 5.7 Knee flexor muscles (distal). Normal mean intensity and timing during free walking (quantified electromyogram). Intensity as a percent of maximum manual muscle test value (%MMT) indicated by height of gray area. The dark gray area indicates the activity pattern of the majority of the subjects. The light gray area indicates less frequent activity. Vertical bars designate the gait phase divisions. N = samples included in data.

Functional Interpretation

The knee has three functional obligations during walking. Two occur during stance: shock absorption as the limb is loaded and extensor stability for secure weight bearing. In swing the knee must rapidly flex for limb advancement. The relationships between motion and muscle action relate to these demands.

Muscular control of the knee for stance begins in terminal swing (Figure 5.10). At that time, two muscle groups are activated: the hamstrings and vasti components of the quadriceps. Throughout stance, the knee moves from a position of stability at initial contact to one of instability as the limb is loaded, and then reverts to a stable posture in single stance. The stimulus for this variation in stability is the changes that occur in body vector alignment. The period of greatest challenge is weight acceptance.

Knee Flexor Muscles

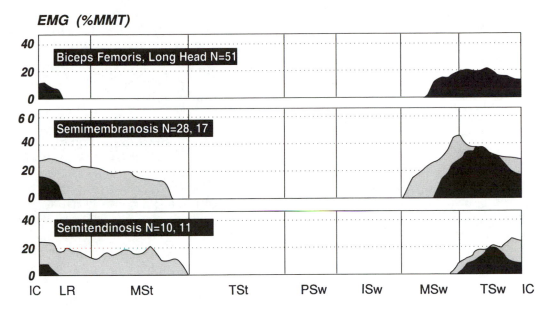

Figure 5.8 Hamstring muscles as knee flexors. Normal mean intensity and timing during free walking (quantified electromyogram). Intensity as a percent of maximum manual muscle test value (%MMT) indicted by height of gray area. The dark gray area indicates the activity pattern of the majority of the subjects. The light gray area indicates less frequent activity. Vertical bars designate the gait phase divisions. N = samples included in data.

Knee Flexor Muscles

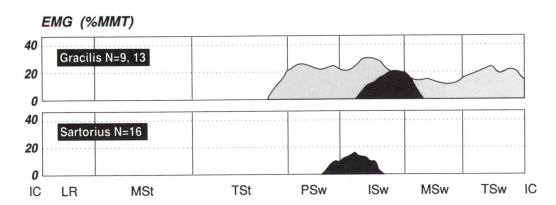

Figure 5.9 Combined knee and hip flexor muscles. Normal mean intensity and timing during free walking (quantified electromyogram). Intensity as a percent of maximum manual muscle test value (%MMT) indicated by height of gray area. The dark gray area indicates the activity pattern of the majority of subjects. The light gray area indicates less frequent activity. Vertical bars designate the gait phase divisions. N = samples included in data.

Knee Function by Gait Phases

Correction of the motion, muscle function and demand vectors that occur in each gait best clarifies the complexity of knee function during walking. The balance between demand and response becomes evident.

Terminal Swing.

Motion: Knee extension

Functions: Complete step length. Prepare for stance

To prepare the limb for stance, the knee flexion used in swing must be reversed to extension. Direct quadriceps activity is required to lift the weight of the tibia and foot as the femur is angled forward 30° in space (Figure 5.10). All four vasti are involved in terminal swing knee extension. It once was assumed that this could be accomplished passively, but the demands are too stringent. Time is limited (0.1 sec), and a secure position of knee extension is needed for initial contact. Dynamic EMG studies confirm participation by the quadriceps (vasti). The rectus is not used because further hip flexion is undesirable. Excessive knee extension is prevented by antagonistic action of the hamstrings, which also are acting to decelerate the hip. At the knee, this muscle action supplements the small resistance provided by the weight of the lower leg and foot. The effect of the hamstring muscle force at the knee will be no more than half that at the hip because of the shorter functional lever available.

Initial Contact.

Motion: Extended knee posture

Function: Stabile weight-bearing

At the time the foot strikes the floor, the knee is in a stable position (Figure 5.11). The knee is extended (−2 to 5° flexion) and two extensor mechanisms are active. First is the favorable alignment of the floor impact vector. The immediate floor reaction force creates a vertical vector anterior to the knee axis. Second is active muscular control. The vasti are active as a result of their role in terminal swing. The upper gluteus maximus/iliotibial band system also was activated in late terminal swing. Continued low-level action (15% MMT) by the hamstring serves as a useful protective flexion force.

Loading Response.

Motion: Knee flexion (15°)

Function: Shock absorption

Dropping body weight on the limb promptly disrupts the knee's initial stability. The knee flexion that follows loading the limb, however, provides valuable shock absorption. The motion is initiated by the heel rocker action that results from floor contact by the heel. This rolls the tibia forward and places the body vector posterior to the knee joint. A flexor moment is created (Figure 5.12). Continuing hamstring muscle activity (10% MMT) accentuates the flexor thrust. Prompt response by the vasti muscles limits the arc of knee flexion to approximately 18°. The quadriceps has functioned eccentrically to restrain (decelerate) but not totally prevent knee flexion. This action serves as a shock absorber. The joint is protected from the deleterious force of full floor impact by

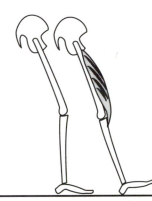
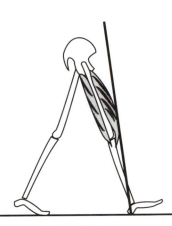

Terminal Swing   **Initial Contact**   **Loading Response**

Figure 5.10 Terminal swing knee control: Quadriceps activity to complete knee extension.

Figure 5.11 Initial contact knee control: Anterior and posterior stabilization by the quadriceps and hamstrings. The anterior vector presents an extensor torque.

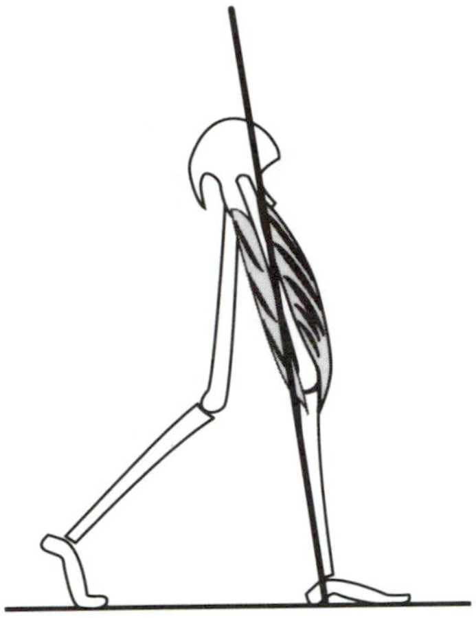

Figure 5.12 Loading response knee control: Quadriceps extension versus the posterior vector. Hamstring activity is waning.

having the heel rocker partially redirect the force into the contracting, yet yielding, quadriceps muscle mass. As a result, the peak vertical force is only 120% of body weight (Figure 3.29).

The early termination of hamstring activity by mid loading response implies that the role of these muscles was primarily protection from potential hyperextension. By their alignment these muscles also assisted in the initiation of knee flexion. As knee flexion continues well past the relaxation of the hamstrings, the dominant flexor mechanism appears to be the heel rocker.

The loading response phase thus challenges knee stability as the mechanisms that provide shock absorption also create an unstable weight-bearing posture. Strength of the quadriceps response is critical to establishing a secure limb.

A second shock-absorbing mechanism also challenges knee stability. The hind foot valgus that occurs in early stance initiates an internal rotation torque on the tibia, which ascends to the knee. Excessive rotation within the joint may be opposed by the external rotational pull of the tensor fascia lata and biceps femoris during the heel support period of loading response (Figure 5.13).

In the coronal plane the knee experiences an adduction torque (Figure 5.14). This persists throughout stance, though it is most marked during loading response when the rapidly unloaded side of the body drops in a momentarily uncontrolled fashion. Brief activity by the long head of the biceps and the gluteus maximus tension on the iliotibial band provides a lateral counterforce to stabilize the knee during the high-stress period of limb loading. Further stabilization depends on tensor fascia lata muscle action, which is highly variable among subjects.

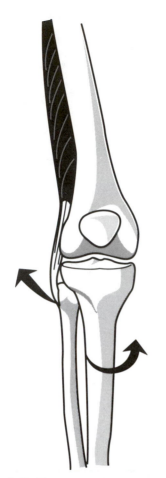

Figure 5.13 Biceps restraint of passive internal rotation.

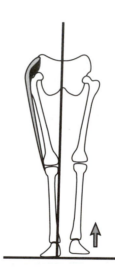

Figure 5.14 Iliotibial band as a lateral restraint of the adduction torque.

Mid Stance.

Motion: Knee extension

Function: Stable weight bearing

Stance stability is optimum when the knee is extended. Attaining this posture, however, involves several steps. The quadriceps is not the only source of knee extensor control.

As total body weight is transferred onto the flexed knee at the onset of single limb support, there is an additional 5° of knee flexion. The quadriceps react to inhibit further flexion by increased intensity of the vasti.

Further demand on the quadriceps is minimized by the tibial stability gained through the action of the soleus (Figure 5.15). This allows the femur to advance at a faster rate than the tibia. Momentum from the contralateral swinging limb provides a passive force replacing the quadriceps as the means of progressively reducing knee flexion.

By 20% in the gait cycle the tibia is vertical, knee flexion is reduced to 12°, the soleus is actively restraining the tibia (20% intensity), the swing limb is advancing ahead of the stance limb and the quadriceps have relaxed. While the gastrocnemius is also active, its intensity builds slowly. This probably reflects the muscle's knee flexion potential, which would be an added quadriceps burden until a source of passive stability has been established.

As the knee extends and the ankle dorsiflexes, the body mass moves forward, bringing its vector closer to the knee joint axis. By the middle of the mid stance phase (22% GC), the vector is in line with the knee axis. It then moves slightly anterior to the knee joint center and provides a small passive extensor force. Continuing knee stability relies on passive knee extension by body alignment. There is no further action by the vasti, and the accelerative phase of swing limb advancement is terminating.

The coronal plane adduction vector persists through mid stance, though it is less than initial force in loading response. The body's center of gravity shifts laterally 2cm, while the feet follow a path 4cm from the midline. Hence, body weight never moves a sufficient distance to have it lie directly over the supporting foot. As a result, the body weight vector remains on the medial edge of the knee (2.5cm from its center). This increases the force on the medial portion of the knee and also necessitates extrinsic lateral support, as the collateral ligament is small. Despite this apparent asymmetry in forces, none of the lateral musculature that have direct effect on the knee remain active during mid stance. An available source of lateral stability, however, is iliotibial band tension through the activity of the hip abductors.

Terminal Stance.

Motion: Completion of knee extension

Function: Stable weight bearing. Further stride length

Three mechanisms contribute to knee extension stability during terminal stance. Strong ankle plantar flexion provides a stable tibia over which the femur continues to advance. Swing limb momentum continues as the leg moves farther ahead of the body center. The forefoot rocker facilitates forward fall of the body vector over the leg (Figure 5.16). In this manner the body vector remains slightly anterior to the knee joint axis for passive extensor stability. Restraint of hip hyperextension by the tensor fascia lata also tenses the iliotibial band to provide indirect knee extension. The sum of these various extensor mechanisms have the potential to create undesirable knee hyperextension. To avoid strain, the popliteus and gastrocnemius provide a flexor action posteriorly. This is the time the popliteus starts increasing its activity (15% MMT). The gastrocnemius already is contracting vigorously (70% MMT) in its role as an ankle stabilizer. While the intensity of the gastrocnemius is much greater, the deep popliteus has the advantage of lying on the joint capsule.

By the end of terminal stance, the knee begins to flex. Several factors contribute. Tibial stability is lost by the body vector moving so far forward on the metatarsal joint that there is nothing to restrain forward rotation of the foot. The posterior muscles that initially were preventing hyperextension over a stable tibia now are free to initiate knee flexion. This logically is a mechanism to unlock the knee to start the large arc of flexion needed in initial swing. The five degrees (5°) attained before end of single limb support are significant considering the total arc of flexion that is needed and the short time available.

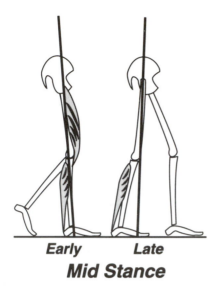

Figure 5.15 Mid stance knee control: (Early) quadriceps continues. (Late) passive extension by an anterior torque over a tibia stabilized by the soleus.

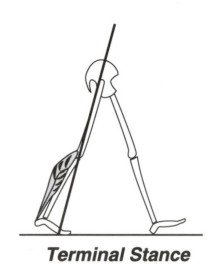

Figure 5.16 Terminal stance knee control: Passive extensor vector over a tibial stabilized by the soleus. At the end of the phase, advancement of the tibia and foot moves the knee axis anterior to the vector, initiating flexion.

Pre-Swing.
Motion: Passive knee flexion
Function: Prepare for swing
As a means of preparing the limb for swing, three mechanisms are used to gain adequate knee flexion during this short pre swing phase. Advancement of the center of pressure (base of the vector) to the distal side of the MP joints removes the force that previously held the mid-foot close to the floor. With foot stability lost, the tibia is free to roll forward. Residual tension in the previously strongly active plantar flexor muscles combined with their continuing low level of action accelerate heel rise and tibial advancement. There is direct knee flexor muscle action by the gastrocnemius (25% MMT). Also, this is the period of peak popliteus action (25% MMT). Rapid transfer of body weight to the other foot frees the limb to respond to such destabilizing forces. The result is 40° of passive knee flexion, which prepares the limb for easy toe clearance in swing. When knee flexion proceeds faster than unloading of the limb, the rectus femoris responds (Figure 5.17). This muscle serves to decelerate hip hyperextension and excessive knee flexion simultaneously. As the average intensity of rectus femoris activity is 10% MMT, the demand obviously is mild. Occasionally the vastus intermedius also responds briefly.[6]

Initial Swing.
Motion: Knee flexion
Function: Foot clearance for limb advancement
Knee flexion is the essential motion to lift the foot for limb advancement. The

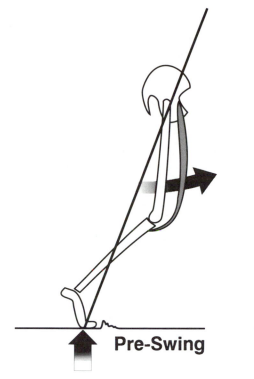

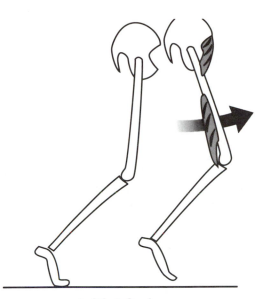

Figure 5.17 Pre-swing knee control: Excessive passive flexion (arrow) restrained by rectus femoris (occasionally a vastus responds).

Figure 5.18 Initial swing knee control: Flexion augmented by forward thigh momentum (arrow) and flexor muscle action biceps femoris, short head).

trailing posture of the limb at the end of pre-swing combined with knee flexion places the toe in an equinus position (i.e., toe down). This adds foot length to the distance between the hip and toe. Consequently, the trailing limb is functionally longer than the standing distance between hip and floor. Mere ankle dorsiflexion is insufficient to lift the toe for unobstructed limb advancement. The necessary additional lift must be supplied by knee flexion of 60°. This is the critical action that assures foot clearance of the floor as the limb swings forward from its trailing posture.

Three mechanisms are used to gain the necessary arc of knee flexion in initial swing (60°) (Figure 5.18). Timing as well as magnitude of motion is critical. Appropriate pre-swing knee flexion (40°) is the first component. Second is momentum initiated by rapid hip flexion. This quickly advances the femur, while tibial inertia leads to knee flexion.[13] The third factor is active knee flexion by the short head of the biceps femoris. There is also variable, low-level assistance from the sartorius and gracilis muscles, which simultaneously flex the hip and knee. If these actions threaten excessive knee flexion then the tibia is pulled forward by brief rectus femoris action, which also assists hip flexion. A brief burst of peak rectus femorus (RF) action (20% MMT) occurs at the onset of initial swing. Then it drops to a 5% level and ceases by the end of the phase.

This complex mode of lifting the foot presents a functional paradox. The objective is toe clearance of the floor, yet knee flexion rather than ankle dorsiflexion is the essential action. Also, attaining adequate knee flexion depends more on other events than direct knee muscle action.

Mid Swing.

Motion: Passive knee extension

Function: Limb advancement

Once the foot has moved forward of the hip joint, knee position does not contribute to the threat of foot drag on the floor. The need for acute flexion has subsided. Thus, this is an appropriate moment to begin knee extension both to complete limb advancement and to prepare for eventual floor contact (Figure 5.19).

No muscle action is needed since the trailing posture of the shank makes gravity an available force once the knee flexor muscles relax. Momentum generated by the continuing hip flexion supplements the pull of gravity on the tibia. These forces reach a balance once the tibia becomes vertical.

Terminal Swing.

Motion: Knee extension

Functions: Limb advancement. Prepare for stance

Knee extension at this time can be considered completion of swing or preparation for stance. The mechanics involved were described at the beginning of the interpretive section.

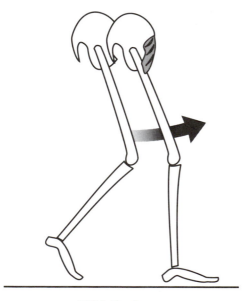

Mid Swing

Figure 5.19 Mid swing knee control: Passive extension as flexors relax and thigh advances (arrow).

Conclusion

The knee is the key to stance stability, and the quadriceps is the most direct source of extensor control. During walking, however, the quadriceps is only used to restrain the shock-absorbing flexion during the loading response. Other mechanisms are employed to attain optimum extension in single stance. Tibial stability by the soleus is a major determinant. Iliotibial band tension is a useful adjunct.

In swing the knee uses a larger arc of motion during walking than any other joint. Sixty degrees of flexion are needed to assure toe clearance of the floor. Again, the necessary knee function is attained by multiple mechanisms rather than just direct knee muscle action. Pre-swing ankle plantar flexor muscle action, hip flexion and tibial inertia are the major determinants of initial swing flexion. The local knee flexors have a minor role. Consequently, knee function involves the entire limb in both stance and swing.

References

1. Adler N, Perry J, Kent B, Robertson K: Electromyography of the vastus medialis oblique and vasti in normal subjects during gait. *Electromyogr Clin Neurophysiol* 23:643-649, 1983.
2. Boccardi S, Pedotti A, Rodano R, Santambrogio GC: Evaluation of muscular moments at the lower limb joints by an on-line processing of kinematic data and ground reaction. *J Biomech* 14:35-45, 1981.
3. Brinkmann JR, Perry J: Rate and range of knee motion during ambulation in healthy and arthritic subjects. *Phys Ther* 65(7):1055-1060, 1985.
4. Cappozzo A, Pedotti A: A general computing method for the analysis of human locomotion. *Biomech* 8:307-320, 1978.
5. Chao EY, Laughman RK, Schneider E, Stauffer RN: Normative data of knee joint motion and ground reaction forces in adult level walking. *J Biomech* 16(3):219-233, 1983.
6. Close JR, Inman VT: *The Pattern of Muscular Activity in the Lower Extremity During Walking: A Presentation of Summarized Data. Prosthetic Devices Research Project, University of California, Berkeley, Series 11, Issue 25. Berkeley, The Project, 1953.*
7. Eberhart HD, Inman VT, Bressler B: The principle elements in human locomotion. In Klopsteg PE, Wilson PD (Eds): *Human Limbs and their Substitutes.* New York, Hafner Publishing Company, 1968, pp. 437-471.
8. Gyory AN, Chao EY, Stauffer RN: Functional evaluation of normal and pathologic knees during gait. *Arch Phys Med Rehabil* 57(12):571-577, 1976.
9. Inman VT, Ralston HJ, Todd F: *Human Walking.* Baltimore, MD, Williams and Wilkins Company, 1981.
10. Kadaba MP, Ramakaishnan HK, Wootten ME, Gainey J, Gorton G, Cochran GVB: Repeatability of kinematic, kinetic and electromyographic data in normal adult gait. *J Orthop Res* 7:849-860, 1989.
11. Kettelkamp DB, Johnson RJ, Smidt GL, Chao EY, Walker M: An electrogoniometric study of knee motion in normal gait. *J Bone Joint Surg* 52A(4):775-790, 1970.
12. Levens AS, Inman VT, Blosser JA: Transverse rotation of the segments of the lower extremity in locomotion. *J Bone Joint Surg* 30A(4):859-872, 1948.
13. Mansour JM, Audu ML: Passive elastic moment at the knee and its influence on human gait. *J Biomech* 19(5):369-373, 1986.

14. Murray MP, Drought AB, Kory RC: Walking patterns of normal men. *J Bone Joint Surg* 46A(2):335-360, 1964.
15. Skinner SR, Antonelli DJ, Perry J, Lester DK: Functional demands on the stance limb in walking. *Orthopedics* 8(3):355-361, 1985.
16. Woollacott MH, Shumway-Cook A, Nashner LM: Aging and posture control: changes in sensory organization and muscular coordination. *Int J Aging Hum Dev* 23(2):97-114, 1986.

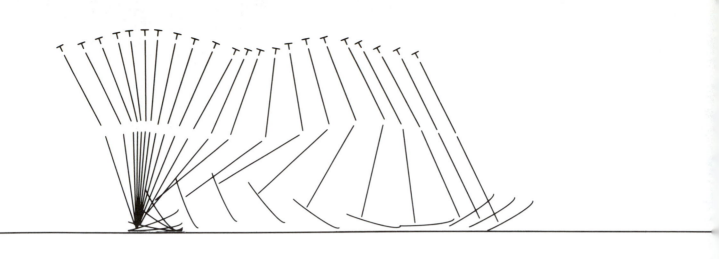

Chapter 6

Hip

Function at the hip differs from the other joints in several respects. The hip represents the junction between the passenger and locomotor units. As a result, it is designed to more overtly provide three-dimensional motion with specific muscle control for each direction of activity. Sagittal plane motion (progression) involves the largest arc, while muscular requirements are brief. In the coronal plane, motion is limited, but the muscular demands are substantial. Transverse rotation remains a subtle event.

The functional focus of the hip musculature also varies with the period in the gait cycle. During stance, the primary role of the hip muscles is stabilization of the superimposed trunk. In swing, limb control is the primary objective.

Motion

Clinically, it is customary to define the joint's motion by the path of thigh displacement from the vertical. In addition there is an arc of pelvic tilt that may either add to or subtract from the arc of hip motion created by thigh displacement.

Instrumented motion analysis generally measures total pelvic-femur angle. In considering the mechanics of walking, thigh and pelvis motions should be judged separately During normal function the ranges of pelvic motion are quite small.

The coronal and transverse plane motions recorded during stance tend to be identified as pelvic motion, yet the hip joint is the site of this action. In this text such events will be described under both topics: hip and pelvis.

Sagittal Plane Motion

The hip moves through only two arcs of motion during a normal stride: extension during stance and flexion in swing (Figure 6.1). The exchange of motion from one direction to the other is gradual, occupying a whole gait phase for each reversal. A normal arc of hip motion averages 40°,[5,8,9,12,16] though one study identified a 48° range.[6] Precise definition of the limits of motion vary with the recording technic used. Some investigators consider maximum hip extension as zero (0°) and note maximum hip flexion as 40°.[5,8]

A technic that is more consistent with clinical practice is to consider the vertical thigh in quiet standing to be the zero position.[9,12,16] Using the latter reference posture results in the peaks of hip motion being 10° extension and 30° flexion (Figure 6.1).

Independent analysis of the pattern of normal thigh extension and flexion

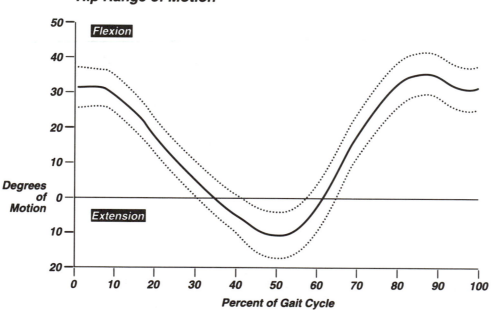

Figure 6.1 Hip motion. Normal range during free walking. Black line = the mean, dotted lines = 1 standard deviation.

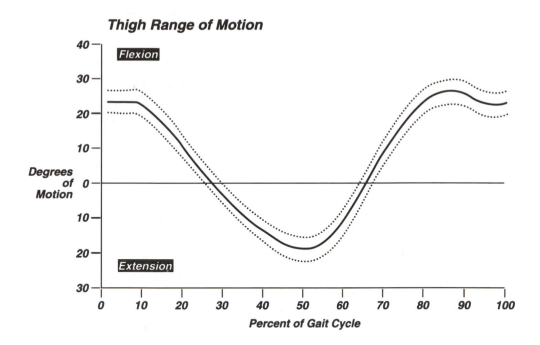

Figure 6.2 Thigh motion. Normal range during a free stride. Black line = the mean, dotted lines = 1 standard deviation.

relative to the vertical plane more clearly identify the contribution of the thigh to stride length. The pelvis is treated as a separate segment, riding on top of a thigh that is rotating over the supporting foot during stance.

At initial contact, the thigh is flexed 20° (Figure 6.2) from the vertical. During the loading response, thigh position is relatively stable, perhaps losing 2° or 3° of flexion. With the onset of mid stance, the hip progressively extends. Continuing at the same rate in terminal stance, the thigh reaches neutral alignment at the 38% gait cycle point. The thigh then assumes a posteriorly aligned posture with peak hip extension (10°) or a trailing thigh of 20° occurring as the other foot contacts the ground (50% GC).

During pre-swing the hip reverses its direction of movement and begins flexing. A neutral position of the hip (0°) is reached at the end of the stance period (60% GC), while the thigh still shows a few degrees of extension. The motion toward flexion continues through the first two phases of swing. During initial swing, the hip attains a large portion of its flexion range with the thigh at 15°. In mid swing the final 10° are accomplished. The final 25° flexed position of the thigh is maintained within five degrees through terminal swing.

These thigh motions have been modified by 3° or 4° of tilt of the pelvis.[7,12] As the pelvis alternately follows the swing limb on one side and then the other, each position changes twice in one stride. Hence, upward tilt of the pelvis increases the thigh angle in early mid stance and again in initial swing. Conversely, a downward tilt of the pelvis increases thigh extension in terminal stance and terminal swing.[12]

Table 6.1

Sagittal Plane Thigh Versus Hip Motion

	Thigh	Hip	Gait Cycle
Flexion	20°	30°	0 %
	25°	35°	85 %
Extension	20°	10°	50 %

Clinically, it is very important to separate motion of the thigh from that of the pelvis, as they respond differently to the various types of pathology that modify the patients ability to walk. By relating the position of the thigh to the axis vertical to the horizon, the displacement of the limb in space is defined independent of pelvic motion. For normal walking, this excludes the mean 10° anterior pelvic tilt from the measurement. Thigh flexion at initial contact is correspondingly reduced to 20°, and extension in terminal stance is increased to 20° (Figure 6.2).

Coronal Plane Motion

The hip moves through a small arc of adduction and abduction as the unloaded side of the pelvis follows the swinging limb. This action begins with the onset of stance. At initial contact, the hip is adducted about 10° in the coronal plane due to the anatomical angle between femur and tibia. Superimposed on this posture is a small arc of passive motion. Adduction occurs during loading response (5°).[15] This reverses to neutral in mid and terminal stance. Then in initial swing, relative hip abduction occurs (5°). The small arcs represent the mean value for both men and women.[12,13]

Transverse Plane Motion

During each stride the limb moves through an arc of internal rotation followed by a similar arc of external rotation. Pelvis and thigh skeletal pins demonstrated that at initial contact the limb is neutral. Peak internal rotation occurs at the end of the loading response (CTO), and maximum external rotation is found at the end of pre-swing (ITO).[10] The total arc of transverse hip motion averages 8°. When this arc is added to the pelvic motion (7.7°), total thigh rotation averages 15°. Surface markers show a similar arc of hip motion, though there is great variability in actual values among the different gait laboratories.[2]

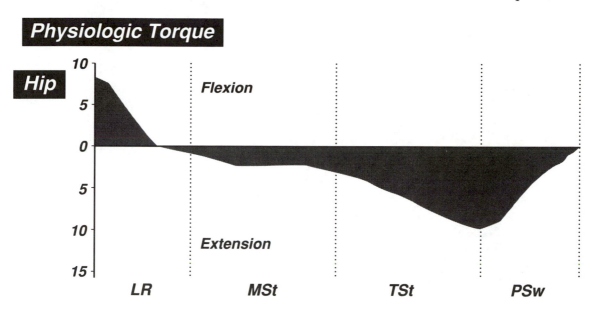

Physiologic Torque

Figure 6.3 Hip torques: Normal weight-bearing pattern generated by the sagittal vector during walking. The early high flexion torque at the onset of stance quickly decreases, crossing the 0 line to become an extensor torque in late mid stance. Deviation of the shadow from 0 indicates the magnitude of the torque in physiological units (Body weight/leg length). LR = loading response, MSt = mid stance, TSt = terminal stance, PSw = pre-swing.

Body Weight Vector

As the trunk advances over the supporting foot, the weight line vector changes its relationship to the hip joint in both the sagittal and coronal planes. Both patterns of resulting torque are functionally significant.

Sagittal Torque

Throughout stance the body weight vector moves backward from an initial position anterior to the hip joint. Peak torque at the hip occurs at the onset of limb loading (Figure 6.3).

Immediately following initial contact, the abrupt drop of body weight onto the foot generates a significant vertical vector (60% body weight) that is very anterior to the hip joint (Figure 6.4a). The effect is an immediate peak flexor torque during the first 2% of the gait cycle. The magnitude of this instantaneous peak is 6.9 BWLL units[17] or 35 Nm.[3] As the initial inertia is replaced with the developing shear forces, the vector rapidly realigns itself with the body center and moves backward toward the hip. This causes an abrupt decline in the flexor torque during the rest of loading response, even though there is an increasing vertical force (Figure 6.4b).

Near the end of the loading response (7% GC) the hip torque reverses from flexion to extension (Figure 6.5). The extensor alignment continues at a low

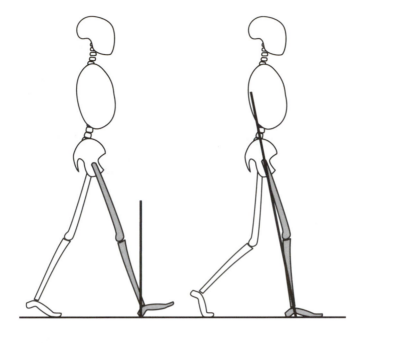
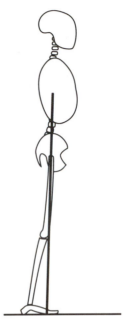

Figure 6.4 Hip vector alignment in early stance (vertical line): (a) Initial contact. The anterior vector signifies a flexor torque. Short line = low force. Distance from hip = long lever arm. (b) Loading response. Vector close to hip joint, flexor torque small.

Figure 6.5 Hip vector in mid stance at joint center, no torque generated.

intensity (2.3 BWLL) through a mid stance and then progressively increases during terminal stance to a peak value of 10.0 anatomical units at the 49% GC point. During pre-swing the torque progressively decreases, reaching zero by the end of stance.

Coronal Plane Torque

Initial floor contact is accompanied by a brief and small laterally directed vector. As the limb is loaded the vector promptly reverses to a medial alignment. Throughout the rest of the stance period, this adducting vector is maintained. Basically the alignment is between the center of the foot and the midpoint of the pelvis. Torque in the coronal plane terminates in pre-swing with the onset of double limb support. The magnitude of the medial vector reflects the vertical floor reaction force generated throughout stance. Hence, its contour is similar to the sagittal force pattern (Figure 3.29).

Muscle Control

During stance the primary muscles controlling the hip are the extensors and abductors. In swing it is the flexors. The adductors tend to participate during the intervals of exchange between swing and stance. Inability to isolate the deep external rotators has prevented definition of their timing. Internal rotation is provided secondarily, as the muscles also perform their primary function.

Extensor Muscles

Action of the hip extensor muscles occurs from late mid swing through the loading response. The five muscles involved are selective in their timing (Figure 6.6).[7,11]

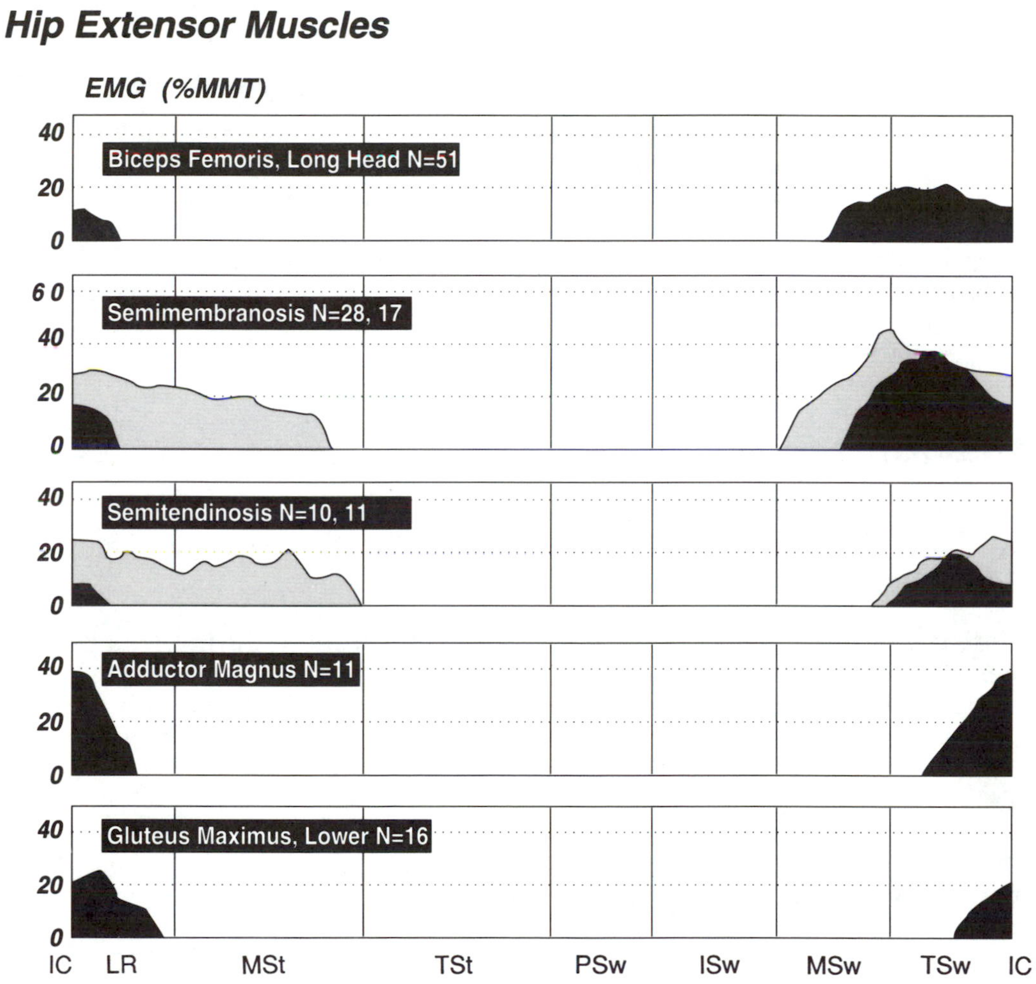

Hip Extensor Muscles

Figure 6.6 Hip extensor muscles. Normal mean intensity and timing during free walking (quantified electromyogram). Intensity as a percent of maximum manual muscle test value (% MMT) indicated by height of gray area. Vertical bars designate the gait phase divisions.

Hamstrings. The semimembranosis, semitendinosis and long biceps femoris begin contracting in late mid swing (80% GC). All three muscles rapidly increase the intensity of their action, reaching peak effort early in terminal swing (semimembranosis 30% and biceps femoris 20% MMT). This is followed by semi-relaxation to a 10% level just before initial contact. The medial hamstrings may act similar to the biceps, followed by rapid relaxation before the end of the phase (8% GC). All three hamstrings cease to be active during the rest of the gait cycle.

Adductor Magnus. Near the end of terminal swing the adductor magnus begins to contract and progressively increases its intensity throughout the phase. With initial contact there is a further increase to 40% MMT. During loading response, the adductor magnus remains moderately active for 7% of the gait cycle and then relaxes. No further activity occurs throughout the stride.

Gluteus Maximus. Functionally the muscle divides into two halves. The upper half acts as an abductor while the lower half serves as a hip extensor. Lower gluteus maximus action begins with the end of terminal swing. With initial contact the muscle quickly increases in intensity to reach a 25% effort level in mid loading response. Following this peak the lower gluteus maximus rapidly decreases its activity level to less than 10% GC by the end of loading response (10% GC). Hence, functional effectiveness has essentially ended at this time.

Abductor Muscles

The hip abductors are the other major muscle group functioning during the initial half of stance. Three muscles are involved, gluteus medius, tensor fascia lata and the upper gluteus maximus (Figure 6.7).

Gluteus Medius. The pattern of gluteus minimus activity during walking has been identified as being similar to that of the medius.[1] Detailed analysis of the medius/minimus muscle complex, however, has been limited to the medius. Gluteus medius activity begins at the end of terminal swing and the intensity of abductor muscle action quickly increases to a 20% MMT peak immediately after initial contact that persists through mid stance.[11]

The upper gluteus maximus follows a similar pattern. Beginning in terminal swing (95% GC), the intensity rapidly rises during loading response (20% MMT) and continues through mid stance.

Tensor fascia lata muscle activity varies between its posterior and anterior portion. Posterior fiber action of moderate intensity (25% MMT) occurs at the onset of the loading response.[14] In contrast, the anterior fibers don't become active until terminal stance and the level of effort is lower (10% MMT).[7,11]

Hip Abductor Muscles

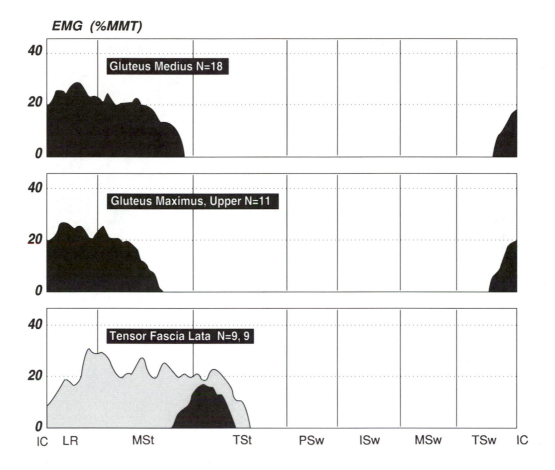

Figure 6.7 Hip abductor muscles. Normal mean intensity and timing during free walking (quantified electromyogram). Intensity as a percent of maximum manual muscle test value (% MMT) indicated by height of gray area. Vertical bars designate the gait phase divisions.

Flexor Muscles

Normal persons walking at their preferred speed may display no significant flexor muscle action after the initiating first step (i.e., less than 5% MMT). This was true for approximately half of the subjects studied. A change in velocity to either a faster or slower pace introduces a consistent pattern of muscular effort, however. This will be the model used to define the role of the hip flexor muscles in walking (Figure 6.8).

Flexor muscle action begins in late terminal stance and continues through initial swing into early mid swing. During this interval there is sequence of

EMG (%MMT)

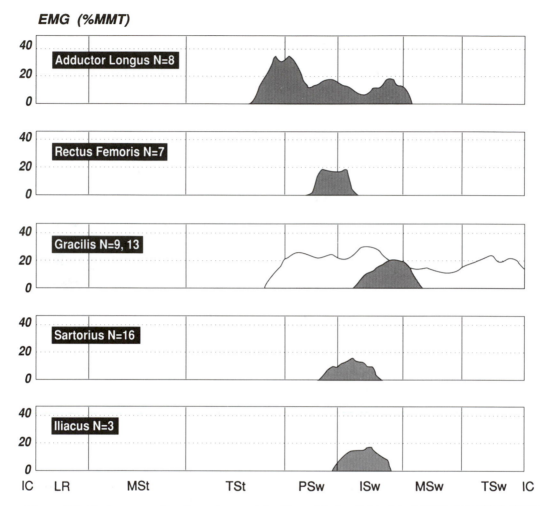

Figure 6.8 Hip flexor muscles. Normal mean intensity and timing during free walking (quantified electro-myogram). Intensity as a percent of maximum manual muscle test value (% MMT) indicated by height of gray area. Vertical bars designate the gait phase divisions.

muscle action. The adductor is both the first and most persistent hip flexor. Its onset is in late terminal stance, and the muscle remains active into initial swing. Probably adductor brevis function is similar to that of the adductor longus, but inability to confirm EMG isolation prevents verification of this assumption. Next is the rectus femoris with a brief period of action in pre-swing and early initial swing. Rectus femoris participation is inconsistent with only half of the subjects showing any action during free gait. The iliacus, sartorius and gracilis have similar periods of action throughout initial swing. EMG studies of the psoas indicate its action during gait is similar to that of the iliacus.[4]

Mid swing activity of the hip flexor muscles is infrequent, and none normally occurs in terminal swing.

Adductor Muscles

Among the major adductor muscles only the actions of the adductors longus and magnus and the gracilis can be defined by dynamic EMG (Figure 6.9). The actions of these muscles already have been described under their roles as a hip flexor (adductor longus and gracilis) and extensor (adductor magnus).

Functional Interpretation

The three-dimensional demands imposed on the hip joint during stance as the trunk remains erect and the limb progresses over the foot are very dependent on its ball and socket contour. Stabilizing the trunk mass over the hip also introduces a high demand for muscular control in the stance period. It is significant, however, that energy is saved by substituting passive forces for direct muscular effort after the insecurity of loading the limb is controlled. The second demand on the hip musculature, that is, to initiate limb advancement, is less intense. Only the mass of

Hip Adductor Muscles

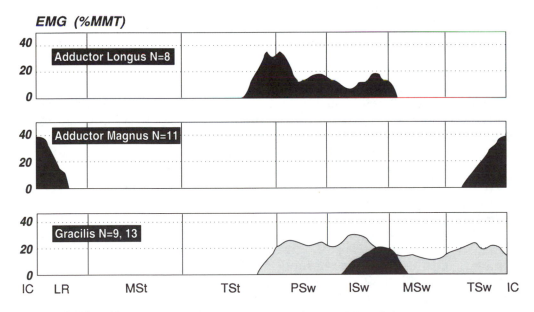

Figure 6.9 Hip adductor muscles. Normal mean intensity and timing during free walking (quantified electromyogram). Intensity as a percent of maximum manual muscle test value (% MMT) indicated by height of gray area. Vertical bars designate the gait phase divisions.

the limb must be controlled. Again, momentum is available to lessen direct muscular input. Consequently, the interplay between motion and muscular control varies considerably throughout the gait cycle.

Hip Function by Gait Phases

Correlation of the motion, muscle function and demand vectors that occur in each gait aids in the understanding of the complexity of hip function during walking. The balance between demand and response becomes evident.

Initial Contact.
Posture: Hip flexion at 30° (thigh forward)
The 30° flexed position of the hip at the moment of initial floor contact represents an optimum compromise between the potential instability from horizontal shear (the foot sliding forward) of a longer step and stability induced by the vertical force of limb loading. Body weight is directed toward the ground, while a significant element of progression is preserved. On a theoretical basis, having the limb in a 25° diagonal posture makes the potential vertical force twice the shear component. Hence, the opportunity for weight-bearing stability exceeds the probability of the limb sliding forward.

At the moment of floor contact, however, the hip is in an unstable position. With the thigh in a flexed position and forward momentum in the trunk, advancement of the limb has been interrupted by floor friction. This places the body vector well anterior of the hip joint at the moment of floor contact (Figure 6.10). Hence, the dynamic control occurring in terminal swing is essential for stability at the moment of floor contact.

Loading Response.
Action: Sagittal and coronal positions are maintained
Weight-bearing stability during limb loading is challenged by three situations. These are a 30° flexed posture at the hip, anterior location of the body vector and forward momentum in the trunk (Figure 6.11).

Hip stability is maintained by action of all five hip extensors, though they contribute at different intensities because of their varying effects at the knee (Figure 6.6). The lower gluteus maximus and adductor magnus provide the most direct response as they act only at the hip joint (i.e., single joint muscles). Activity of the hamstrings is reduced because of the flexor effect at the knee. The more prolonged action of the semimembranosis suggests an internal rotation role to assist in advancement of the contralateral pelvis. At the knee, continued semimembranosis action would also introduce active knee internal rotation. Our early finding of more intense activity by the long head of the biceps femoris did not persist when the study sample was enlarged. This suggests a possibility of prolonged biceps femoris, long head (BFLH) action to protect the anterior cruciate knee ligament, but it is not a standard function.

As a result of the interplay between hip and knee demands, the gluteus

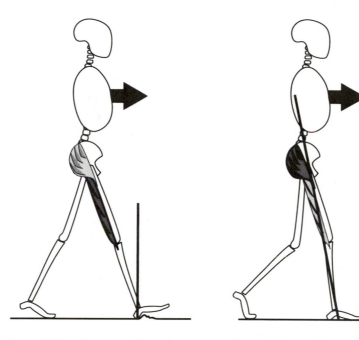

Figure 6.10 Initial contact hip extensor muscle action restrains flexor momentum (arrow and vector line). Hamstrings muscles and gluteus maximus active.

Figure 6.11 Loading response hip extensor action. Vector close to hip and posterior to knee. Hamstring action reduced, gluteus maximus activity increased.

maximus and adductor magnus increase their activity during early loading response to a 30% effort level, while the hamstrings reduce their intensity.

Hip extensor stabilization of the trunk also contributes to limb stability. By tying the femur to the pelvis, forward momentum of the trunk mass indirectly draws the thigh backward, thereby, extending the knee.

The hip extensor muscles cease their activity by the end of loading response as a result of two factors: vector realignment and a passive extensor effect initiated by the heel rocker. The body vector rapidly retreats from its initial anterior position to realign itself close to the hip joint. While there is a persistent flexor torque, it is more representative of the high ground reaction force than the vector's moment arm.

Passive hip extension follows the propagation of limb progression from the heel rocker to the femur by the quadriceps (Figure 6.12). As the vasti act to restrain knee flexion, their origin also pull the femur forward with the advancing tibia. Inertia delays the advancement of the pelvis, causing relative extension at the hip. With the introduction of passive hip extension, direct muscular control is no longer needed and the muscles relax.

In the coronal plane, rapid transfer of body weight onto the loading limb demands active lateral stabilization of the pelvis over the hip. The base of the body vector shifts to the supporting foot while the controlling C/G is in the midline of the body. Weight transfer also reduces the support for the contralateral side of the pelvis. The effect is a large medial (i.e., adductor)

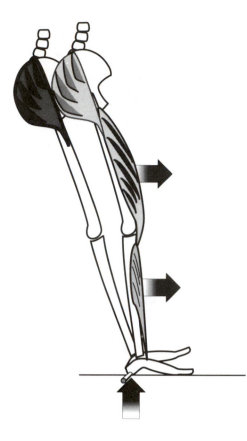

Figure 6.12 All hip extensor action terminates early in loading response (pale GMax). Heel rocker advances tibia, quadriceps advances thigh, extending hip against inertia of the pelvis and trunk.

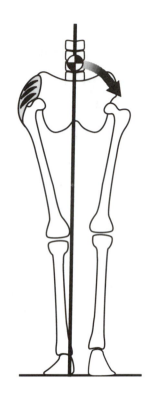

Figure 6.13 Coronal muscle control of hip. Adducting midline torque (arrow) restrained by hip abductor muscles.

torque at the hip that causes the unsupported side of the pelvis to drop (Figure 6.13). To stabilize the pelvis (and secondarily the trunk), the abductor muscles (gluteus medius, upper gluteus maximus and posterior tensor fascia lata) react promptly and with considerable intensity (35% MMT). This is the interval of greatest abductor muscle action. The intensity of the response is stimulated by two situations: speed with which the muscles must act and a high mechanical demand (muscle moment arm is only 67% of body weight vector lever).

Internal rotation in the transverse plane is a third action being initiated during the loading response. There are two causes. The change in support from the trailing limb to the forward foot starts forward rotation of the ipsilateral side of the pelvis. Also, the limb internally rotates as a result of the subtalar joint reaction to heel loading. Hip rotation is decelerated by the external rotational effect of gluteus maximus activity.

Mid Stance.

Action: Progressive hip extension

As the limb rolls forward over the supporting foot during mid stance, the hip moves from its 30° flexed posture toward extension in the sagittal plane. This places the body vector at the hip joint center. By the end of mid stance, the sagittal plane vector has moved posterior to the hip center. Both alignments remove the need for further extensor muscle action (Figure 6.14).

After the major abductor muscles have returned the pelvis to neutral alignment in the coronal plane, little additional force is needed. Thus, the gluteal muscles relax and the tensor fascia lata muscle takes over (Figure 6.7).

Terminal Stance.

Action: Hyperextension of the hip

As body weight rolls forward over the forefoot rocker, it puts the limb a trailing posture. With the pelvis and trunk remaining erect, the body vector moves posterior to the hip joint, and the thigh is pulled into full extension and then hyperextension (Figure 6.15). The anterior portion of the tensor fascia lata responds for two purposes. Its flexor role restrains the rate and extent of passive hip extension. Also, this muscle action provides the low level of abduction force that continues to be needed. The amount of hip hyperextension is slightly reduced (3°) by an anterior tilt of the pelvis.

The low level of abductor muscle activity presents a bit of a paradox as the medial vector continues through the entire single support period. The answer probably lies in the body's lateral shift pattern. By the middle of mid stance (25% GC), the body's center of gravity is at its most lateral point. Then, it begins to retreat back toward the midline. This introduces passive abduction and correspondingly reduces the need for direct muscle action. Energy is conserved by the larger muscles (gluteus medius and upper gluteus) relaxing, and the smaller tensor fascia lata is sufficient for continued support.

Pre-Swing.

Action: Hip flexion to neutral

Hip flexion in pre-swing appears to be a reaction to two events. First there are the ankle mechanics that advance the tibia. While inducing knee flexion, they also carry the thigh forward. Rectus femoris restraint of the knee motion would provide direct hip flexion, as well (Figure 6.16).

The second thigh-advancing maneuver is response of the adductor muscles to decelerate the passive abduction caused by weight transfer to the other foot. The presence of a hyperextending stretch on the hip joint capsule would stimulate the iliacus muscle to provide active protection from excessive strain. Through these various mechanisms the hip regains a neutral alignment. Because hip motion is rather rapidly reversed from extension into flexion, the pre-swing phase also has been called the interval of limb acceleration.

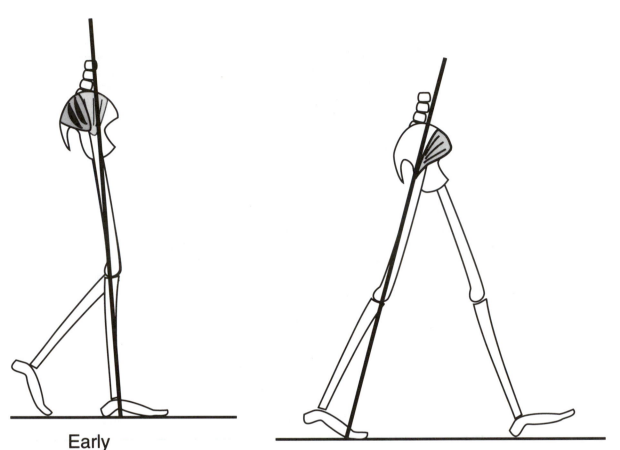

Early
Mid Stance

Terminal Stance

Figure 6.14 Mid stance needs no hip extensor control as vector posterior to hip joint. Gluteus medius coronal plane control still active.

Figure 6.15 Terminal stance hip control by tensor fascia lata restraining posterior vector.

Initial Swing.

Action: Hip flexion

Momentum generated in pre-swing continues into initial swing. At the normal person's free walking speed, limb advancement may be passive as a result of the pre-swing mechanics. This is supplemented by direct hip muscle action as needed. Being unloaded, the limb rapidly advances 20 within 0.1 sec (10% of the gait cycle). Walking faster or slower stimulates dependence on the iliacus (Figure 6.17). Two muscles that commonly display small levels of activity are the gracilis and sartorius. The gracilis provides adduction, internal rotation and flexion. Simultaneous sartorius activity provides counterforces of abduction and external rotation as it assists in flexion. The final three-dimensional path of the limb in initial swing could represent the balance

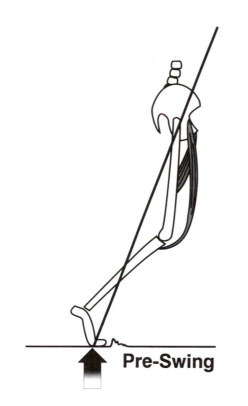

Pre-Swing

Figure 6.16 Pre-swing hip flexion being initiated by adductor longus and rectus femoris (if active). Vector posterior to knee and at hip axis.

between these two muscles. The gracilis and sartorius also induce knee flexion as they act at the hip. Generally, this is a desirable synergy in initial swing. When tibial inertia causes excessive knee flexion, response of the rectus femoris preserves accelerated hip flexion while correcting the knee motion. Because of the varying needs for three-dimensional control of a dangling limb and the interactions of hip and knee motion, the pattern of hip flexor activity varies considerably among individuals.

Mid Swing.

Action: Continuing hip flexion

The limb advances an additional 10 by a continuation of the action occurring in initial swing. This is a period of virtually passive hip flexion. Recordable muscle action may be absent or minimal and occur among any of the flexors (Figure 6.8). Momentum persisting from the initial flexor effort is the prime mover.

Terminal Swing.

Action: Cessation of hip flexion

Terminal swing is the transitional phase between swing and stance. Hip muscle action at this time prepares the limb for stance by stopping further flexion. Strong action by the hamstring muscles is the controlling force. All

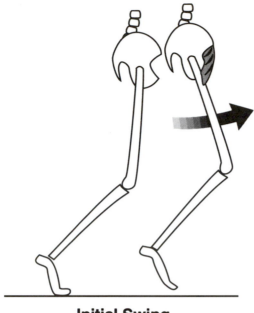

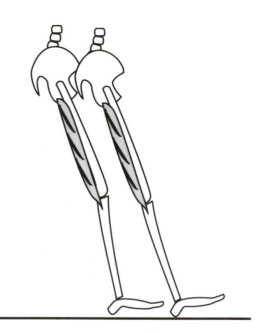

Initial Swing

Terminal Swing

Figure 6.17 Initial swing hip control with flexion (arrow) being stimulated by iliacus muscle.

Figure 6.18 Terminal swing cessation of hip flexion by hamstring muscle action.

three hamstrings participate at a 20% MMT intensity (Figure 6.18). Imbalance in the size of the muscles probably is responsible for the mild internal rotation that occurs. The medial muscle mass (semimembranosis and semitendinosis) is approximately 50% larger than the long head of the biceps.[18] Preferential use of the hamstring muscles rather than the single joint hip extensors (gluteus maximus and adductor magnus) indicates the advantage of simultaneous deceleration at the knee, otherwise the thigh would be restrained while the shank was free to respond to the existing momentum and quadriceps pull. The reduction of hamstring muscle activity and the end of terminal swing and the accompanying onset of the gluteus maximus and adductor magnus indicate a need for hip extension by less involvement of the knee.

The onset of gluteus medius action in terminal swing counteracts the earlier adducting of the hip flexors influences. As a result of these many actions, the limb is optimally positioned for initial contact and the beginning of another weight-bearing interval.

Conclusion

Hip motion during the stance period allows the pelvis and trunk to remain erect while the limb rolls forward over the supporting foot. The hip extensor muscles have two functions. First is to decelerate the limb's momentum in terminal swing to prepare for stance. Secondly, they act to restrain the forward momentum in the pelvis and trunk as the limb is loaded. The abductor muscles act to counteract contralateral pelvic drop induced by the medial alignment of body weight. During swing, the hip flexors advance the limb, but the demand is low.

References

1. Basmajian JV, Deluca CJ: *Muscles Alive: Their functions revealed by electromyography.* 5th edition, Baltimore, Williams & Wilkins, 1985, pp. 19-64.
2. Biden E, Olshen R, Simon S, Sutherland D, Gage J, Kadaba M: Comparison of gait data from multiple labs. *Transactions of the Orthopaedic Research Society* 12:504, 1987.
3. Boccardi S, Pedotti A, Rodano R, Santambrogio GC: Evaluation of muscular moments at the lower limb joints by an on-line processing of kinematic data and ground reaction. *J Biomech* 14:35-45, 1981.
4. Close JR: *Motor Function in the Lower Extremity: Analyses by Electronic Instrumentation.* Springfield, Charles C. Thomas, Publisher, 1964.
5. Dettmann MA, Linder MT, Sepic SB: Relationships among walking performance, postural stability and assessments of the hemiplegic patient. *American Journal of Physical Medicine* 66(2):77-90, 1987.
6. Gore DR, et al.: Walking patterns of men with unilateral surgical hip fusion. *J Bone Joint Surg* 57A(6):759-765, 1975.
7. Inman VT, Ralston HJ, Todd F: *Human Walking.* Baltimore, MD, Williams and Wilkins Company, 1981.
8. Johnston RC, Smidt GL: Measurement of hip-joint motion during walking; evaluation of an electrogoniometric method. *J Bone Joint Surg* 51A(6):1083-1094, 1969.
9. Kadaba MP, Ramakaishnan HK, Wootten ME, Gainey J, Gorton G, Cochran GVB: Repeatability of kinematic, kinetic and electromyographic data in normal adult gait. *J Orthop Res* 7:849-860, 1989.
10. Levens AS, Inman VT, Blosser JA: Transverse rotation of the segments of the lower extremity in locomotion. *J Bone Joint Surg* 30A(4):859-872, 1948.
11. Lyons K, Perry J, Gronley JK, Barnes L, Antonelli D: Timing and relative intensity of hip extensor and abductor muscle action during level and stair ambulation: an EMG study. *Phys Ther* 63:1597-1605, 1983.
12. Murray MP, Drought AB, Kory RC: Walking patterns of normal men. *J Bone Joint Surg* 46A(2):335-360, 1964.
13. Murray MP, Kory RC, Sepic SB: Walking patterns of normal women. *Arch Phys Med Rehabil* 51:637-650, 1970.
14. Pare EB, Stern JT Jr, Schwartz JM: Functional differentiation within the tensor fascia lata. A telemetered electromyographic analysis of its locomotor roles. *J Bone Joint Surg* 63A:1457-1471, 1981.
15. Saunders JBdeCM, Inman VT, Eberhart HD: The major determinants in normal and pathological gait. *J Bone Joint Surg* 35A(3):543-557, 1953.
16. Skinner HB, Abrahamson MA, Hung RK, Wilson LA, Effeney DJ: Static load response of the heels of SACH feet. *Orthopedics* 8:225-228, 1985.
17. Skinner SR, Antonelli D, Perry J, Lester DK: Functional demands on the stance limb in walking. *Orthopedics* 8(3):355-361, 1985.
18. Weber EF: Ueber die Langenverhaltnisse der Fkeuscgfaserb der Muskeln im Allgemeinen. *Math-phys Cl*, Ber. Verh. K. Sachs. Ges. Wissensch., 1851.

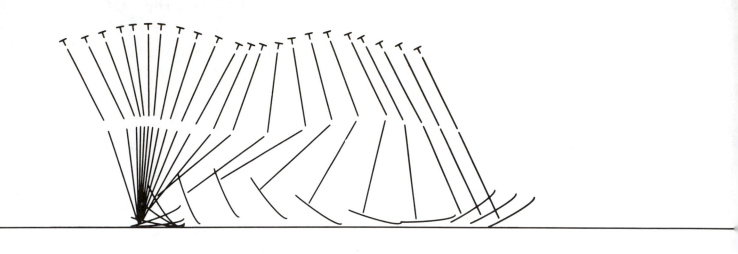

Chapter 7

Head, Trunk and Pelvis

The axial segment of the body consists of three rigid structures (head, thorax and pelvis) separated by two mobile areas (cervical and thoracolumbar spines). Functionally, the head and neck (cervical spine) are considered one unit resting on top of the trunk. Definition of the trunk is inconsistent. By common usage the term *trunk* has at least two meanings. The word may refer to all body segments between the base of the neck and the hip joints (except the arms) or represent just the lumbar and thoracic segments. This latter interpretation is more useful for gait analysis because the thoracolumbar trunk (TL) and the pelvis have different functional obligations leading to dissimilar motion patterns. The lumbosacral joint is the dividing point.

Gait Dynamics

Motion

While the neck allows the head to move independently to expand one's field of vision, during normal gait the head and trunk travel as a unit. Neither segment displays any visually apparent change in position except vertically. In this direction the segments move with the body's center of gravity as it follows the mechanics of the limbs. Instrumented analysis, however, has registered small arcs of displacement in both the sagittal and coronal planes. Minor arcs of motion also occur at the pelvis.

Total Axial Displacement. Throughout the gait cycle the HAT deviates from the mean line of progression in all three planes (vertical, lateral, progressional). Each displacement pattern is a sinusoidal curve, but the individual characteristics differ for each direction of motion.

Vertical displacement of the sacrum, trunk and head is equal with each segment and follows a double sinusoidal path. The average amount of vertical change is 4.5cm[11] or 2.5cm up and an equal amount downward (Figure 7.1).[7] There are two cycles of downward and upward displacement in each stride. These reflect the mechanics of the right and left steps. The movement of C_7 and L_3 is equal. Peak downward deviation occurs in loading response (6% GC) and in pre-swing (56% GC). Both of these phases are periods of double limb support. Each descent is followed by a progressive rise above the mean level. These occur in the two single support intervals: terminal stance (34% GC) and late mid

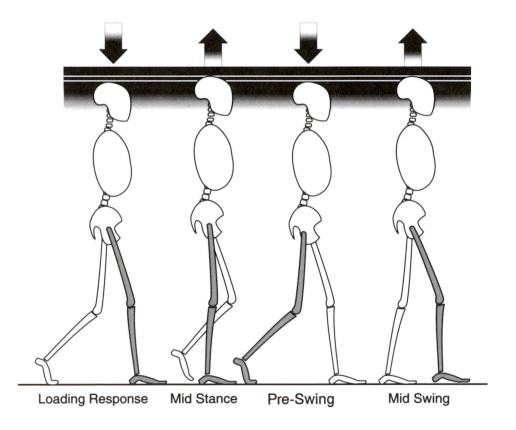

Loading Response   Mid Stance   Pre-Swing   Mid Swing

Figure 7.1 Vertical displacement of trunk during a stride indicated by head height. Lowest in double support (loading response and pre-swing). Highest in mid single stance (mid stance and contralateral mid swing).

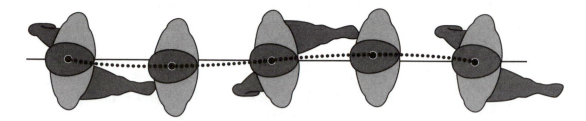

Figure 7.2 Lateral displacement of trunk during a stride (indicated by head location). Midline during double limb support (Figures 1,3,5). Displace to right with right single stance (Figure 2). Displace to left with left single stance (Figure 4).

swing (84% GC). The amount of displacement varies with the subject's walking speed.

The rate of vertical displacement also varies. Initial contact is followed by rapid upward acceleration, which peaks (0.31 gravity) at 5% GC and then quickly dissipates. A minor and brief second wave follows (10% GC). Subsequently, there is a relatively consistent downward acceleration that is maximal (0.08g) at the 50% gait cycle point. Thorstensson found the amount of vertical trunk excursion varies with gait velocity, ranging from 2.7cm at 90m/min to 6.8cm at 150m/min.[9]

Lateral displacement is also the same for all of the axial segments, averaging 4.5cm for the total arc between maximum right and left deviations. In the lateral direction, however, the path is a single sinusoid for each gait cycle (Figure 7.2).[11] Motion of the axial segments is toward the side of the supporting limb. From an initial neutral point at the onset of the stance phase, the segments reach maximum ipsilateral displacement at the 31% point in the gait cycle, that is, the onset of terminal stance. This is followed with a gradual return to neutral (50% GC). The head, trunk and sacrum then deviate toward the other side. Maximum contralateral displacement occurs at the 81% point in the stride. This mid swing time correlates with contralateral terminal stance.

Progressional displacement of the axial segments (HAT), measured during treadmill walking, shows a relationship to gait velocity that follows a double sinusoidal curve. During the first third of each step cycle, the axial segments advance faster than the mean gait velocity. The deviation is greatest for the sacrum (23cm/sec), moderate at the thorax (T10 = 14cm/sec) and least at the head (2cm/sec). The difference between HAT advancement and average progression is maximal at the 15% and 55% points in the stride. Then, the rate of axial segment advancement slows until it is proportionally less than the mean gait progression, being 15, 8, and 2cm/sec respectively, at the 45% and 95% points in the gait cycle. These differences in the rates of segment advancement result in the greatest rate of forward motion occurring at the sacrum and the least at the head (Table 7.1).

Changes in gait velocity alter the segment displacement pattern. Slow walking causes a greater deviation (+30%), while the difference is 20% less with a fast gait compared to free speed walking.

Table 7.1

**Segment Progression Compared to Mean Gait Velocity
(Gait Cycle Timing and Magnitude of Displacement)**

	FASTER	SLOWER
Sacrum	(S_2) +19% (2.6cm)	–12%
Trunk	(T_{10}) +10% (1.8cm)	–7%
Head	+ 2% (0.5cm)	–2%

Pelvis

During each stride the pelvis moves asynchronously in all three directions. The site of action is the supporting hip joint. All the motion arcs are small, representing a continuum of postural change (Figure 7.3). The individual arcs are as follows.

Sagittal:	Anterior/posterior tilt (4°)[5,6]
Coronal:	Contralateral drop/rise (7°)[7]
Transverse:	Posterior/anterior rotation (10°)[6,7]

Motion at the junctions of the pelvic bones and sacrum (sacroiliac [SI] joint) has not been noted during walking. The larger effort of sitting up from a reclining position may involve 0.5cm of sacroiliac motion.[12] This is an inconstant finding, however, as fusion of part or all the SI joint is common. Mobility of the symphysis pubis has not been studied. It is assumed to allow minute degrees of rotation and translation.[12]

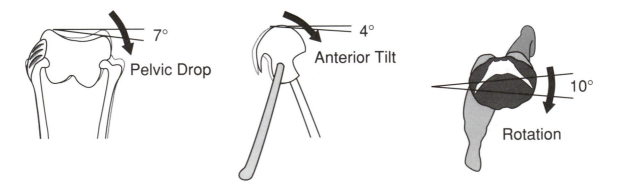

Figure 7.3 Motions of the pelvis during walking: Contralateral pelvic drop (7°), anterior tilt (4°), transverse rotation (10°).

Vector Pattern

During quiet standing, alignment of the body vector in the head passes approximately 1cm anterior to the ear hole (Figure 7.4).[1] It can be assumed this also is true during free walking, as the head only deviates 2% from the mean rate of progress. Further analysis of the body vector location relates to the pelvis.

Sagittal Plane

The precise relationships between the body vector and the center of the pelvis have not been defined. Gross analysis of mean visible vector records indicates the following vector pattern.

At the time of initial contact, the floor impact vector lies anterior to the

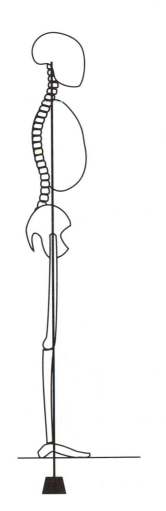

Figure 7.4 Quiet standing alignment of body vector to trunk (anterior to L₃). (Adapted from Asmussen E. The weight-carrying function of the human spine. *Acta Orthop Scand* 29:276-280. 1960.)

pelvis. During loading response, the vector rapidly moves posteriorly toward the center of the pelvis. Gradual posterior displacement continues through the rest of stance. By pre-swing, the vector is in the area of the sacrum.

Coronal Plane

The body vector lies in the midline of the pelvis throughout the gait cycle. Two brief exceptions occur at the onset of loading response and pre-swing when there is a momentary deviation lateral to the hip joint being loaded.[2]

Muscle Control

Stabilization of one vertebral segment on the other within the spine is provided by the musculature contained within the trunk. Gross alignment is accomplished by the long muscles arising from the pelvis. Basic stability of the HAT unit depends on muscular control of the pelvis at the hip.

Pelvis

Two muscle groups, the abductors and extensors of the hip are the primary source of pelvic control. The low intensity of trunk muscle action does not appear to effect the motion of the pelvis.

Action of the hip abductor muscle is the only type of pelvis control that has been specifically identified (Figure 6.7). The upper gluteus maximus and gluteus medius have a similar pattern of action.[4] Onset is in late terminal swing (95% GC) and continues into the middle of mid stance (24% GC). The low level of activity following onset (5%) rises with initial contact and reaches peak intensities of 30 to 35% MMT during loading response (4% to 8% GC). Then the muscles return to their former low level of action (5% to 10% MMT) until they relax in mid stance.

Trunk

Stabilization of the normally aligned trunk requires minimal muscular action during quiet standing. Walking introduces phasic muscle activity. The lumbar and thoracic components of the erector spinae act synchronously.[8,10] Their prime activity occurs at the time of contralateral initial contact, that is, peak action is at 50% GC of the ipsilateral reference stride. The muscles begin their activity in late terminal stance (40% GC), peak at 50% GC and continue through pre-swing. (This timing is related to the contralateral limb's phases of terminal swing and loading response). Ipsilateral action is less intense. Beginning in terminal swing (90% GC), a low peak action (10% MMT) occurs during loading response (5% GC) or mid stance (15% GC).

The large lumbar intrinsic group (multifidus) is bilaterally active at the time of each heel strike (right and left). Ipsilateral peak activity tended to be greater than the contralateral effort (30% versus 20% MMT).[8] Action of rotatores and the quadratus lumborum is similar to that of the multifidi.[10] The activity of these localized muscles coincide with the terminal swing and loading phase action of both the ipsilateral (90-12% GC) and contralateral limbs (45-62% GC).

The abdominal muscles have two patterns of action. Activity of the external oblique muscles is an intermittent, low-intensity (5% MMT) pattern throughout stance. Peak action at a 10% MMT intensity occurs during late mid swing and early terminal swing (75-90% GC). The rectus abdominis has a low level of continuous action.

Study of the trunk muscles during treadmill walking showed a similar pattern of extensor muscle action. Abdominal muscle activity, however, was reversed, with the rectus abdominis being more phasic. This may represent a response to the extensor thrust of the moving platform.[10]

Functional Interpretation

During walking, displacement and acceleration of the axial segments (HTP) reflect the action of the limbs in swing and stance. Consequently the greatest amount of motion occurs at the pelvis. Two mechanisms are in effect, the impact of limb loading and the drag of the contralateral swinging limb. Motion in the plane of progression is stimulated by the change in momentum induced by foot floor contact and the height of the HAT center of gravity. Pelvic motion is initiated by the base of the trunk mass (sacroiliac joint) being eccentric to the center of the supporting hip joints. Movement of the pelvis is restrained by the hip muscles, while the back and abdominal musculature control the alignment of the trunk over the pelvis. Activity of the erector spinae and intrinsic muscles during limb loading and later action of the abdominal muscles decelerate the passive forces reflected to the trunk.

The muscles serve two functions: shock absorption and preservation of upright trunk stability. With only five lumbar segments available to dissipate the sacral motion compared to 17 intervertebral joints in the thoracic and cervical segments to preserve head neutrality, it is evident that the major dynamic effects of walking are experienced by the lumbar spine.

Initial Contact

At the onset of stance, the pelvis is level in both the sagittal and coronal planes and transversely rotated forward about 5°.[3] Loading the limb introduces changes in all three directions.

Loading Response

Weight acceptance by the limb is accompanied by progressional (forward) displacement of the sacrum (S_2), which is twice as great as that occurring at the trunk (T_{10}). The difference in acceleration is 73%. Further intervertebral deceleration removes virtually all progressional effects on the head.[10]

Simultaneous unloading of the opposite limb removes the support for that side of the pelvis, leading to a rapid contralateral pelvic drop. When the focus is on the ipsilateral limb, the motion is described as relative elevation of that side of the pelvis, because unloading the opposite limb has allowed the midpoint of the pelvis to drop. Lateral drop of the contralateral side of the pelvis during loading response is the motion of concern. The rapid drop of the pelvis is decelerated by the hip abductor muscles (gluteus medius and upper gluteus maximus).

The back muscles respond to both of these events. Bilateral intrinsic extensor (multifidus and rotatores) and quadratus lumborum action decelerates the forward displacement of the trunk. Activity of the erector spinae (large, extrinsic extensors) is greater on the contralateral side in response to the pelvic drop. The ipsilateral erector spinae action contributes to decelerating trunk progression. With sacral displacement exceeding that of the trunk, the result is slight lumbar extension associated with a minor forward lean.

Transfer of body weight to the stance limb also frees the unloaded side of the pelvis to begin rotating forward in the transverse plane. External rotation incidental to extensor stabilization of the hip by the gluteus maximus and biceps femoris provides an antagonistic force, while prolonged action of the semimembranosus enhances pelvic rotation.

Mid Stance

Vertical and progressional displacement of the trunk return to neutral, while lateral displacement continues. Transverse rotation and lateral tilt of the pelvis also return to neutral by the middle of mid stance. Lacking any local destabilizing forces, the trunk muscles are quiet. By the end of this phase the HAT is maximally displaced toward the supporting limb. During the latter half of this phase, the pelvis begins to reverse its transverse alignment.

Terminal Stance

Progression of the sacrum and other axial segments now is slower than the mean walking speed. At the same time there is increasing forward acceleration of the supporting limb throughout this phase, which reaches its peak at the end of single limb support. The accelerating mechanism is forward roll of the supporting limb over the forefoot rocker.

At the onset of terminal stance the supporting limb is vertical. This combined with heel rise results in peak elevation of the body axis in early terminal stance (34% GC). Further forward roll of the limb lowers the sacrum, trunk and head. Inertia delays the response of the axial segments that introduces a relative hyperextension effect and anterior tilt of the pelvis. The trunk is stabilized by the flexor action of the rectus abdominis. Reduced participation of the oblique abdominal muscles is consistent with their less effective flexor action.

Pre-Swing

Total axis motion is the same as that occurring in loading response, except for the fact that it reflects the effects of the contralateral limb. In this second double support period, the head, trunk and sacrum again descend to their lowest level. As the limb is unloaded, the pelvis on that side rapidly drops below the body line, creating an ipsilateral tilt of 5°. The pelvis also is released to rotate forward in the sagittal plane.

Initial Swing and Mid Swing

This is a quiet transition period comparable to contralateral mid stance. Transversely, the pelvis regains its neutrally aligned posture. Both posterior tilt (symphysis up) and forward rotation begin.

Terminal Swing

At the onset of this phase, the axial segments are at their highest level. This represents the terminal stance posture of the contralateral limb. A progressive drop from this level then follows. As the pelvis continues to follow the swinging limb, the ipsilateral drop persists and a 3° anterior tilt (symphysis down) develops. The pelvis also is maximally rotated forward (5°).

Conclusion

Movement of the head, neck, trunk and pelvis is secondary to the function of the lower limbs. The significant events are the impact of loading, the changing alignment of the stance and swing limbs, and the loss of bilateral support for the pelvis. Action by the trunk and hip muscles decelerates the imposed forces. As a result all motions are small. Also, both the magnitude and acceleration of displacement are least at the head.

References

1. Asmussen E: The weight-carrying function of the human spine. *Acta Orthop Scand* 29:276-280, 1960.
2. Boccardi S, Pedotti A, Rodano R, Santambrogio GC: Evaluation of muscular moments at the lower limb joints by an on-line processing of kinematic data and ground reaction. *J Biomech* 14:35-45, 1981.
3. Inman VT, Ralston HJ, Todd F: *Human Walking*. Baltimore, MD, Williams and Wilkins Company, 1981.

4. Lyons K, Perry J, Gronley JK, Barnes L, Antonelli D: Timing and relative intensity of hip extensor and abductor muscle action during level and stair ambulation: an EMG study. *Phys Ther* 63:1597-1605, 1983.
5. Mooney V: Special approaches to lower extremity disability secondary to strokes. *Clin Orthop* 131:54-63, 1978.
6. Murray MP, Drought AB, Kory RC: Walking patterns of normal men. *J Bone Joint Surg* 46A(2):335-360, 1964.
7. Saunders JBdeCM, Inman VT, Eberhart HD: The major determinants in normal and pathological gait. *J Bone Joint Surg* 35A(3):543-557, 1953.
8. Sisson G, Perry J, Gronley J, Barnes L: Quantitative trunk muscle activity during ambulation in normal subjects. *Trans Orthop Res Soc* 10:359, 1985.
9. Thorstensson A, Nilsson J, Carlson H, Zomlefer MR: Trunk movements in human locomotion. *Acta Physiol Scand* 121:9-22, 1984.
10. Waters RL, Morris J, Perry J: Translational motion of the head and trunk during normal walking. *J Biomech* 6:167-172, 1973.
11. Waters RL, Morris JM: Electrical activity of muscles of the trunk during walking. *J Anat* 111(2):191- 199, 1972.
12. Weisl H: Movements of the sacro-iliac joint. *Acta Anat* 23:80-91, 1955.

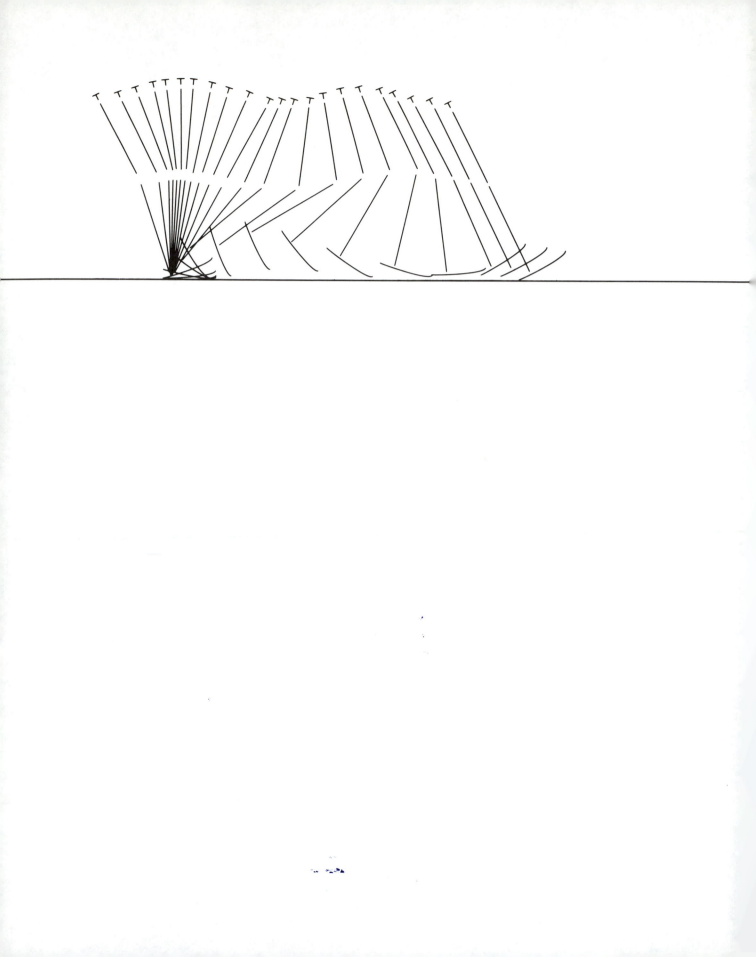

Chapter 8

Arm

Reciprocal arm swing spontaneously occurs during walking. Elftman calculated the angular momentum of the arm swing in the three functional planes and found the pattern was opposite to that of the rest of the body.[2] He concluded that this allowed the lower legs to perform their necessary motion without imparting marked rotation to the body. The significance of this calculation is challenged by the results of energy cost analysis. Testing subjects walking with their arms free to swing and with them bound showed no differences in oxygen usage.[7] These two findings suggest arm swing may be useful, but it is not an essential component of walking.

Gait Mechanics

Motion

During a stride, each arm, reciprocally, flexes and extends for a total arc of arm displacement of 30°[5] or 40°[3] (Figure 8.1). Timing between the two arms is a 50% offset in

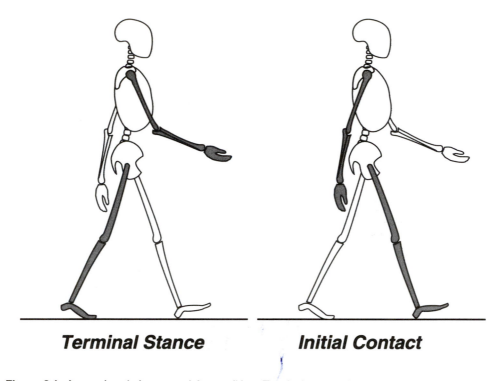

Terminal Stance   **Initial Contact**

Figure 8.1 Arm swing during normal free walking. Terminal stance (maximum forward swing). Initial Contact (maximum backward swing).

the cycle, with the peak displacement in either direction occurring at initial contact. During the stance period from initial contact until contralaeral toe-off, the arm, measured as displacement of the wrist, completes an arc of approximately 20° of flexion. Then, with the onset of contralateral stance, arm motion reverses toward extension reaching a position 9° behind the vertical.[3] While both investigators reported good consistency in the total arc of motion, there was considerable variation among individuals in the amount of flexion and extension used.[3,4] Walking fast increases the total arc of motion by using greater shoulder extension and elbow flexion, while the other arcs are unchanged.[5]

At either free or fast walking, as the arm swings forward and back, the shoulder and elbow move through different arcs of motion.

Shoulder. From a position of maximum extension (8°) at the onset of stance, the shoulder flexes to a position of 24° flexion by the end of terminal stance (contralateral initial contact time) (Figure 8.2). After holding this position of peak flexion momentarily, the shoulder then extends throughout the swing phases.

Elbow. Moving in the same direction as the shoulder, the elbow also goes through an equivalent arc of flexion and extension during each stride.[5] The

ARM

Motion

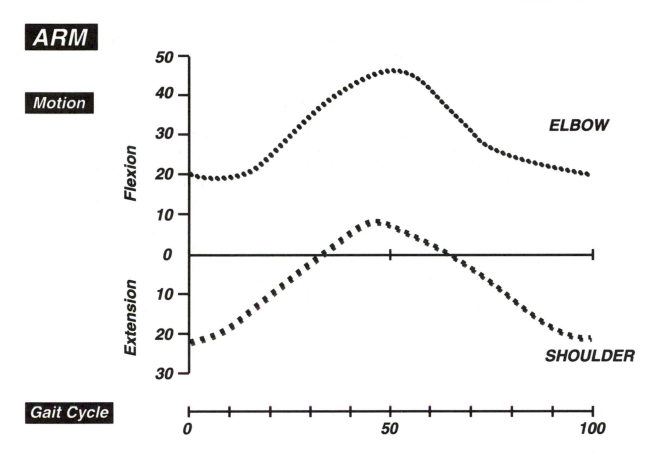

Figure 8.2 Arcs of elbow and shoulder motion during arm swing while walking. Horizontal scale indicates % gait cycle beginning with initial contact (0). (Adapted from Murray MP, Sepic SB, Barnard EJ. Patterns of sagittal rotation of the upper limbs in walking. *Phys. Ther.* 47:272-284, 1967.)

elbow, however, never extends beyond 20° flexion. As a result, maximum flexion is 44° by the time of contralateral floor contact (Figure 8.2).

Phasing of arm motion during walking is quite distinct. At initial contact the ipsilateral arm is maximally extended at both the shoulder and elbow. Following a brief delay (5% GC) the shoulder progressively flexes. There is a greater delay in the onset of elbow flexion that may relate to the maximally extended position being 20° flexion. Movement at the elbow toward greater flexion begins in mid stance. Maximum shoulder flexion of 24° is reached near the end of terminal stance (45% GC), and slightly later (55% GC) the elbow completes its flexor action of 44°. Contralateral foot/floor contact at the onset of pre-swing stimulates both the shoulder and elbow to reverse their motion toward extension. This motion continues throughout the swing period. The elbow reaches its maximally extended position of 20° flexion by mid swing, while the shoulder continues extending until its final posture of 8° extension is attained as the ipsilateral heel contacts the floor once again. The phasic correlation of peak arm motion with floor contact by the ipsilateral or contralateral foot is very consistent, with the majority of the subjects exhibiting less than a 0.1 second deviation.

Muscle Control

Only one study has assessed the electromyographic pattern of the shoulder muscles during walking.[3] Five of the twelve muscles recorded showed activity.

Judging from this single study, the supraspinatus and upper trapezius are the most active. Their onset is just after initial contact, and the action continues until the end of terminal swing, with only scattered short periods of rest (Figure 8.3).

Middle and posterior deltoid action are synchronous. Their activity begins just before the end of flexion and continues throughout extension. During the rest of the stride these two muscles are silent.

The upper latissimus dorsi and teres major complex exerts two bursts of activity. Both relate to shoulder extension. Their periods of action are at the end of extension (loading response) and at the onset of extension (pre-swing). None of the other muscles participate in the arm swing of walking (anterior deltoid, infraspinatus, sternal and clavicular heads of the pectoralis major, rhomboids, biceps and triceps).

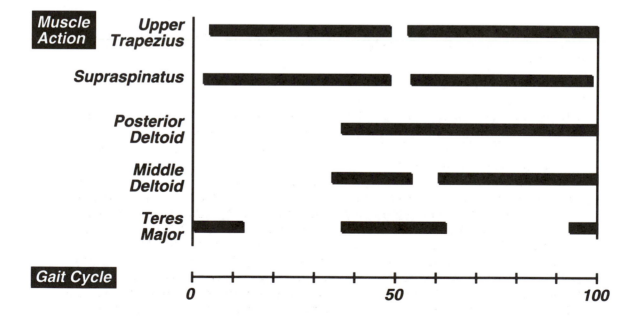

Figure 8.3 Timing of the muscles related to arm swing during walking. Horizontal distance is one gait cycle beginning with initial contact. (Adapted from Fernandez-Ballestreros ML, Buchthal F, Rosenfalck P. The pattern of muscular activity during the arm swing of natural walking. *Acta Physiol Scand* 63:296-310, 1965.)

Functional Interpretation

The shoulder presents three functional patterns during walking: flexion, extension and support of a dependent arm. Each has a specific pattern of muscular activity.

Support of the arm is provided at both the scapula and the humerus. The upper trapezius actively supports the scapula. It is logical to assume the levator scapulae also is contributing as it is a larger suspensory muscle, and significant EMG in quiet standing has been demonstrated. Humeral support is the role of the supraspinatus.[1] The horizontal alignment of the supraspinatus allows it to draw the humeral head into the socket as it also lifts the humerus.[6]

Extension of the shoulder and deceleration of flexion are dynamic events under distinct control by the posterior deltoid (and teres major). Simultaneous timing of the middle deltoid activity contributes to better abduction of the arm, so it will clear the body while following the pull of the extensor muscles.

In contrast, the flexion component of arm swing during walking appears to be purely passive. Currently there is no evidence of flexor muscle activity (anterior deltoid, clavicular pectoralis major or biceps).[3] One can only speculate on the role of the coracobrachialis, as its actions during walking have not been studied.

The role of arm swing is indicated by the timing of the active component. Dynamic arm extension occurs at the same time the leg is swinging forward. Each extremity (arm and leg) also moves through a 30° arc. Hence, the arm is providing a purposeful counterforce to minimize the rotatory displacement of the body by the locomotor mechanics of the legs, just as Elftman calculated.[2] Actively holding the arm back at the beginning of limb loading (the first 5% of the gait cycle) may be a second deliberate, dynamic stabilizing maneuver.

References

1. Basmajian JV, Bantz FT: Factors preventing downward dislocation of the adducted shoulder joint: an electromyographic and morphological study. *J Bone Joint Surg* 41A:1182- 1186, 1959.
2. Elftman H: The functions of the arms in walking. *Hum Biol* 11:529-536, 1939.
3. Fernandez-Ballesteros ML, Buchtal F, Rosenfalck P: The pattern of muscular activity during the arm swing of natural walking. *Acta Physiol Scand* 63:296-310, 1965.
4. Freeborn C: Analog recording of myoelectric signals. *Trans Orthop Res Soc* 6(1):297-298, 1981.
5. Murray MP, Sepic SB, Barnard EJ: Patterns of sagittal rotation of the upper limbs in walking. *Phys Ther* 47(4):272-284, 1967.
6. Perry J: Biomechanics of the shoulder. In Rowe CR (Ed): *The Shoulder.* New York, Churchill Livingstone, 1988, pp. 1-15.
7. Ralston HJ: Effect of immobilization of various body segments on the energy cost of human locomotion. Proc. 2nd I.E.A. Conf., Dortmund. *Ergonomics* 53, 1965.

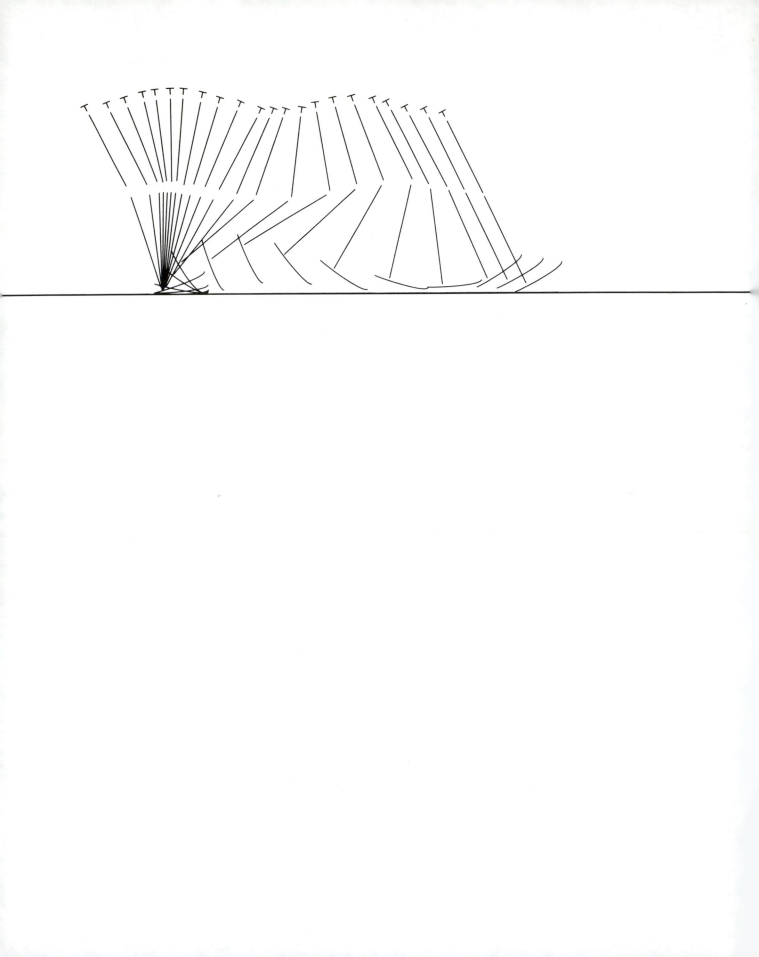

Chapter 9

Total Limb Function

The multiple phases of gait represent the serial patterns of motion and muscle control used at the trunk, hip, knee, ankle and foot to advance the body over the supporting limb. In the preceding chapters, function at each joint has been detailed. Now, it is appropriate to integrate these actions in to a concept of total limb function.

Initial Contact

Interval: 0-2% GC.
Critical event:
Floor contact by the heel. To initiate an optimum heel rocker, the ankle is at neutral, knee extended and hip flexed.

At the moment the foot strikes the ground, the limb is optimally positioned to initiate both progression and knee stability. The ankle is in neutral dorsiflexion, the knee extended and the hip flexed approximately 30° (Figure 9.1). Floor contact is made by the heel. The impact of striking the floor creates a momentary, abrupt vertical floor reaction force as the body freely falls about 1cm.

The alignment of the force line (vector) with the joints introduces three positions of instability (ankle, hip and trunk) and one stable relationship (knee). At the ankle, the vector with its base in the heel creates a torque that opposes the ankle's dorsiflexed position. The knee is provided passive stability by the anterior alignment of the vector. Both the hip and trunk experience flexor torques due to the anterior location of the vector.

The pattern of muscle activity present at the time of initial contact anticipates the controls needed as the limb is loaded. At the hip both extensor groups, that is, the hamstrings and single joint muscles (gluteus maximus and adductor magnus), are active to restrain the flexion torques present. Quadriceps action at the knee is unnecessary at the moment of initial contact, as a passive extensor torque is provided by the anterior vector. Its existence reflects an overlap between terminal swing and loading response when quadriceps action is vital. Simultaneous activity of the hamstring provides a counterforce to prevent knee hyperextension. The foot is supported at neutral by the action of the pretibial muscles. Both the ankle and subtalar joints are stabilized by the combined activity of the tibialis anterior (inversion) and the long toe extensors (extensor digitorium longus [EDL] and extensor hallucis longus [EHL] as evertors).

Loading Response

Interval: 0-10% GC.
Critical events:
Restrained knee flexion. Shock absorption is provided by the quadriceps limiting the arc of knee flexion. This muscular action also maintains weight-bearing stability at the knee.
Restrained ankle plantar flexion. The heel rocker continues body progression, while also contributing to shock absorption.
Hip stabilization. An erect posture of the trunk is preserved.

Loading response is the phase of greatest muscular activity, since demands in all three planes must be controlled. The three arcs of motion that accompany limb loading provide shock absorption to lessen the effect of rapid weight transfer, and thigh retraction adds to knee stability. These actions are knee flexion to 18°, 10° of ankle plantar flexion and subtalar valgus. All are stimulated by the body weight vector being located in the heel. At the same time, motion at the hip is minimized to stabilize the trunk over the weight accepting limb.

Sagittal plane motions are initiated by the heel rocker. Transfer of body weight onto the stance limb, with the heel as the only area of support, drives the forefoot toward the floor. The resulting motions are ankle plantar flexion and knee flexion (Figure 9.2).

Ankle plantar flexion is initiated by the vector being based in the heel. This motion contributes to shock absorption by allowing the tibia to drop slightly in a controlled manner as the pretibial muscles decelerate the rate of ankle motion. The

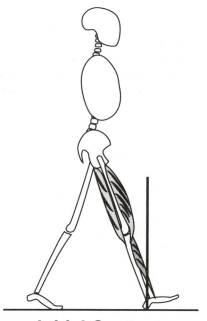

Initial Contact

Figure 9.1 Initial Contact: Heel contact with hip flexed, knee extended and ankle dorsiflexed. Vector anterior, activity of quadriceps, hamstrings and pretibial muscles.

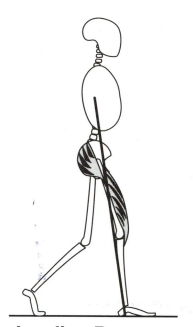

Loading Response

Figure 9.2 Loading Response (end of phase): Hip and knee flexed, foot flat. Vector anterior to hip, posterior to knee and at ankle. Activity of gluteus maximus and quadriceps.

amount of ankle plantar flexion allowed (10°) reduces the degree of tibial advancement and the resulting knee flexion by providing earlier forefoot contact.

Knee flexion is introduced by pretibial muscle action to restrain the rate of foot drop that also draws the tibia forward of the body weight line. Flexion of the knee is accentuated by the inertia of the thigh causing the femur to lag behind. With the knee passively unlocked by the heel rocker, further flexion of the knee is encouraged by the low level of hamstring action that is present. The flexed posture of the hip adds to the knee flexor thrust by the load of body weight on the proximal end of the femur. Knee motion is limited to 15° by the rapidly increased activity of the quadriceps. The result is sufficient knee flexion to absorb the shock of limb loading while the stability needed for secure weight bearing is preserved. Peak quadriceps action is about 30% of the maximum manual muscle test strength. This knee control is provided by the four vasti. The rectus femoris component of the quadriceps seldom participates as its hip flexion action would merely add to the demands on the hip extensors that are actively restraining a passive flexor torque.

In addition to restraining passive knee flexion, the quadriceps produces an anterior shear force that is resisted passively by the anterior cruciate ligament. This anterior drawer is lessened dynamically by the antagonistic posterior force of the hamstring muscles. All three hamstrings are active. Ideal protection of the anterior cruciate would seem to need dominance of the biceps femoris long head to add external rotation to the flexor action, but the most protracted hamstring action is by the semimembranosus.

The hip, being flexed 30°, experiences a flexor torque as the limb is loaded and the body vector is anterior to the joint. A quick and strong (30% MMT) response by the gluteus maximus and adductor magnus prevents further flexion. This hip extensor control is assisted by the continuing low level of hamstring action. Flexion of the trunk on the pelvis is resisted by brief action of the lumbar extensor muscles. These muscles are assisted by the pelvic stabilization provided by the action of the hip extensor muscles.

Coronal plane demands at the hip and knee relate to the strong adduction torque that follows the rapid transfer of body weight onto the limb. The stimulus is the drop of the unloaded side of the pelvis. The torque is greater at the hip than knee because the lever arm between the body vector and joint line is longer. These demands continue throughout stance.

At the hip, the contralateral pelvis drop is limited to 5° by the strong response of the hip abductor musculature (gluteus medius/minimus, upper gluteus maximus and tensor fascia lata). Calculations of the abductor muscle force supporting the pelvis average 1.5 times body weight (range 1.02 to 1.8 x BW).[1-3]

The adductor torque at the knee is restrained largely by the iliotibial band. This may be a passive event that accompanies the contralateral pelvic drop, or it can be dynamic as both the gluteus maximus and tensor fascia lata muscle insert into the band. There is the possibility of further dynamic lateral protection of the joint during the period of biceps femoris long head action, but this usually is brief.

Coronal plane action at the foot is subtalar joint valgus. This adds another shock-absorbing motion by allowing the talus to drop slightly. The rate of subtalar valgus is restrained by the action of the tibialis anterior and tibialis posterior.

Transverse plane rotation relates to events at both the foot and hip. The primary effect of the subtalar valgus is internal rotation of the talus. As the ankle follows the talus, better alignment of the ankle axis with the path of progression is gained. The accompanying rotation of the tibia introduces an internal rotation torque at the knee. Deceleration of knee rotation by an external rotatory force depends on the availability of iliotibial band tension and biceps femoris long head action.

Transverse rotation at the hip generally is defined as anterior pelvic rotation. The presence of a dynamic transverse rotatory action at the hip is implied by the difference in the duration of the medial and lateral hamstrings. Semimembranosus action persists throughout the loading response (and into mid stance), while the long head of the biceps femoris ceases early. The result is an imbalance toward internal rotation. This would assist advancement of the other limb in its pre-swing phase. At the knee, there are two mechanisms for internal rotation of the tibia: the remote effects of subtalar valgus and semimembranosus muscle action. Counterforces for external rotation would follow tension of the IT band and biceps femoris action. Consequently, little motion actually occurs.

Mid Stance

Interval: 10-30% GC.
Critical Events:
Restrained ankle dorsiflexion. The ankle rocker motion allows forward progression. Triceps surae muscle action to restrain the rate of tibial advancement is a major determinant of knee stability.

Knee extension. Progressive straightening of the knee increases weight-bearing stability of the limb.

Hip stabilization in the coronal plane. Abductor muscle action stabilizes the pelvis in a level posture. This provides an appropriate base for an upright alignment of the trunk.

This phase is the time when the body weight line changes its anterior/posterior alignments at each joint (Figure 9.3). As the limb rolls forward over the supporting foot, the critical site for dynamic stability shifts from the knee to the ankle. The intense muscle action at the hip and knee that was present during loading response rapidly terminates by early mid stance. Limb stability becomes dependant on the actions of the soleus augmented by the gastrocnemius. The significant factors are vector alignment and progressional momentum. During mid stance, the vector becomes anterior to the ankle and knee, and posterior to the hip.

Contralateral toe-off transfers total body weight to the mid stance limb.

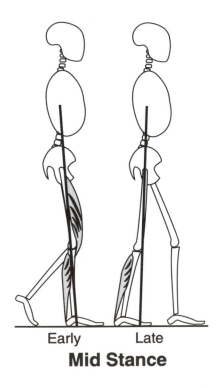

Early   Late

Mid Stance

Figure 9.3 Mid Stance: Early interval has body over mid foot with limb vertical, ankle neutral and foot flat. Vector minimally displaced from joint centers. Quadriceps and soleus muscle activity. Late interval has body over forefoot with continued heel contact. Ankle dorsiflexed. Vector anterior to knee and ankle. Soleus (and gastrocnemius only extensor muscles active).

Progressional momentum from the contralateral swinging limb and residuals from the heel rocker draw the ankle into dorsiflexion. Advancement of the tibia from its position of 7° PF at the moment of contralateral toe-off is more rapid during the first half of mid stance. Neutral alignment is reached by the 20% point in the gait cycle. During the last half of mid stance, only 4° dorsiflexion occurs. This difference in the rate of ankle dorsiflexion represents the relative anterior alignment of the vector and the early response of the soleus muscle. Once both the vector and tibial alignments are anterior to the vertical midline, there is a strong stimulus for the soleus to stabilize the tibia for weight-bearing stability of the limb. The gastrocnemius tends to begin about 5% later in the gait cycle, and its intensity rises more slowly. These modifications are consistent with the knee flexion action of the gastrocnemius and the corresponding knee position.

At the knee, the added load of single limb support introduces a small increase in knee flexion to 18° at the onset of mid stance, since the vector is still posterior to the joint. Beyond this point, there is progressive extension of the knee as the femur advances over the tibia that has been restrained by the soleus muscle. Action of the quadriceps continues until the vector is anterior to the knee. During this time, the vasti are pulling the femur forward. This could be considered as a contribution to progression.

The hip continually reduces its flexed posture, moving from the initial 30° flexion to 10°. However, direct muscle control of the ongoing hip extension is minimal. During early mid stance there is a low level semimembranosus EMG and a continuing contribution by the posterior gluteus medius. Further hip extension is gained indirectly from the quadriceps pull on the femur and displacement of the vector posterior to the hip joint. The timing of this later event depends on the relative verticality of the trunk over the pelvis. The recorded hip flexion (10°) represents the inclusion of anterior pelvic tilt, as the thigh has attained a neutral posture by the end of mid stance.

Terminal Stance

Interval: (30-50% GC).
Critical Events:
Heel rise. The forefoot rocker allows body weight to advance beyond the area of support. Dynamic stabilization of the ankle is an essential element of heel rise.
Free forward fall of the body. This is the major component of progression. It also creates instability in sagittal plane balance.

Provision of a forefoot rocker for the final phase of progression is the contribution of terminal stance to both progression and stability (Figure 9.4). As the body rolls forward over the forefoot, the ankle dorsiflexes to 10° and the heel rises as the knee completes its extension and the thigh reaches a trailing alignment.

Advancement of the trunk moves the vector to its most anterior alignment at the ankle and the trailing posture of the limb allows body weight to drop at an accelerated rate that increases the vertical ground reaction force. The result is a large ankle dorsiflexion torque that requires strong gastrosoleus muscle action to stabilize the tibia at the ankle. Stability at the knee and hip is gained passively from the actions of the soleus on the tibia.

At the end of terminal stance, rotation of the foot/ankle complex on the forefoot rocker advances the knee center to and then slightly ahead of the vector. This unlocks the extended knee and flexion begins. Gastrocnemius muscle tension at this time may be a factor in initiating knee flexion.

Pre-Swing

Interval: 50-60% GC.
Critical event:
Knee flexion. Most of the knee flexion range used in initial swing is attained during this final phase of stance. The energy for knee flexion is the release of potential energy through indirect reactions from actions at the hip and ankle.

The large arc of knee flexion that will be needed in swing is initiated during this phase of double limb support (Figure 9.5). As the ankle plantar flexes 20°, there is 40° knee flexion and hip flexion to neutral. Advancement of the vector to the metatarsophalangeal joint and unloading of the limb by weight transfer to the other extremity free the foot to roll into a high heel rise. This moves the tibia anterior to the vector and causes the unrestrained knee to flex and the thigh to advance. The accompanying ankle plantar flexion maintains limb length and the height of the pelvis. Muscle action during this pre-swing period is limited. Soleus and gastrocnemius muscle activity decreases in intensity to match the reduction in weight-bearing demand of double limb support as the other limb is loaded. There is a similar, rapid decrease by the flexor hallucis longus. If knee flexion threatens to become excessive, the rectus femoris responds. This restrains the knee while assisting hip flexion. Advancement of the thigh (hip flexion) from its trailing position reflects a flexor action of the adductor longus muscle as it contracts to restrain the passive abductor torque that is developing. With the rapid transfer of body weight onto the other limb, displacement of the pelvis precedes that of the trunk. This aligns the coronal vector lateral to the hip joint axis, creating an abductor torque that must be restrained to preserve weight-bearing balance. The anteriormedial alignment of the adductor longus results in a flexor as well as adduction torque, and both are desirable.

The actions occurring during pre-swing commonly are called *push-off* and it is assumed the body is driven forward. More accurately, this is *push-off of the limb*, with the action providing the force that advances the limb in swing.

Initial Swing

Interval: 60-73% GC.
Critical Events:
Knee flexion. Foot clearance of the floor is dependent on adequate knee flexion rather than ankle position because the trailing posture of the limb spontaneously places the foot in a toe down posture.

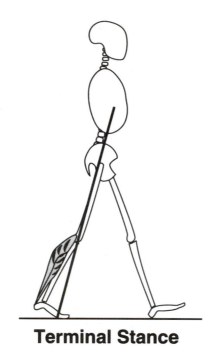

Terminal Stance

Figure 9.4 Terminal Stance: Heel rise with ankle dorsiflexion, knee and hip extended. Vector anterior to knee and ankle, posterior to hip. Soleus and gastrocnemius are the active extensors.

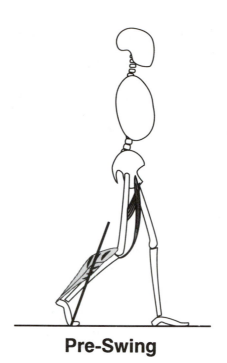

Pre-Swing

Figure 9.5 Pre-Swing: Metatarsophalangeal joints dorsiflexed, ankle plantar flexed, knee flexed hip at neutral. Vector at MtP joint, posterior to knee, magnitude reduced. Calf muscle action weak. New activity by adductor longus and rectus femoris.

Hip flexion. Rapid advancement of the thigh contributes a significant propelling force.

Toe rise signals the advancement of the unloaded limb. Knee flexion increases to 60° to lift the foot above the ground. The ankle only partially reduces its plantar flexion (10°). Hip flexion advances the thigh 20° (Figure 9.6). At the hip and knee, muscle action during initial swing is variable. The most consistent knee flexor is the short head of the biceps femoris. Because the two heads of the biceps share the same tendon, this action often is erroneously attributed to the lateral hamstring (biceps, long head). Such action, however, would inhibit hip flexion as the long head of the biceps also is a hip extensor. EMG recordings clearly differentiate the action of the two biceps muscles. Combined hip and knee flexion may be gained by low levels of sartorius or gracilis activity. Independent hip flexion is provided by the iliacus in the majority of subjects during free walking and regularly when the pace is fast or slow.

Pretibial muscle action (tibialis anterior and the long toe extensors) is brisk during initial swing as the muscles begin lifting the foot. The limited motion that is accomplished reflects the inertia that must be overcome.

Mid Swing

Interval: 70-85% GC.
Critical events:
Ankle dorsiflexion. Active control of the ankle enables the foot to clear the floor.
 Hip flexion. Limb advancement is continued actively.

Floor clearance now is dependent on ankle and hip position. The ankle dorsiflexes to neutral and the hip attains 30° flexion. Knee flexion decreases to 30° (Figure 9.7).
Muscle control at the ankle is a low-intensity continuation of the brisk action of the tibialis anterior, EHL and EDL begun in initial swing. Hip flexor muscle action is minimal. Knee extension is purely passive. At the end of mid swing the hamstrings begin their action that will become intense in terminal swing.

Terminal Swing

Interval: 85-100% GC.
Critical events:
Hip deceleration. Further hip flexion (i.e., thigh advancement) is inhibited.
Knee deceleration. Hyperextension of the knee is avoided.
 Knee extension. This provides a position of passive knee stability in preparation for accepting body weight.
 Ankle dorsiflexion. A neutral position is maintained to put the foot in the desired position for floor contact.
This is the transition phase between swing and stance. Advancement of the thigh is stopped while the knee continues to extend to neutral (0-5° flexion) (Figure 9.8). The ankle remains at neutral (or may drop into 5° plantar flexion).
Muscle activity is intense. During the first half of terminal swing, all three hamstrings (semimembranosus, semitendinosus and biceps femoris, long head) contract vigorously (30% MMT) to restrain hip flexion. Their simultaneous knee flexor action avoids excessive hyperextension from tibial momentum acting on a stationary femur. Then, the hamstrings rapidly reduce their action to a 10% or 5% MMT intensity. At this time the quadriceps (vasti) become active to complete knee extension. Activity of the pretibial muscles is also brisk to assure continued ankle dorsiflexion. As a result of this combination of muscle action the limb is optimally poised for the onset of weight bearing as the next initial contact occurs.

Summary

Walking is a pattern of motion under muscular control. The relative significance of the events occurring during each stride is best summarized by the sequence of muscular action. Phasing within the stride displays the gross control requirements. The timing of peak muscle activity accentuates their

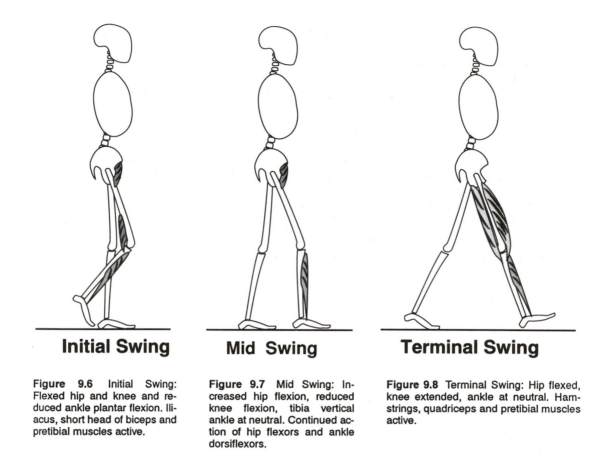

Initial Swing

Mid Swing

Terminal Swing

Figure 9.6 Initial Swing: Flexed hip and knee and reduced ankle plantar flexion. Iliacus, short head of biceps and pretibial muscles active.

Figure 9.7 Mid Swing: Increased hip flexion, reduced knee flexion, tibia vertical ankle at neutral. Continued action of hip flexors and ankle dorsiflexors.

Figure 9.8 Terminal Swing: Hip flexed, knee extended, ankle at neutral. Hamstrings, quadriceps and pretibial muscles active.

unique responsibility for the limb's function. Such information groups the muscles according to three basic functions; stance, swing and foot control.

Stance Muscle Control Pattern

During the stance phases of gait, the controlling muscles are dedicated to providing weight bearing stability, shock absorption and progression over the supporting foot in a manner that conserves energy. With one exception the responsible muscles are the extensors of the limb. Basically they act to restrain the torques created by falling body weight. The extensor muscle follows a dedicated sequence of action that begins in terminal swing and continues through terminal stance (Figure 9.9, Table 9.1). Three functional synergies are performed: swing-to-stance transition (terminal swing), weight acceptance (loading response) and progression over the supporting foot (mid and terminal stance).

Terminal Swing. The three hamstrings (semimembranosus, semitendinosus, biceps femoris long head) follow their activation in late mid swing with a rapid rise to peak intensity in the early part of terminal swing. The accompanying

Extensor Muscle Sequence for Stance

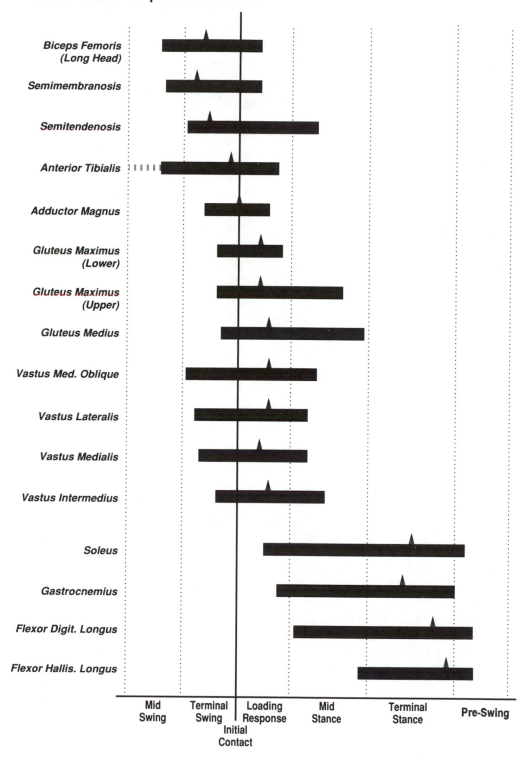

Figure 9.9 Extensor muscle sequence for Stance.

Table 9.1

Extensor Muscle Sequence for Stance
% Gait Cycle

Muscle	On	Off	Peak
BFLH	82	5	92
SMEMB	83	5 (28)	90
STEND	88	18 (31)	93
ANT TIB	82	9	98
ADD MAG	92	7	0
GLUT MAX L	95	10	5
GLUT MAX U	95	24	5
GLUT MED	96	29	7
VMO	88	18	7
VL	90	16	7
VML	91	16	5
VI	95	20	7
SOL	6	52	40
GAST	9	50	38
FDL	13	54	45
FHL	28	54	48

change in joint motion is deceleration of hip flexion while the knee continues to extend. This prepares the limb for stance by limiting the thigh position to 30° flexion and prevents knee hyperextension. In late swing, the hamstrings reduce the intensity of their action to avoid flexing the knee. After this strong effort, the hamstrings significantly reduce their intensity in late terminal swing to avoid introducing knee flexion.

In preparation for stance three other muscle groups begin their activity in late terminal swing. The two singleton hip extensors (adductor magnus and lower gluteus maximus) become active as the hamstrings regress. By crossing only the hip joint these muscles continue deceleration of the femur without having a flexor influence on the knee. Activation of the four vasti (lateralis, intermedius, medialis longus and medialis oblique) counteracts the flexor effect of the hamstrings to assure full knee extension for initial contact. Reactivation of the pretibial muscles (tibialis anterior and long toe extensors) positions the foot for the later heel rocker action.

Loading Response. With floor contact, action of the single joint hip extensors (adductor magnus and lower gluteus maximus) rapidly reaches peak intensity and this level of effort continues into early loading response. Through their insertion on the femur the adductor magnus and lower gluteus maximus impart an extensor effect on the knee as well as at the hip. The hip abductor muscles (upper gluteus maximus and gluteus medius) enhance femoral stability as they respond to the contralateral drop of the pelvis. Also, the upper gluteus maximus has a direct extensor action on the knee through its insertion into the iliotibial band.

Pretibial muscle (tibialis anterior and long toe extensors) action reaches its peak intensity in the early part of loading response to restrain the rate of passive ankle plantar flexion. This provides a heel rocker to initiate knee flexion for shock absorption during weight acceptance.

The four vasti (lateralis, intermedius, medialis longus and medialis oblique) rapidly increase their action to peak intensity. Their function is to limit the knee flexion that was initiated by the heel rocker and assure stable weight acceptance. Once this initial knee flexion wave has been restrained at the onset of mid stance, the vasti promptly relax.

Thus, the hip and knee extensors are serially activated during the terminal swing and loading response phases to end swing limb advancement and assure stability as body weight is transferred to the limb. Shock absorption is provided by the heel rocker stimulus and vasti restraint of the resulting knee flexion. Progression is preserved by the heel rocker mechanics under control of the pretibial muscles. Having accomplished their tasks, the hip and knee extensor and pretibial muscle groups relax.

Mid Stance and Terminal Stance. While there is a brief period of vastus muscle action at the knee during early mid stance, to assist knee extension, the primary responsibility for limb control is transferred to the ankle extensor muscles to provide graded progression over the supporting foot. For the rest of the weight-bearing period, the ankle plantar flexor muscles assume full responsibility for limb stability.

The soleus muscle is first to be activated. Once the foot becomes stable as a result of forefoot contact creating a foot flat posture in late loading response, the tibia becomes the moving segment. Soleus action provides a plantar flexor force to restrain the rate of tibial advancement. Two functions are accomplished. Passive knee extension is induced by having the tibia move forward more slowly than the femur. This also assists hip extension. As a result there is no need for action by either the hip or knee extensors. Secondly, increasing intensity of soleus action parallels the demand torque of body weight advancing over the foot. Peak soleus muscle action occurs near the end of terminal stance. This is in response to two demands. The body weight vector has advanced to the forefoot, creating a strong dorsiflexor torque which must be restrained if weight bearing stability is to be preserved. Secondly, heel rise requires a strong plantar flexor torque to support body weight. The intensity of soleus action rapidly recedes once the other foot contacts the floor.

Gastrocnemius muscle activation soon follows that of the soleus and its increase in effort is similar. Presumably the delay relates to the knee flexor action of the gastrocnemius.

The final source of sagittal limb control is the toe flexors. It starts with the flexor digitorum longus in mid stance when body weight follows the foot's midline. Then, the flexor hallucis becomes active as body weight rolls toward the first metatarsal phalangeal joint. Action of the toe flexors enlarges the forefoot support area by incorporating the base of the first phalanx with the metatarsal heads. Rapid transfer of body weight to the other foot with the onset of double limb support in pre-swing terminates the action of the plantar flexors. The new task is limb advancement.

Swing Muscle Control Pattern

Limb advancement relies on two patterns of muscle action. The transition from stance to swing is accomplished in pre-swing. This is followed in initial swing with a near mass synergy of flexor muscle action that lifts and advances the limb (Figure 9.10, Table 9.2). The effects of the initial swing effort continue through mid swing with minimal additional muscular action.

Pre-Swing. The adductor longus muscle becomes active in pre-swing to restrain the abducting torque at the hip created by body weight falling toward the other limb. Its anteriormedial alignment also produces hip flexion and this appears to be its main role as peak adductor longus effort occurs near the end of pre-swing. The result is reversal of hip motion from hyperextension toward flexion.

Rectus femoris activation often occurs in late pre-swing. Its role is deceleration of excessive knee flexion when the passive events are overly effective. The hip flexor capability of the rectus femoris also assists limb advancement.

The ability of these hip flexors to influence limb advancement is augmented by the passive events that are also occurring. With the onset of double stance, the limb is rapidly unloaded. Limb stability is further interrupted by the foot being released as the body vector advances to the MP joint. This allows the limb's potential energy to become kinetic energy and the tibia falls forward, creating knee flexion which also advances the thigh. Residual tension in the gastrosoleus and toe muscles augment knee flexion by adding to tibial and foot advancement around the point of toe contact. This mild plantar flexor force also assists balance as toe contact is maintained by ankle plantar flexion.

The pretibial muscles (anterior tibialis and long toe extensors) become active in the latter half of pre-swing and rapidly increase their intensity to nearly peak effort. This dorsiflexion action counteracts the residual ankle plantar flexion.

All these actions prepare the limb for swing during this terminal double support period. Stance stability has been disrupted, a large arc of knee flexion has been provided and the muscular control to reverse ankle motion has been activated. These actions display a mini-flexor synergy with simultaneous action by the hip flexors and ankle dorsiflexors while passive knee flexion is supported.

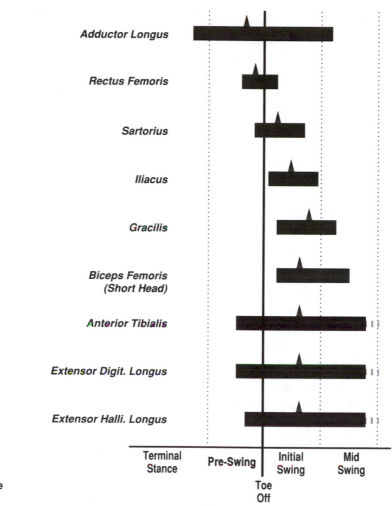

Figure 9.10 Flexor Muscle
Sequence for Swing

Initial Swing. The nearly simultaneous activation of the sartorius, iliacus and gracilis and the early development of peak intensity, advances the thigh. Accompanying action by the biceps femoris short head (BFSH) augments the knee flexion component of the initial swing hip and knee flexor synergy to lift the foot for limb advancement. The slight delay in the peak effort of the BFSH compared to the timing of the hip flexors is consistent with the increasingly horizontal alignment of the tibia, creating a greater demand torque and accentuating the foot's greater equinus position. Use of the three hip flexor muscles is inconsistent among individuals and is of low intensity. It appears that the momentum gained in pre-swing often is sufficient to continue thigh advancement through initial and mid swing. Biceps femoris

Table 9.2

Flexor Muscle Sequence for Swing
% Gait Cycle

Muscle	On	Off	Peak
ADD LONG	46	77	58
RF	57	65	60
SART	60	71	65
ILIACUS	63	74	68
GRAC	65 (47)	78 (4)	72
BFSH	65	81	70
ANT TIB	56	8	70
EDL	56	12	70
EHL	58	10	70

action, to assure adequate knee flexion for toe clearance, is a consistent finding. Its peak activity occurs at the moment of maximum swing phase knee flexion.

Increasing intensity of the pretibial muscles (anterior tibialis, extensor hallucis, extensor digitorum longus) lifts the foot from its previously plantar flexed position. Peak swing phase intensity of this muscle group is similar to the other limb flexors. Their strong activity, however, is more sustained, having started in pre-swing and continuing throughout initial swing.

Limb advancement and toe clearance of the floor is thus accomplished by two flexor muscle synergies. Limb preparation is provided in the double support interval of pre-swing by the first group of muscles, acting primarily at the hip and ankle. A second group of muscles assures completion of limb advancement by the actions in initial swing.

Mid Swing. Inconsistent continuation of the gracilis is the only hip muscle action occurring at this time, even though advancement of the thigh continues. Residual momentum from initial swing appears to be sufficient.

Control at the ankle also is variable. While peak ankle dorsiflexion is reached in mid swing, the mean EMG pattern shows a significant reduction in the intensity of ankle dorsiflexor activity, particularly the inverting anterior tibialis and extensor hallucis longus. Often the muscles are silent in mid swing. Again this implies that momentum generated by the vigorous muscle action in initial swing is sufficient to meet the mid swing demands. Toe clearance of the floor is provided with the minimal amount of muscular effort.

Thus, the pattern of swing phase muscle control differs from the actions during stance. The demands of swing stimulate a nearly synergistic action of the limb flexors. In contrast the stance requirements at the hip, knee and ankle are sequential, though overlapping participation by the muscles.

Intrinsic Foot Muscle Control

The sequence of muscular control for the intrinsic foot joints reflects the demands made by body weight rolling across the foot (Figure 9.11, Table 9.3). Torques imposed on the subtalar, midtarsal and metatarsal joints are restrained

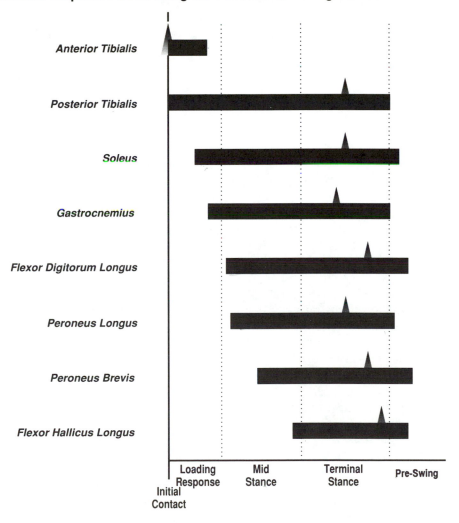

Figure 9.11 Muscle Sequence Controlling the Foot Joints During Stance

Table 9.3

Muscle Sequence Controlling the Foot Joints
% Gait Cycle

Muscle	On	Off	Peak
ANTTIB	0	9	0
PTIB	0	50	40
SOL	6	52	40
GAST	9	50	38
FDL	13	54	45
PL	14	51	40
PB	20	55	45
FHL	28	54	48

in a timely manner by the inverting, plantar, and everting muscle groups. As all of the foot muscles except the intrinsic also cross the ankle, their two functions (ankle and foot control) must be differentiated.

Loading Response. Peak tibialis anterior muscle action following initial contact in synergy with the long toe extensors, reflects their role at the ankle. The larger mass of the tibialis anterior, however, also contributes an inversion force during this heel support period. This acts to restrain the eversion torque created at the subtalar joint.

Tibialis posterior activation at initial contact adds a more dedicated inversion torque. Its initial peak action in early loading response is specifically related to subtalar deceleration. Following a variable level of action during mid stance, the increasing intensity of posterior tibialis activity to a peak in terminal stance indicates a high demand for subtalar joint control. During this period of forefoot support the tibialis posterior is actively inverting the subtalar joint to lock the mid tarsal joints.

Soleus onset in late loading response adds an inversion force for subtalar control incidental to its primary role at the ankle. The nearly simultaneous activation of the gastrocnemius, which has a mild eversion torque, supports the interpretation that ankle control is the primary objective of these muscles.

Mid and Terminal Stance. Flexor digitorum longus activation in early mid stance is a response to loading of the forefoot. With the toes stabilized by floor contact, the flexor digitorum longus provides a plantar flexor force across the arch to oppose the dorsiflexion moment being imposed on the mid tarsal joints. The intensity progressively increases in response to the higher demands of advancing body weight across the foot. Peak action occurs in late terminal stance and then recedes as unlocking the knee also reduces the dorsiflexion strain on the mid foot.

Peroneus longus onset in early mid stance identifies the need for first ray stabilization to counteract the lift effect of the inverting (soleus and posterior tibialis) muscles on forefoot position. Peroneus brevis activation, which quickly follows that of the PL, adds a more direct eversion force for lateral foot stability. This is needed as increasing intensity of the inverting muscles introduces imbalance. Total forefoot contact is, thus, assured. The onset of flexor hallucis longus in late mid stance anticipates heel rise and the need to stabilize the first metatarsophalangeal joint for weight-bearing. Stable toe contact also enlarges the area of support for the forefoot rocker action. Transfer of body weight to the other limb in pre-swing terminates the action of these muscles.

References

1. Inman VT: Functional aspects of the abductor muscles of the hip. *J Bone Joint Surg* 29(3):607-619, 1947.
2. McLeish RD, Charnley J: Abduction forces in the one-legged stance. *J Biomech* 3:191-209, 1970.
3. Merchant AC: Hip abductor muscle force. An experimental study of the influence of hip position with particular reference to rotation. *J Bone Joint Surg* 47A:462-476, 1965.

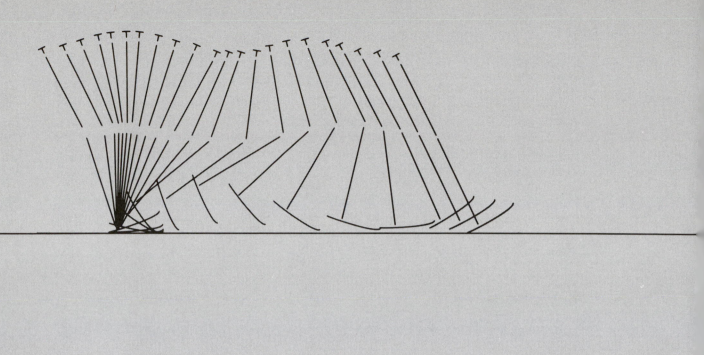

Pathological Gait

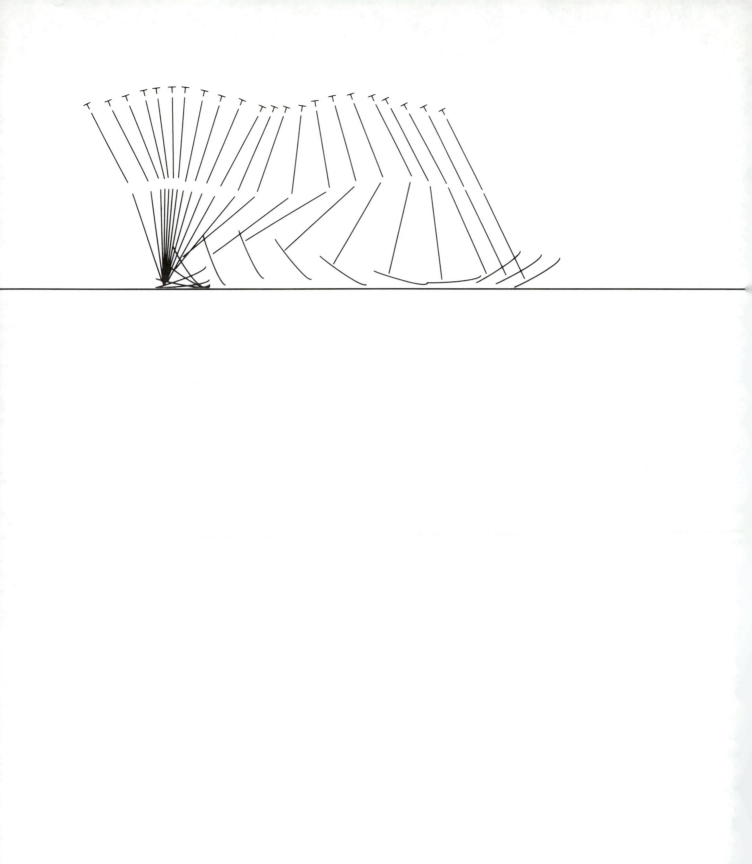

Chapter 10

Pathological Mechanisms

While the long list of diseases that impair patients' ability to walk may differ markedly in their primary pathology, the abnormalities they impose on the mechanics of walking fall into four functional categories. These are deformity, muscle weakness, impaired control and pain. Each category has typical modes of functional impairment. Awareness of these characteristics allows the examiner to better differentiate primary impairment from substitutive actions.

Deformity

A functional deformity exists when the tissues do not allow sufficient passive mobility for the patients to attain the normal postures and ranges of motion used in walking. Contracture is the most common cause. Abnormal joint contours and ankylosis (bony rigidity) also may occur.

A contracture represents structural change within the fibrous connective tissue component of muscles, ligaments or joint capsule following prolonged inactivity or scarring from injury.[1,3,6,13] Relative density, as well as maturity of the connective tissue leads to two clinical contracture patterns: elastic and rigid.

An elastic contracture is one that yields to forceful manual stretch such as using one's whole triceps and shoulder strength (Figure 10.1). The force of two fingers is sufficient to move any normal joint through its full range. Failure to sense the stretch force required causes the examiner to miss the contracture. An elastic contracture presents a confusing picture during walking. In swing the limitations of the contracture will be apparent as the muscles are not programmed to pull harder. Then, during stance, body weight will stretch the tissues so that passive mobility may appear normal or just slightly delayed.

A rigid contracture is one that resists all stretching efforts. Its effect will be consistent throughout the stride. Each joint presents a specific problem.

At the ankle, a plantar flexion contracture obstructs progression of the limb over the supporting foot during stance (Figure 10.2). Depending on its severity, it may affect all the stance phases or just the later ones. In swing a plantar flexion contracture at the ankle inhibits floor clearance.

A knee flexion contracture blocks progression during stance by inhibiting the advancement of the thigh (Figure 10.3a). In addition, it increases the level of muscular activity required to stabilize the knee (Figure 10.3b). In contrast,

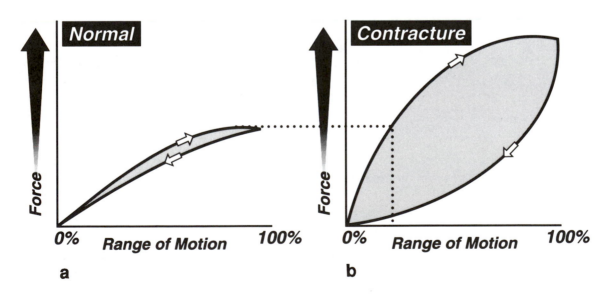

Figure 10.1 Energy absorption by tissues during passive motion. Black lines = force involved. Tissue stiffness indicated by width of space between flexion (up) and extension (down) force curves. (a) Normal tissue flexibility takes minimal energy. (b) Contractures absorb greater energy proportional to their tissue stiffness.

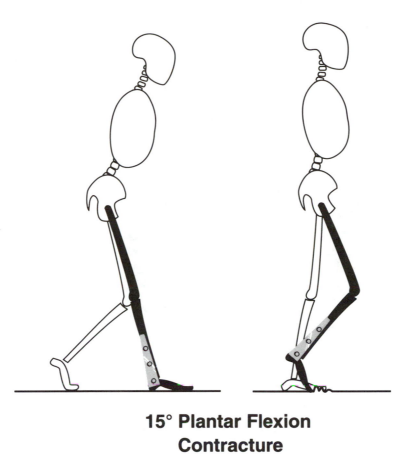

15° Plantar Flexion
Contracture

Figure 10.2 Plantar flexion contracture. In stance, tibial advancement is blocked by contracture at ankle (rigidity indicated by bolted plate). Swing requires increased hip flexion for floor clearance.

an extension contracture increases the energy cost of walking by the additional body maneuvers required for floor clearance during swing.

Hip stability during stance is impaired by a flexion contracture. The trunk is placed forward of the vertical midline (Figure 10.4). This introduces additional strain on the back and hip extensors.

Muscle Weakness

The patient's problem is insufficient muscle strength to meet the demands of walking. Disuse muscular atrophy as well as neurological impairment may contribute to this limitation. When the cause is a lower motor neuron disease or muscular pathology (poliomyelitis, Guillain-Barre' syndrome, muscular dystrophy, primary muscular atrophy), the patients have an excellent capacity to substitute. With normal sensation and selective

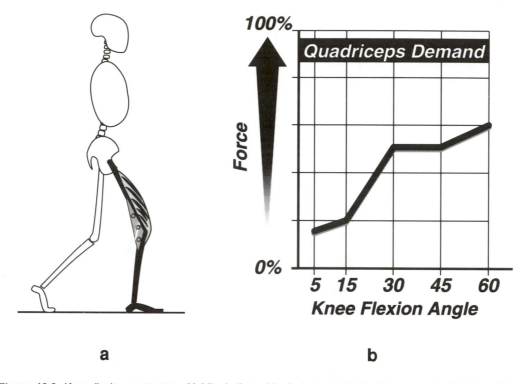

a   b

Figure 10.3 Knee flexion contracture (rigidity indicated by bolted plate). (a) Advancement of thigh inhibited. (b) Demand on quadriceps increased with each greater degree of fixed knee flexion. (Adapted from Perry J, Antonelli D, Ford W. Analysis of knee-joint forces during flexed knee stance. *J Bone Joint Surg*, 57A:961-967, 1975.)

neuromuscular control, patients with *just* muscle weakness can modify the timing of muscle action to avoid threatening postures and induce protective alignment during stance. Similarly, they find subtle ways to advance the limb in swing. Each major muscle group has a postural substitution. Patients also reduce the demand by walking at a slower speed.

If the multiplicity of muscle involvement or a contracture prevents the essential substitutions, the muscles may be suddenly overwhelmed. This is almost an all-or-none situation, that is, either the joints are or are not stable at any one moment. Because the patients do so well when they can substitute, clinicians tend to expect too much from a weakened muscle.

Predictions of walking ability are also obscured by the inability of manual muscle testing to identify the upper levels of normal strength. At the knee, a grade 5 (maximum examiner resistance) represents only 53% of nonparalytic normal (Figure 10.5).[2] A similar grade at the hip is 65% of normal. Manual testing of ankle plantar flexion strength assesses only 18% of a person's ability to do a single, complete heel rise. Today, assessing the quality of a heel rise has been replaced with the number of repetitions that can be done. Recent research showed that normal plantar flexor capability

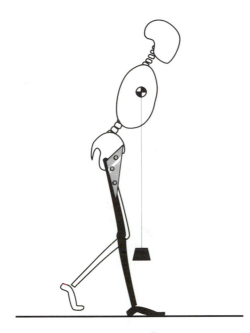

Hip Flexion Contracture

Figure 10.4 Hip flexion contracture (rigidity indicated by bolted plate). To place body center of gravity (vector) over supporting foot, limb must retract and trunk lean forward.

included being able to perform 20 full heel rises.[7] Weakness is displayed by a lesser number (10 for grade 4 and 1 for grade 3).

The earliest display of weakness (grade 4 or Good) represents 40% of normal strength.[12] Grade 3 (Fair) is approximately 15% of normal. During normal walking, muscles function at a fair plus (3+) level.[11] This effort, averaging about 25% of normal strength, allows adequate reserve so fatigue is avoided. Patients with only fair plus (3+) strength will have no endurance or reserve, since they must be functioning at a 100% level. Hence, strength testing must be judged critically and put in perspective of the testers' limitations. When patients meet the normal manual tests, instrumented strength testing is needed to define their true capability. Otherwise, subtle yet significant limitations will be missed.

Sensory Loss

Proprioceptive impairment obstructs walking because it prevents the patient from knowing the position of the hip, knee, ankle or foot and the type of contact with the floor. As a result, the patient does not know when it is safe to transfer body weight onto the limb. Persons with intact motor control may substitute by keeping the knee locked or hitting the floor with extra vigor to emphasize the moment of contact. The mixture of sensory impairment and

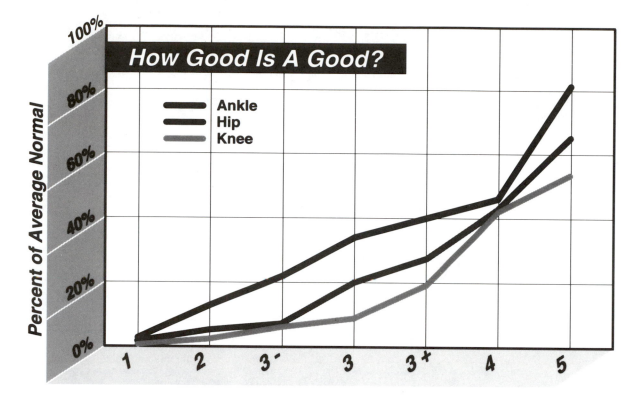

Figure 10.5 Relative value of a manual muscle test for the lower limb extensor muscles (percent of true normal). For all muscles grade 4 = 40 % normal. Grade 5 varies between 50% (knee) and 80% (ankle). At the lesser grades the three muscle also differ. (Adapted from Beasley WC. Quantitative muscle testing; principles and application to research and clinical services. *Arch Phys Med Rehabil.* 42:398-425, 1961.)

muscle weakness prevents rapid substitution. Hence, even with moderate sensory impairment, walking is slow and cautious. When there is a greater deficit, the patient will be unable to use his available motor control because he cannot trust the motions that occur.

As sensory impairment is not visible, it tends to be ignored. Also, proprioceptive grading is quite crude. There are only three grades: absent, impaired and normal. A grade of normal should not be given unless the responses are rapid as well as consistently correct. Hesitation, as well as the occasional error, is a sign of impairment. A slow response is equivalent to not having sufficient time to catch an overly flexed knee or inverted foot during walking. Consequently, the assessment of proprioception must be critical.

Pain

Excessive tissue tension is the primary cause of musculoskeletal pain. Joint distension related to trauma or arthritis is the common situation. The physiological reactions to pain introduce two obstacles to effective walking: deformity and muscular weakness.

Deformity results from the natural resting postures of a swollen joint. Experimentally, this has been shown to be the position of minimal intra-articular pressure with movement in either direction increasing the joint tension.[5] For the ankle, the minimal pressure posture is 15° plantar flexion (Figure 10.6). The knee has an arc between 30° and 45° flexion (Figure 10.7), while the hip's position of least pressure is 30° flexion (Figure 10.8). These minimal intra-articular pressure findings also identify the joint position where the capsule and ligaments are loosest. One can consider these to be the postures that will be assumed by any resting joint.

Muscle weakness occurs secondary to the pain of joint swelling causing reduced activity. Experimental distention of the knee with sterile plasma increased intra-arterial pressure, while quadriceps activation became progressively more difficult.[4] After the pressure prevented all muscle action, anesthetizing the joint restored full quadriceps function (Figure 10.9). This reaction indicated that there is a feedback mechanism designed to protect the joint structures from destructive pressure. Patients display the cumulative effect of this protective reflex as disuse atrophy. During gait analysis, the examiner should expect less available strength and increased protective posturing when the joints are swollen.

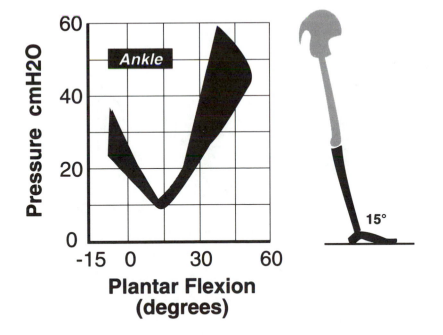

Figure 10.6 Ankle intra-articular pressure of a swollen joint through its range. Minimum pressure at 15° plantar flexion represent the joint's natural resting position (greatest capacity). (Adapted from Eyring EJ and Murray WR. The effect of joint position on the pressure of intra-articular effusion. *J Bone Joint Surg.* 47A:313-322, 1965.)

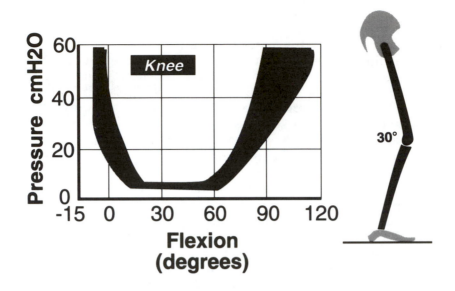

Figure 10.7 Knee intra-articular pressure of a swollen joint through its range. Minimum pressure at 30 flexion represent the joint's natural resting position (greatest capacity). (Adapted from Eyring EJ and Murray W. The effect of joint position on the pressure of intra-articular effusion. *J Bone Joint Surg.* 47A:313-322, 1965.)

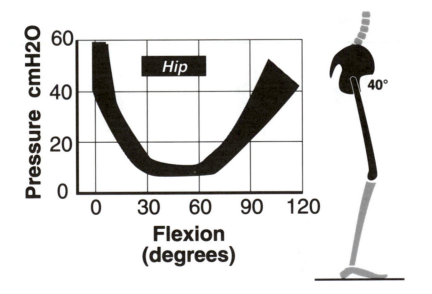

Figure 10.8 Hip intra-articular pressure of a swollen joint through its range. Minimum pressure at 30 flexion represent the joint's natural resting position (greatest capacity). (Adapted from Eyring EJ and Murray W. The effect of joint position on the pressure of intra-articular effusion. *J Bone Joint Surg.* 47A:313-322, 1965.)

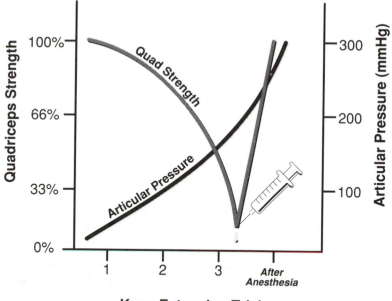

Figure 10.9 Quadriceps inhibition with knee joint distension. Quadriceps strength (top curve) decreases as articular pressure is increased (bottom curve). Injection (syringe) of an anesthetic into swollen joint restores full quadriceps strength (vertical line).

Impaired Motor Control (Spasticity)

Patients with a central neurological lesion (brain or spinal cord) that results in spastic paralysis develop five types of function deficits in varying mixtures and to differing extents.[9,10] The basic effect is an overreaction to stretch (i.e., spasticity). Selective control is impaired. Primitive locomotor patterns emerge. Muscles change their phasing. Proprioception may be altered. In addition, muscular control is altered by limb position and body alignment. The most common causes of a *spastic* gait are cerebral palsy, strokes, brain injury, incomplete spinal cord injury and multiple sclerosis.

Spasticity obstructs the yielding quality of eccentric muscle action during stance. The presence of spasticity is readily apparent when a quick stretch induces clonus (Figure 10.10a). Hypersensitivity of the muscles to slow stretch, however, may be missed (Figure 10.10b). Soleus and gastrocnemius spasticity lead to persistent ankle plantar flexion. Progression is obstructed by loss of the ankle rocker and inability to rise on the metatarsal heads for the forefoot rocker. The persistent knee flexion that follows hamstring spasticity limits the effectiveness of terminal swing and restricts thigh advancement in stance. Hip flexor spasticity similarly restricts progression in mid and terminal stance, while sustained quadriceps action inhibits pre-swing preparation for limb advancement.

RESPONSE TO STRETCH

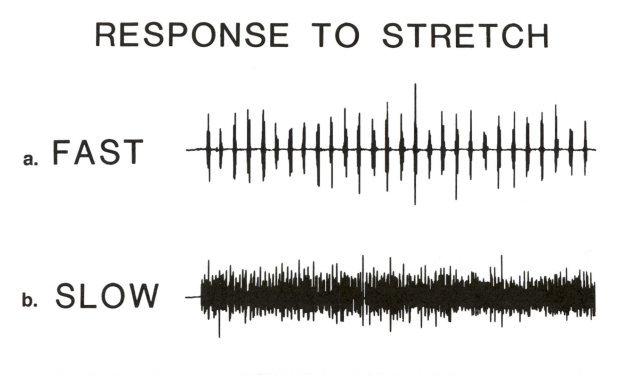

a. FAST

b. SLOW

Figure 10.10 Spastic muscle response to stretch (EMG). (a) Fast stretch elicits clonus. (b) Slow stretch generates sustained muscle action.

The lack of selective control prevents the patient from controlling the timing and intensity of muscle action. This deficit is displayed as weakness similar to a flaccid paralysis, except the reflexes are intact. While the whole limb generally is involved, the control loss is more severe distally.

Primitive locomotor patterns commonly become an alternate source of voluntary control. They allow the patient to willfully take a step by using a mass flexion pattern, that is, the hip and knee flex simultaneously while the ankle dorsiflexes with inversion (Figure 10.11a). Stance stability is attained through the mass extensor pattern. Now the hip and knee extensors and the ankle plantar flexors act together (Figure 10.11b). Inability to mix flexion and extension eliminates the motion patterns that allow a smooth transition from swing to stance (and vice versa). Also, the primitive patterns do not let the patient vary the intensity of muscle action occurring during the different phases of gait. A further problem is the incompleteness of the patterns that result in insufficient strength.

Inappropriate phasing results from the sum of the control errors and spasticity. As a result, the action of any muscle may be prolonged or curtailed, premature or delayed, continuous or absent.

The patients' ability to substitute is proportional to the amount of selective control and the acuity of their proprioception. Generally, only the mildly involved persons are capable of accommodating to their lesions.

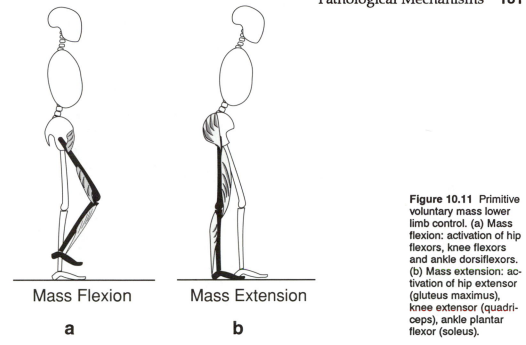

Mass Flexion

a

Mass Extension

b

Figure 10.11 Primitive voluntary mass lower limb control. (a) Mass flexion: activation of hip flexors, knee flexors and ankle dorsiflexors. (b) Mass extension: activation of hip extensor (gluteus maximus), knee extensor (quadriceps), ankle plantar flexor (soleus).

Hemiplegia, by having one side intact, offers the best opportunity. Paraplegia from incomplete spinal cord injury is the next most versatile lesion. Spastic quadriplegia is the most disabling.

Each patient is a unique mixture of the above control dysfunctions.[8] The general rules merely describe the gross picture. Dynamic electromyography is the only means of accurately defining the pattern of muscle dysfunction that is contributing to the individual patient's gait errors.

References

1. Abrahamson MA, Skinner HB, Effeney DJ, Wilson LA: Prescription options for the below-knee amputee: a review. *Orthopedics* 8:210-220, 1985.
2. Beasley WC: Quantitative muscle testing: principles and applications to research and clinical services. *Arch Phys Med Rehabil* 42:398-425, 1961.
3. Breakey J: Gait of unilateral below-knee amputees. *Orthot and Prosthet* 30:17-24, 1976.
4. deAndrade MS, Grant C, Dixon A: Joint distension and reflex muscle inhibition in the knee. *J Bone Joint Surg* 47A:313-322, 1965.
5. Eyring EJ, Murray WR: The effect of joint position on the pressure of intra-articular effusion. *J Bone Joint Surg* 46A(6):1235-1241, 1964.
6. Gage J, Fabian D, Hicks R, Tashman S: Pre- and postoperative gait analysis in patients with spastic diplegia: a preliminary report. *J Pediatr Orthop* 4:715-725, 1984.
7. Mulroy SJ, Perry J, Gronley JK: A comparison of clinical tests for ankle plantar flexion strength. *Trans Orthop Res Soc* 16:667, 1991.
8. Noyes FR, Grood ES, Perry J, Hoffer MM, Posner AS: Kappa delta awards: pre- and postoperative studies of muscle activity in the cerebral palsy child using dynamic electromyography as an aid in planning tendon transfer. *Ortho Rev* 6(12):50-51, 1977.

9. Perry J, Giovan P, Harris LJ, Montgomery J, Azaria M: The determinants of muscle action in the hemiparetic lower extremity (and their effect on the examination procedure). *Clin Orthop* 131:71-89, 1978.

10. Perry J, Hoffer MM, Giovan P, Antonelli D, Greenberg R: Gait analysis of the triceps surae in cerebral palsy. *J Bone Joint Surg* 56A:511-520, 1974.

11. Perry J, Ireland ML, Gronley J, Hoffer MM: Predictive value of manual muscle testing and gait analysis in normal ankles by dynamic electromyography. *Foot and Ankle* 6(5):254-259, 1986.

12. Sharrad WJW: Correlations between the changes in the spinal cord and muscular paralysis in poliomyelitis. *Proc R Soc Lond* 40:346, 1953.

13. Waters RL, Perry J, Antonelli D, Hislop H: Energy cost of walking of amputees: the influence of level of amputation. *J Bone Joint Surg* 58A:42-46, 1976.

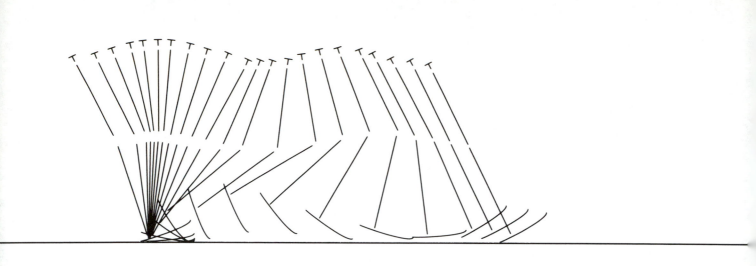

Chapter 11

Ankle and Foot Gait Deviations

Ankle

Terminology

Clinical visibility of some gait errors at the ankle have introduced the terms *equinus* for toe walkers and *drop foot* for the flaccid foot in swing. They, however, do not cover all the situations involving excessive plantar flexion. Similarly, the opposite term of *calcaneus* has limitations when one considers all of the possibilities for excessive ankle dorsiflexion. Further confusion in terminology is added by the fact that normal ankle function involves alternate arcs of dorsiflexion and plantar flexion. Consequently, the same gait error could be classified as *excessive plantar flexion* or *inadequate dorisflexion*. This is particularly true for those phases where neutral ankle alignment is expected and the common functional error is failure to fully dorsiflex the foot from a previous planter flexed posture. Conversely, during those gait phases where some degree of plantar flexion is normal, failure to attain the appropriate arc can be either *inadequate plantar flexion* or *excessive dorsiflexion*.

A preliminary trial with such duplicative terminology proved very confusing. As a result, all the functional errors at the ankle will be classified as either *excessive plantar flexion* or *excessive dorsiflexion*.

A second concern is the extent of the motion variability that is normal. At the ankle one standard deviation from the mean averages 5°. As the arcs of normal ankle motion are small, yet functionally critical to either progression or stability, in some situations a 5° error is clinically significant. This is particularly true for the heel and ankle rockers. Consequently, the mean normal values represent optimum function, and deviations from this imply a subtle error that must be related to the actions occurring elsewhere in the limb.

Excessive Ankle Plantar Flexion

During stance the primary functional penalty of excessive ankle plantar flexion is loss of progression. This leads to a shortened stride length and reduced gait velocity. Stability also is threatened by the difficulty of attaining an upright posture.

In swing, excessive plantar flexion obstructs limb advancement. Commonly this is avoided by substitutive actions that require increased limb or body effort. Throughout swing, the minimal penalty is a shortened step caused either by delayed floor clearance or the initiation of an effective substitution.

Plantar flexion of the ankle below neutral alignment introduces a functional error in five of the eight gait phases. These diagnostic phases are initial contact, mid stance, terminal stance, mid swing and terminal swing (Figure 11.1). As the other three phases in the gait cycle normally involve 10°-20° of plantar flexion, only arcs in excess of this would indicate a functional error. Loading response, initial swing and pre-swing are the less demanding phases.

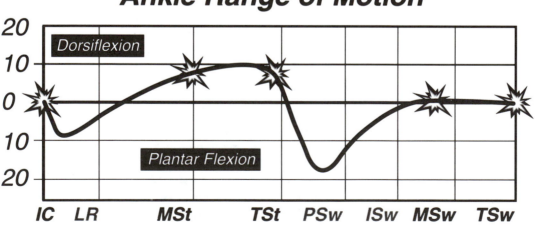

Figure 11.1 Gait phases where excessive ankle plantar flexion is most significant.

Phasic Effects of Excessive Ankle Plantar Flexion

Initial Contact. Two abnormal modes of floor contact may result from excessive ankle plantar flexion: low heel and forefoot (toe). Their differences relate to the knee position established during terminal swing.

Low heel contact occurs when the foot strikes the floor with the ankle in 15° PF and the knee fully extended. While the heel still initiates floor contact, the foot is nearly parallel with the floor (Figure 11.2a).

Forefoot contact represents a mixture of ankle equinus and knee flexion. Either joint may have the greater deformity, or they can be similar. A 20° posture at each joint is sufficient to place the forefoot lower than the heel at the time the floor is contacted (Figure 11.2b).

Loading Response. The action that accompanies loading the limb varies with the cause of excessive ankle plantar flexion and the mode of initial contact. Normal initial heel contact can be followed by *instantaneous* foot drop when pretibial control of the heel rocker is weak.

Low heel contact markedly reduces the heel rocker, as the foot has only a 10° arc rather than the usual 25-30° to travel. Consequently, the knee flexion thrust is markedly reduced.

Forefoot contact can result in three loading patterns, depending on the cause of the excessive ankle plantar flexion (Figure 11.3). If there is good ankle mobility the foot will rapidly drop onto the heel while the tibia stays vertical (Figure 11.3a). Rigid plantar flexion can lead to two possible reactions. The heel off posture may continue (Figure 11.3b). Otherwise, the tibia is driven backward as the heel drops to the floor (Figure 11.3c).

Mid Stance. Excessive plantar flexion in mid stance inhibits tibial advance-

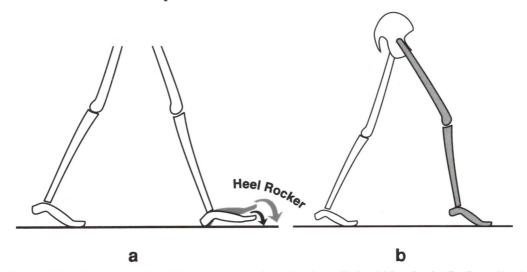

a   **b**

Figure 11.2 Initial contact gait deviations from excessive ankle plantar flexion (a) Low heel strike (loss of heel rocker). (b) Forefoot contact.

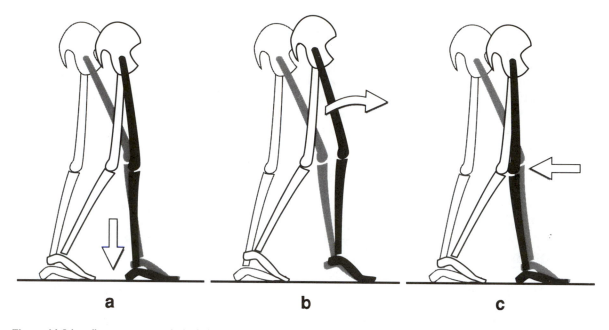

Figure 11.3 Loading response gait deviations from excessive ankle plantar flexion. (a) Forefoot contact with rapid drop to foot flat by a flexible ankle. (b) Forefoot contact sustained. (c) Forefoot contact drop to foot flat with rigid ankle plantar flexion.

ment. If a foot flat contact continues the tibia advances only to the extent of the available passive range. Any limitation that restricts dorsiflexion to less than 5 by the 30% point in the gait cycle represents an abnormal restraint. With loss of the ankle rocker, progression is proportionally limited, leading to a short step length by the other limb.

Patients have three characteristic substitutions for their loss of progression. These include premature heel-off, knee hyperextension and forward trunk lean (Figure 11.4). All represent efforts to move the trunk forward over the rigid equinus. Which measure is used varies with the patient's gait velocity and knee mobility. A mixture of the three adaptations is also common.

Premature heel rise (Figure 11.4a) is the mechanism used by vigorous walkers with no other major disability. These patients have the ability to propel themselves from a low heel contact, across an obstructive foot flat posture and onto the forefoot. Now the heel rise occurs in mid rather than terminal stance. Exact timing varies with the magnitude of the plantar flexion contracture and the momentum available. The duration of foot flat is correspondingly limited. The extra time used in this effort results in a moderate reduction in walking speed. A velocity approximating 70% of normal (% N) is common.

Knee hyperextension can overcome the posteriorly aligned tibia when there is sufficient ligamentous laxity (Figure 11.4b). The knee hyperextends as the femur follows body momentum and rolls forward over the immobile tibia. Walking vigor is not a factor in the use of this substitution. It is common with stroke hemiplegia, incomplete spinal cord injury and cerebral palsy. The range of knee

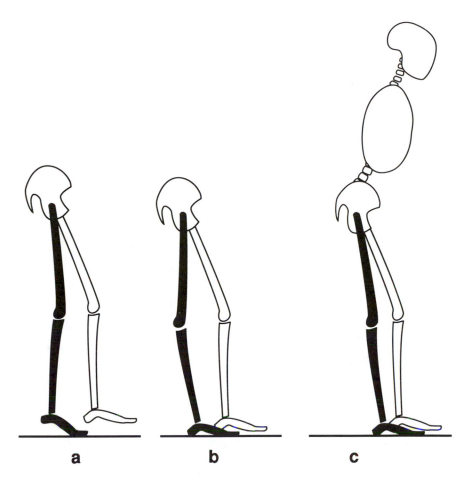

Figure 11.4 Mid stance gait deviations from excessive ankle plantar flexion. (a) Premature heel rise. (b) Foot flat with a posteriorly restrained tibia. (c) Substitution for lack of tibial progression by forward trunk lean. (Note short contralateral step.)

hyperextension can increase in the growing child and in the more vigorous spastic patient. Their dynamics produce sufficient repetitive strain for the tissues to yield.

Forward lean of the trunk with anterior tilt of the pelvis is the final substitution available (Figure 11.4c). This serves more to maintain balance over the plantigrade foot with fixed ankle plantar flexion than to enhance progression. Stance stability is attained, but a significant demand is imposed on the hip and back extensors. These more disabled persons have a very slow gait velocity (15% N). When the patient has persistent forefoot support following limb loading, the ankle rocker is absent. Body weight advances as the patient rolls across the forefoot and the patient proceeds immediately into terminal stance.

Terminal Stance. The effects of excessive plantar flexion on terminal stance gait mechanics depend on the patient's ability to roll onto the forefoot. If the patient

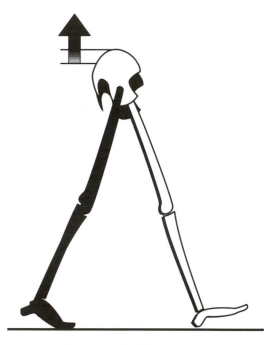

Terminal Stance

Figure 11.5 Terminal stance gait deviation from excessive ankle plantar flexion is an increased heel rise when patient is able to roll onto forefoot.

can not attain a heel rise, the advancement of the body is limited to the extent that knee hyperextension or trunk lean and pelvic rotation improve the forward reach of the opposite limb. In contrast, the vigorous walker who advanced from low heel strike to premature heel rise will have a seemingly normal motion pattern in terminal stance. Excessive heel rise will be an unconscious event (Figure 11.5).

Step length is shortened. The loss may be mild in the vigorous walker but can be severe in patients who never attain good stability on the forefoot.

Pre-Swing. If forefoot support was attained during terminal stance, there will be no significant gait abnormalities in pre-swing. The alignment to initiate knee flexion is present.

Patients who had maintained heel contact throughout terminal stance may develop a late heel rise after body weight has been transferred to the other limb. Otherwise the heel will not rise until the thigh begins to advance for initial swing.

Initial Swing. The diagnosis of excessive ankle plantar flexion in initial swing is hidden by the natural toe down posture of trailing limb alignment. Unless it is extreme, excessive ankle plantar flexion in initial swing has no clinical significance. The trailing posture of the tibia tends to minimize the effect increased ankle plantar flexion has on toe drag.

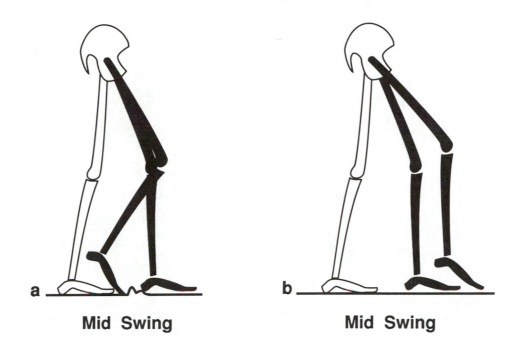

Mid Swing   **Mid Swing**

Figure 11.6 Mid swing gait deviations from excessive ankle plantar flexion. (a) Toe drag is the immediate reaction. (b) Substitution with increased hip and knee flexion is common.

Mid Swing. Excessive plantar flexion in mid swing drops the foot below horizontal. The immediate effect is toe drag on the floor and inhibition of limb advancement (Figure 11.6a). As a result, swing is prematurely terminated unless there is adequate substitution to preserve floor clearance.

The most direct substitution for lack of adequate ankle dorsiflexion in swing is increased hip flexion to lift the limb and, hence, the foot (Figure 11.6b). As the thigh is lifted, the knee flexes in response to gravity. Because displacement at the knee is more conspicuous, it often is erroneously considered to be the primary substitution for a foot drag. Knee flexion without hip flexion, however, would direct the tibia backward and actually increase the foot's equinus posture rather than lift the toe.

The other substitutions used to attain floor clearance relate to a lack of adequate hip flexion. These include circumduction, lateral trunk lean and contralateral vaulting.

Terminal Swing. Excessive ankle plantar flexion in terminal swing seldom interferes with floor clearance because the flexed hip and extended knee place the forefoot above the floor (Figure 11.7). Commonly, a toe drag that is present in mid swing is corrected by the terminal swing lift of the foot. Hence, persistent toe drag indicates a mixture of excessive ankle plantar flexion and inadequate knee extension.

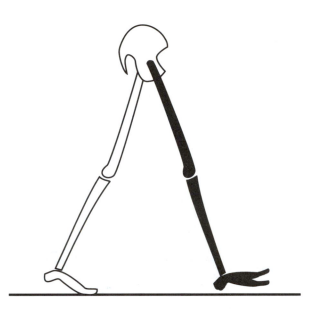

Terminal Swing

Figure 11.7 Terminal swing gait deviation from excessive ankle plantar flexion. The foot is nearly parallel to the floor with the 15° position.

Causes of Excessive Plantar Flexion

Four basic types of dysfunction cause excessive plantar flexion. These are pretibial muscle weakness, plantar flexion contracture, soleus overactivity (spastic or primitive pattern control) and voluntary posturing for a weak quadriceps. Their effects within the gait cycle lead to different patterns of abnormal function (Table 11.1).

Pretibial Muscle Weakness. Failure of the pretibial muscles (primarily the tibialis anterior) to produce an adequate dorsiflexion force allows the foot to fall in an uncontrolled manner. If only the tibialis anterior is lost, the foot drop involves just the medial side of the foot. Continued activity by the extensor hallucis, extensor digitorum longus and peroneus tertius produces a mixture of dorsiflexion and eversion.

The magnitude of passive ankle plantar flexion also varies with the age of onset. Adult acquired disability seldom causes more than a 15° equinus posture. This also is generally true for the foot drop resulting from spastic paralysis (Figure 11.8). In contrast, when flaccid paralysis of the pretibial musculature occurs in early childhood, passive equinus may reach 30°, perhaps more. These differences in magnitude also influence the types of gait errors recorded.

Excessive plantar flexion resulting from inadequate tibialis anterior activity is most apparent and clinically significant in mid swing (Figure 11.6), initial

Table 11.1

Phasic Patterns of Excessive Ankle Plantar Flexion

	IC	LR	MS	TS	PSw	ISw	MSw	TSw
30° Contracture X	X	X	X	X	X	X	X	
15° Contracture X		X	X			X	X	
15° Elastic Ctr X						X	X	
Spastic Calf	X		X	X			X	X
PreTib Weakness	X	X					X	X
Voluntary	X	X						X

Key: X = phases altered by the designated pathology
      IC = initial contact   PSw = pre-swing
      LR = loading response   ISw = initial swing
      MS = mid stance   MSw = mid swing
      TS = terminal stance   TSw = terminal swing

contact (Figure 11.2) and loading response (Figure 11.3). During swing, floor clearance is the problem. In stance, the heel rocker is altered. Following all three situations, the subsequent stance phases will be normal if inadequate pretibial muscle action is the only deficit.

Plantar Flexion Contracture. The phases of gait that are altered by a plantar flexion contracture vary with the magnitude of dorsiflexion lost as well as the rigidity of the tissues. A 15° plantar flexion contracture is most common because that is the position of minimal joint capsule tension.[3] It may be rigid or elastic. An elastic contracture is created by moderately dense tissues that stretch under the force of body weight but hold against manual testing. Other clinical circumstances, however, may introduce greater deformity. Hence, ankle plantar flexion contractures fall into three gross categories: elastic PF 15°, rigid PF 15° and PF 30°. Each modifies different phases of the gait cycle.

30° plantar flexion contracture. Floor contact with a flat foot is possible, but flexing the knee and striking the floor with the forefoot is much more common (Figure 11.2b), because this adaptation facilitates progression. Because the 30° PF deformity exceeds the normal ranges of plantar flexion, there will be abnormal function in each phase of gait. There will be no heel contact in stance even with the slow walker. Instead, the forefoot will be the only mode of support. Stride length will be shortened by the absence of the heel and ankle rockers. Each phase of swing is threatened by toe drag, unless the patient has an adequate substitution.

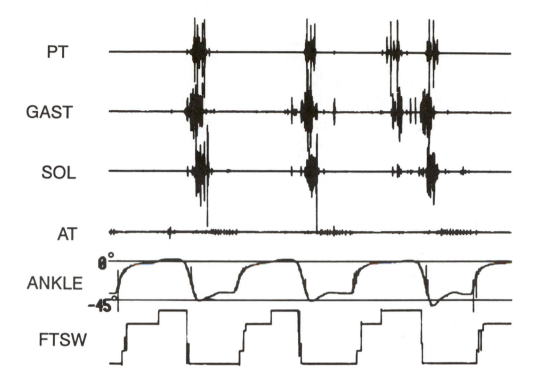

Figure 11.8 Tibialis anterior paralysis as a cause of excessive ankle plantar flexion in swing. The extent of the foot drop (45° PF) suggests a coexisting elastic contracture that partially stretched in stance under body weight.

Rigid 15° contracture. Stiffness of the fibrous tissues determines the effect of the contracture. A rigid contracture can cause deviations in five of the gait phases. The severity of the deviations also varies with the vigor of the patient's walking ability. The typical picture is a low heel mode of initial contact, early foot flat in loading response and lack of tibial advancement in mid stance. In the vigorous walker, the deviations during loading response and mid stance will be obscured by heel-off occurring while the limb is still vertical (i.e., technicaly in mid stance). This represents a premature terminal stance posture. Slow walkers will lack the energy to roll up onto the forefoot. Persistent heel contact and an obstructed ankle rocker terminates the patient's ability to advance. Progression is restricted to the extent of available knee hyperextension.

Subtalar eversion can lessen the apparent amount of plantar flexion through two mechanisms. Dorsiflexion is a normal component of eversion. In addition subtalar eversion unlocks the midtarsal joint, leaving it free to dorsiflex. These actions will reduce the angle between the forefoot and tibia.

In mid swing there will be a toe down foot posture similar to the passive drop foot from pretibial muscle weakness. Toe drag will occur if the patient is unable to substitute.

Elastic 15° contracture. The flexibility of this contracture allows the ankle to yield under body weight (Figure 11.8). As a result, it leads to an inappropriate foot position only at initial contact and in mid swing. During mid and terminal stance, the restraint to tibial advancement presented by the elastic contracture may mimic that of normal soleus activity and thus induces no motion abnormality. With stiffer tissues the rate of tibial advancement is slowed, but this generally is an imperceptible deviation from normal function. A dynamic EMG recording may be needed to differentiate soleus action from contracture. Subtalar substitution also is common.

In mid swing, the elastic contracture will create excessive plantar flexion similar to that of pretibial muscle weakness, as the limited force provided by the dorsiflexor muscles is insufficient to stretch the tissues. Functionally, these muscles are prepared only to rapidly lift the weight of the foot when there is virtually no resistance at the ankle. This effort is equivalent to grade 3 or fair strength.[1] Loading response, however, will not show an uncontrolled drop of the foot.

Because the secondary events are brief, a dynamic EMG recording may be needed to differentiate the effects of an elastic contracture from the lack of pretibial musculature.

Soleus and Gastrocnemius Spasticity. With severe spasticity the soleus and gastrocnemius may be continuously active (Figure 11.9). Then the gait pattern is similar to a plantar flexion contracture of similar magnitude.

More commonly, the excessive action of the triceps surae muscles is a component of the primitive extensor muscle pattern. Terminal swing is the phase in which the primitive extensor pattern starts. As the quadriceps begins its action to extend the knee in preparation for stance, there is synergistic activation of the soleus and gastrocnemius. The ankle moves from a mid swing dorsiflexed posture to about 15° of plantar flexion (see Hemiplegia, Chapter 15). This rigidly plantar flexed ankle posture will affect the patient's gait in each phase of stance, from initial contact through pre-swing.

Initial swing and mid swing are periods of normal ankle dorsiflexion. Activation of the flexor pattern to take a step terminates the extensor muscle action. The ankle promptly dorsiflexes to a near neutral position, which persists

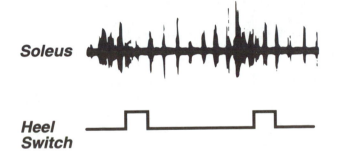

Soleus

Heel Switch

Figure 11.9 Soleus spasticity causing continuous activity through the gait cycle. Clonic beats in swing precede the premature patterned activation (dense area) in stance.

through mid swing. It is this patterned reversal of ankle motion in swing that differentiates the spastic primitive extensor response from a plantar flexion contracture.

Voluntary Excessive Ankle Plantar Flexion. As a means of protecting a weak quadriceps from the usual knee flexion thrust of the loading response, patients with normal selective control deliberately reduce their heel rocker.

Terminal swing is the usual time that the protective mechanics begin. Premature action by the soleus drops the foot into approximately 10° plantar flexion. The gastrocnemius is an inconsistent participant. Tibialis anterior muscle action may continue to control the rate of the foot drop. The low heel strike at initial contact minimizes the heel rocker flexion thrust on the tibia. Loading reponse follows with a rapid ankle plantar flexion leading to foot flat and tibial retraction as the calf muscles continue their strong activity. The soleus dynamically restrains the tibia to preserve an extended knee throughout mid stance and terminal stance action. Muscle intensity is graduated so the soleus and gastrocnemius decelerate, but do not inhibit tibia advancement. The calf muscles yield sufficiently to allow a delayed arc of relative dorsiflexion to preserve progression. As a result, peak dorsiflexion occurs late in pre-swing rather than during terminal stance, and heel contact is continued. The progressive ankle dorsiflexion differentiates the voluntary calf activity from a plantar flexion contracture or soleus spasticity.

During the other gait phases, ankle dorsiflexion is normal. The soleus has relaxed and the pretibial muscles become active.

Excessive Ankle Dorsiflexion

Dorsiflexion beyond neutral is an abnormal event in all of the gait phases except mid stance and terminal stance. Diagnosing excess dorsiflexion during these two stance phases presents a challenge. A five degree deviation can be considered within the normal variance, yet it also may have functional significance as it still leads to considerable tibial tilt.

The term *excessive dorsiflexion* also is used to indicate the lack of normal plantar flexion. This can occur during loading response, pre-swing and initial swing. Excessive dorsiflexion has more functional significance in stance than swing.

Initial Contact. Excessive dorsiflexion at the time the heel contacts the floor is an infrequent finding. When it occurs, it is a position of instability. An exaggerated heel rocker has been established, as the forefoot will be higher above the floor than normal (Figure 11.10).

Loading Response. Two forms of excessive dorsiflexion are possible. There may be an abnormal form of initial contact or inhibition of the normal ankle plantar flexion.

Floor contact with the flat foot has eliminated the 10° plantar flexion that normally accompanies the heel rocker action. This introduces a passive form of excessive dorsiflexion as the limb is loaded. The potential for accelerated tibial advancement has been established.

Fixation of the ankle at neutral (90°) during the heel support period causes the tibia to advance at the same rate as the foot falls to the floor. Consequently the heel rocker effect on the knee is doubled (potentially 30° rather than 15°) (Figure 11.11). There is a corresponding increase in the quadriceps demand.

Mid Stance. Two situations can make excessive dorsiflexion in mid stance functionally significant. First is an accelerated rate of ankle dorsiflexion from its initial position of plantar flexion (Figure 11.12a). As momentum from the swing limb draws the body C/G forward, the tibia follows. While the final position of the ankle may not exceed the normal 10° because that is the limit of the patient's passive range, the patient experiences the instability of excessive dorsiflexion at the onset of single limb support.

The second form of excessive ankle dorsiflexion is a greater than normal angle being attained between the tibia and foot (Figure 11.12b). This is more marked in terminal stance.

Both situations (rate and magnitude) lead to increased quadriceps demand. The lack of tibial control also creates an unstable base for the quadriceps that prevents the muscle from fully extending the knee.

Terminal Stance. Excessive dorsiflexion of the ankle during terminal stance is difficult to identify by observation because two actions tilt the tibia forward. These are heel rise and ankle dorsiflexion. When heel contact continues through terminal stance, the ankle position suddenly becomes visible (Figure 11.13a). Now, even the normal 10° dorsiflexion may appear excessive. Conversely, as

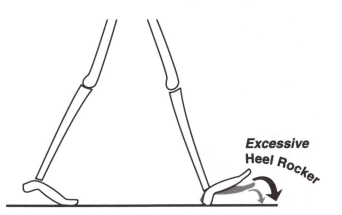

Figure 11.10 Excessive ankle dorsiflexion at initial contact presents a higher heel rocker.

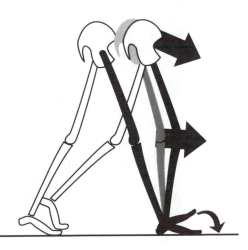

Figure 11.11 Excessive ankle dorsiflexion during the loading response increases the heel rocker, leading to greater knee flexion.

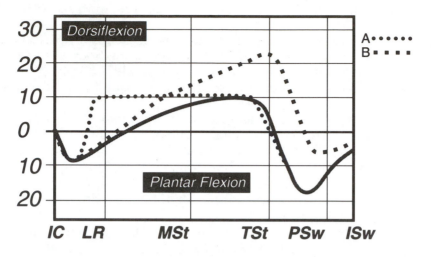

Figure 11.12 Excessive ankle dorsiflexion in mid stance occurs in two action patterns: (a) an abrupt change from LR plantar flexion into dorsiflexion with maintenance of the ankle posture, (b) progressive increase into excessive ankle dorsiflexion throughout mid and terminal stance.

elevation of the foot is more conspicuous than an increase in tibial angle, the combination of heel rise and excessive dorsiflexion masks the change in ankle position (Figure 11.13b).

Pre-Swing. Whenever the normal 20° plantar flexion is reduced, the ankle is in excessive dorisflexion. This most often occurs with prolonged heel contact as the body, by being well forward of the foot, draws the tibia forward once the ankle's passive range has been reached (Figure 11.14).

Initial Swing, Mid Swing and Terminal Swing. Seldom does the foot rise above neutral during swing. The only clinical significance relates to the position the ankle will be in at the time of initial contact.

Causes of Excessive Ankle Dorsiflexion

Two primary conditions lead to excessive dorsiflexion. These are soleus weakness and fixation of the ankle at neutral. Accommodating to a flexed knee during stance is another cause of excessive ankle dorsiflexion. The functional significance of these mechanisms involves different phases in the gait cycle.

Soleus Weakness. Loss of tibial stability during the weight-bearing period is the problem. This leads to increased demand of the quadriceps.

Mid stance advancement of the tibia over the foot rapidly moves the ankle into overt dorsiflexion when the soleus response is inadequate. Basically, the tibia follows the progression of the vector. Thus, there is an excessive ankle

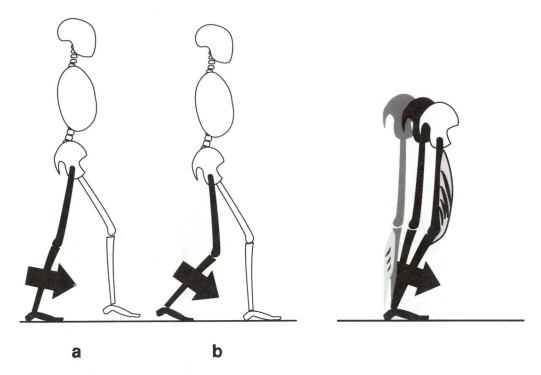

a   **b**

Figure 11.13 Excessive ankle dorsiflexion in terminal stance can be identified by two gait deviations: (a) prolonged heel contact displays the accompanying tibial displacement (arrow), (b) excessive knee flexion combined with a heel rise may mask the additional tibial advancement (arrow).

Figure 11.14 Excessive ankle dorsiflexion in pre-swing represents a loss of the normal plantar flexion. Sustained heel contact also is common.

rocker. Anterior alignment of the tibia perpetuates the flexed knee posture and the need for continued quadriceps support. The quadriceps cannot reestablish knee extension because as it acts to advance the femur the entire proximal body mass (C/G) moves forward (Figure 11.15). This increases the dorsiflexion vector at the ankle, leading to further tibial tilt. Gastrocnemius action contributes a knee flexion effect at the same as it is augmenting the soleus at the ankle.

Terminal stance heel rise also is lost with soleus weakness. This may occur even if the patient had a normal dorsiflexion arc in mid stance because the intensity of muscular effort during terminal stance needs to be twice that of mid stance. Terminal stance knee extension is lost and replaced with persistent flexion.

The common causes of inadequate triceps surae action are primary muscle weakness (disuse or paralysis) and excessive surgical lengthening of a tight Achilles tendon. The undesirable surgical outcome may result from the restoration of normal range when there is not sufficient neurological control to use such mobility advantageously. A second cause of *over lengthening* could be physiological muscle lengthening by the addition of sarcomeres to the muscle fiber chain in response to the repeated eccentric stretch experienced in gait.[4]

There generally is gastrocnemius weakness associated with the lack of

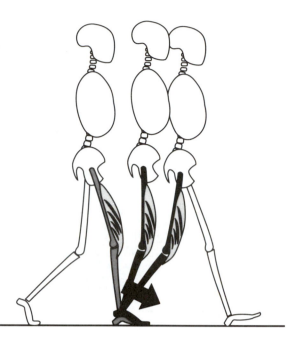

Figure 11.15 Soleus weakness fails to stabilize the tibia, causing sustained knee flexion. Without a stable base the quadriceps cannot extend the flexed knee.

soleus action, but it is does not directly contribute to the excessive ankle dorsiflexion. Gastrocnemius action combined with a weaker soleus can accelerate tibial advancement through its effect at the knee.

Substitution for soleus weakness is difficult as momentum draws the limb forward over the supporting foot throughout stance. If the patient has normal quadriceps strength, no effort is made to accommodate the weak calf. Instead the subject walks with knee flexion. Hence, the need to substitute for excessive dorsiflexion relates to knee control inadequacy (see the knee section). The most common substitution is the reduction of the heel rocker to avoid initiating knee flexion in loading response. As a result, the knee remains extended, and continuation of this posture requires little quadriceps effort during the rest of stance.

Knee recurvatum restrains tibial advancement by aligning the tibia posteriorly. Other measures include the use of shorter steps and a slower walking speed. There is a good correlation between walking velocity and ankle plantar flexor strength.[5]

Ankle Locked at Neutral. Either a pantalar fusion (ankle and subtalar joints) or an orthosis fitted with a locked ankle joint (plantar flexion stop) causes excessive dorsiflexion by obstructing the normal plantar flexion that occurs as the limb is loaded. Right angle rigidity between the tibia and foot increases the heel rocker action (Figure 11.16). The initial early free fall of the foot now carries the tibia with it. As a result, the knee flexes at the same rate as the foot falls, rather than at half of that speed. Quadriceps demand is correspondingly

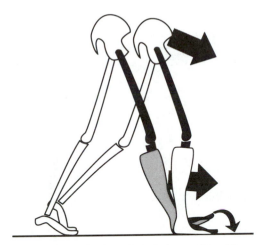

Ankle-Foot Orthosis — Loading Response

Figure 11.16 A rigid ankle-foot orthosis (AFO) or an ankle fusion set at neutral causes excessive ankle dorsiflexion at the loading response. The effect is excessive knee flexion as the tibia follows the tibia.

increased. The ability to tolerate the locked ankle thus depends on quadriceps strength.

A variant of the locked ankle is the solid ankle, cushion heel (SACH) prosthetic foot. While the soft heel is designed to serve as a heel rocker, the transition to forefoot support generates rapid tibial advancement similar to the weak soleus.

Stance Knee Flexion. Persistent knee flexion during the foot flat support period (mid stance) requires ankle dorsiflexion beyond neutral in order to align the body vector over the foot for standing balance. The amount of dorsiflexion required is proportional to the flexed knee posture (Figure 11.17).

Foot Dysfunction

Abnormal function of the foot during walking may be displayed by two situations. These are the pattern of foot contact during the stance phase and malalignment of the foot in swing. The cause may be a reflection of knee and ankle dysfunction or intrinsic foot pathology. Deviations occur in both the sagittal and coronal planes.

Sagittal Plane (Progressional) Deviations

As the body progresses over the supporting foot, the normal sequence of floor contact by the heel, foot flat and forefoot may be altered (Figure 11.18). Each mode of contact can be curtailed, extended or absent. The errors in stance

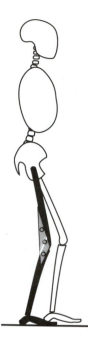

Figure 11.17 Excessive ankle dorsiflexion allows an upright posture in the presence of a fixed knee flexion contracture.

Foot/Floor Contact Patterns

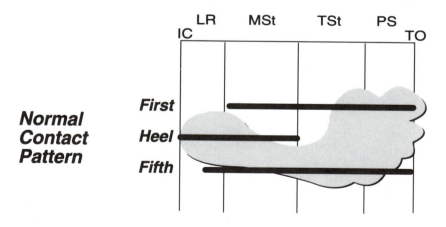

Normal Contact Pattern

Figure 11.18 Normal foot contact pattern.

primarily are identifed by the timing and duration of heel contact. During swing any floor contact is an error. This is commonly called *toe drag.*

Prolonged Heel Only. This is an infrequent finding. The normal loading response pattern of heel-only support is extended into the other stance phases (Figure 11.19). The cause is either a painful forefoot or marked imbalance between the ankle dorsi and plantar flexor muscles. There will be excessive ankle dorsiflexion. The intensity of the pretibial muscles will be increased and that of the plantar flexor muscles reduced.

Premature Heel Off. Loss of heel contact is an abnormal event in initial contact, loading response, and mid stance. The severest disability is the lack of heel contact throughout stance (continuous forefoot support). This is a readily recognized gait deviation (Figure 11.20).

Premature heel rise may develop at any time during the loading response and mid stance phases. Inability to preserve heel contact throughout loading response or mid stance following its initiation at the onset of stance (initial contact) is a subtle deviation. This may be overlooked because heel rise is normal in terminal stance.

Delayed Heel Contact. Although the heel may not be the initial site of floor contact, it often drops to the floor later in loading response or even mid stance.

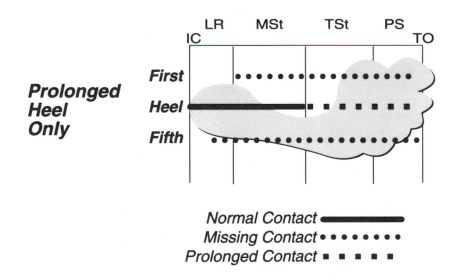

Figure 11.19 Prolonged heel-only floor contact. Foot switches: First (1st Mt), Heel, Fifth (5th Mt). Length of solid line indicates the duration of foot switch activity. Dotted line = lack of normal heel switch activity. Squares = additional switch action.

Foot/Floor Contact Patterns

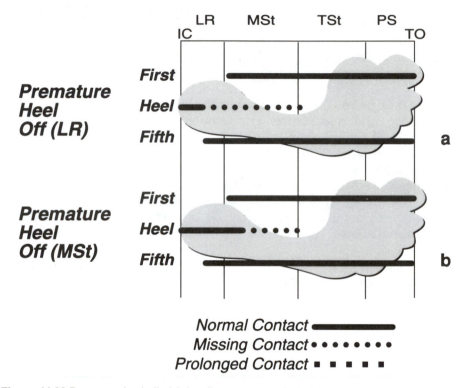

Figure 11.20 Premature heel-off. (a) Loading response deviation. (b) Mid stance deviation. Foot switches: First (1st Mt), Heel, Fifth (5 Mt). Dotted line = lack of normal heel switch activity. Length of solid line indicates the duration of foot switch activity.

This is characteristic of tight tissues (an elastic contracture) yielding as a greater load is applied to the limb later in stance (Figure 11.21).

Prolonged Heel On. Absence of the normal heel rise is an error seen in terminal stance or pre-swing. The lack of heel rise in terminal stance is the more significant deviation, since that is an interval of single limb support (Figure 11.22).

Curtailed Heel Only. While initial contact is made by the heel, the forefoot prematurely drops to the floor. As a result, the heel period of heel-only support is shortened (Figure 11.23). This correspondingly limits the heel rocker action.

Toe Drag. Failure to adequately lift the foot for swing may be a brief or a persistent gait deviation. Toe drag may involve a single phase (initial swing or

Foot/Floor Contact Patterns

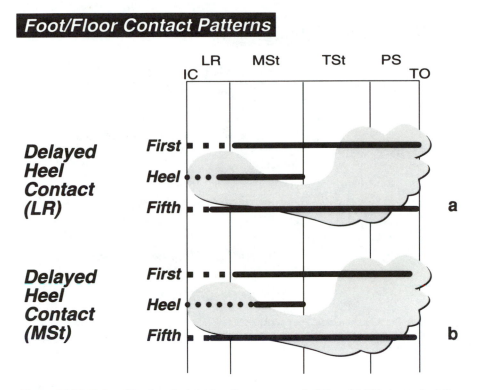

Figure 11.21 Delayed heel contact. (a) Loading response deviation. (b) Mid stance deviation.

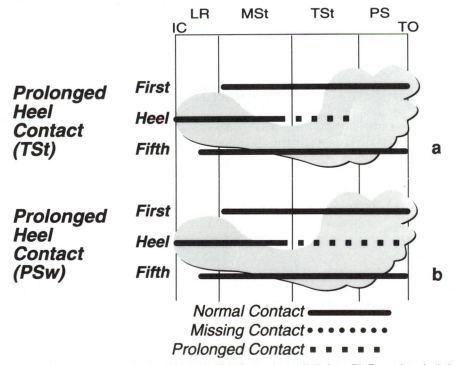

Figure 11.22 Prolonged heel contact. (a) Terminal stance deviation. (b) Pre-swing deviation. Foot switches: First (1st Mt), Heel, Fifth (5th Mt). Dotted line = lack of normal heel switch activity. Squares = additional switch action. Length of solid line indicates the duration of foot switch activity.

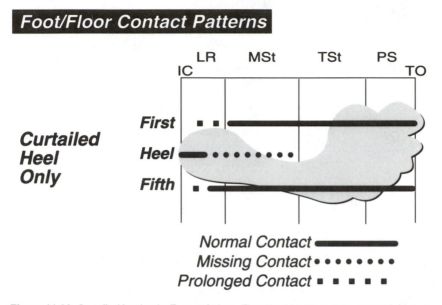

Figure 11.23 Curtailed heel only. Foot switches: First (1st Mt), Heel, Fifth (5th Mt). Dotted line = lack of normal heel switch activity. Squares = additional switch action. Length of solid line indicates the duration of foot switch activity.

mid swing), or it may continue throughout the swing period. Toe drag in initial swing causes tripping. Limb advancement is delayed and this can lead to a fall. Persistent toe drag into mid swing tends to significantly shorten the swing phase.

Causes of Abnormal Floor Contact in the Sagittal Plane

The pattern of foot contact resulting from abnormal mobility or control at the ankle and knee differs with the gait phase in which it occurs.

Initial Contact. Three patterns of initial floor contact are seen. These are called low heel, foot flat and forefoot contact.

Low heel contact occurs with ankle plantar flexion of approximately 15°, while the knee is fully extended. A plantar flexion contracture, tibialis anterior weakness and premature action by the calf muscles are the possible etiologies (Figure 11.2a).

While the heel makes the initial contact, the forefoot is very close to the floor. Hence, the period of heel-only support is abnormally short, leading to an equally brief heel rocker contribution to progression. Visual identification of this gait error requires close observation, because initial contact is by the heel, and the final foot and ankle postures are normal during loading response.

Foot flat contact is caused by a flexed knee rather than excessive ankle plantar flexion. As the forefoot and heel strike the ground simultaneously, the heel-only period is missing. Consequently, there is no heel rocker to induce additional knee flexion. Foot flat contact provides the person with an immediately stable base of support, though the flexed posture requires quadriceps control. The primary pathologies leading to foot flat floor contact are a knee flexion contracture, overactivity of the hamstring muscles and dependence on primitive locomotor control.

Forefoot contact is a form of *premature heel off.* The cause is combined excessive ankle plantar flexion and knee flexion. While 20° deviations at each joint are enough to position the forefoot lower than the heel at the time of initial floor contact, the actual combinations of abnormal posturing vary markedly (Figure 11.2b).

The most common pathology is combined spasticity of the hamstrings and ankle plantar flexors. Persons with extreme ankle equinus (often flaccid paralysis) voluntarily flex their knee to bring the area of floor contact closer to the body vector line for easier weight transfer.

Loading Response. *Curtailed heel-only* time follows two situations: foot slap and delayed heel contact.

Foot slap. Foot slap results from the foot dropping in an uncontrolled fashion following a normal initial heel contact in the presence of a weak tibialis anterior. Low heel contact curtails the time allowed for heel-only support (Figures 11.3 and 11.23).

Delayed heel contact. Having the heel reach the floor after an initial forefoot contact is a common finding in the slower walker with excessive ankle plantar flexion. As the limb is loaded, the plantar flexed ankle creates a rigid reverse rocker that drives the heel to the floor. The nonvigorous walker lacks the momentum to overcome this decelerating situation. As a result, the tibia is driven backward and progression is inhibited.

Premature heel rise. Premature heel rise during loading response generally is a continuation of initial forefoot contact. After a period of heel contact, premature heel rise can begin in loading response when momentum is sufficent to roll the limb onto the forefoot (Figure 11.20a). The cause is either excessive ankle plantar flexion or excessive knee flexion.

Mid Stance.

Premature heel rise. Patients with sufficient walking vigor overcome the loss of tibial advancement from an inadequate ankle rocker by a premature heel rise. Ankle plantar flexion contracture or spastic posturing is the cause (Figure 11.20b).

Excessive knee flexion (inadequate extension) is the second cause of premature heel rise in mid stance. Continued heel contact requires more than normal ankle dorsiflexion. To allow progression of the body, the tibia must advance. Either the ankle provides an increased arc of dorsiflexion or the heel rises.

Premature heel rise also may be voluntary. Deliberate plantar flexion is used to accommodate a short limb. Vaulting by active, excessive ankle plantar flexion raises the body as an assistance in floor clearance by the opposite swinging limb.

Delayed heel contact. The plantar flexion contracture or spasticity that caused an initial heel-off situation yields to body weight in mid stance. The loss of forward momentum may be slight, even imperceptible, in persons with otherwise good walking ability (Figure 11.22).

Terminal Stance and Pre-Swing.

Delayed heel rise (Prolonged heel contact). Advancement of the body mass ahead of the supporting foot normally moves the vector to the forefoot, and the heel rises. Persistent heel contact in terminal stance or pre-swing indicates either plantar flexor muscle weakness or excessive ankle plantar flexion with inhibition of limb advancement in a slow walker.

Delay of heel rise is a more signficant sign of a weak soleus in early terminal stance. The mere trailing posture of the limb will lift the heel once the ankle reaches the end of its passive dorsiflexion range.

Pre-swing is a period of double limb support, and body weight is being rapidly transferred to the forward limb. The reduced demands on the weak soleus may allow the heel to rise as body weight rolls over the forefoot. By the end of stance, knee flexion also will roll the tibia forward enough to lift the heel. Hence, the timing of the delayed heel rise has functional significance.

Knee hyperextension provides a second hinge for body weight progression as the vector moves toward the forefoot. Pre-swing knee flexion is delayed until the foot is completely unloaded, as the backward thrust on the tibia has also locked the knee. This also delays heel-off.

Coronal Plane Deviations

Excessive subtalar inversion and eversion lead to the clinical abnormalities of varus (*excessive inversion*) and valgus (*excessive eversion*). The cause may be either a static deformity or inappropriate muscle action.

Deviations in heel support are only visible by a posterior view of the foot. Forefoot deviations are identified by the floor contact pattern of the metatarsal heads. Particular attention is directed to the first and fifth metatarsals, which represent the outer margins of the forefoot.

Excessive Inversion (Varus). As the insertions of the muscles that can cause excessive inversion vary, either or both forefoot and hindfoot postures can be altered. The deviations of the foot in swing and stance may vary. Varus of the heel is displayed by medial tilt of the calcaneus under the talus. Forefoot varus during stance is characterized by elevation of the first metatarsal head from the floor (Figure 11.24). Arch height also tends to be increased with varus. In addition, the forefoot may be adducted.

Initial contact and loading response. Floor contact by the lateral surface of the heel is normal. Excessive inversion is evident only if there is also involvement of the lateral forefoot. Foot flat contact with inversion involves the heel and fifth metatarsal (H-5) (Figure 11.24a). Equinovarus contact is made by the fifth metatarsal head (Mt 5).

Mid stance. Floor contact is by the heel and fifth metatarsal (H-5), while the ankle continues to provide progression. The conflict between a rigid ankle plantar flexion contracture and the dorsiflexion force of progression tends to accentuate the existing varus. This may result in premature heel-off (Figure 11.20).

Terminal stance and pre-swing. During forefoot support, the natural posterior-lateral obliquity of the metatarsal head axis tends to invert the foot slightly even though all metatarsal heads are contacting the floor (Mt 1-5). Thus, the floor contact of pathological excessive inversion (varus) will not be evident by foot switches unless only the lateral metatarsals are the source of support (Mt 5) (Figure 11.24b).

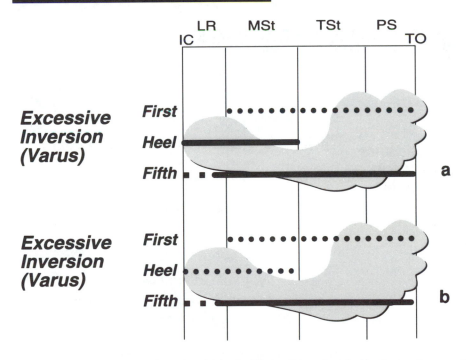

Figure 11.24 Excessive subtalar inversion. (a) Lack of first metatarsal contact and premature onset of fifth metatarsal switch. (b) Contact by fifth metatarsal head only.

Swing. Excessive inversion (varus) of the foot during the three phases of swing tends to be similar. While visually prominent, there is no function significance to swing-phase varus, except at the end of terminal swing. Then, foot posture determines the mode of floor contact.

Excessive Eversion (Valgus). Excessive eversion occurs when forefoot support is only by the medial area. In this circumstance, floor contact is registered by the first but not the fifth metatarsal head (Figure 11.25). Excessive valgus also is indicated by the first metatarsal contacting the ground before the fifth metatarsal. With more extreme collapse, the medial arch also contacts the floor.

Initial contact. Both total heel contact and striking the floor with just the medial undersurface of the heel are abnormal. Generally there is an associated shortened heel-on interval.

Loading response and mid stance. At the end of the heel-only support period, excessive valgus causes foot flat to begin with the first metatarsal head (H-1) (Figure 11.25). This foot posture may continue through mid stance. As body weight advances on to the forefoot, depression of the mid- foot becomes more apparent as subtalar eversion also has unlocked the midtarsal joints, allowing them to sag into dorsiflexion.

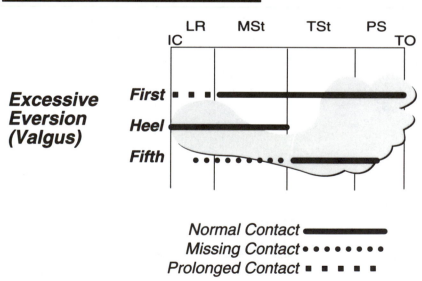

Figure 11.25 Excessive subtalar eversion. Foot switches: First (1st Mt), Heel, Fifth (5th Mt). First, Heel and Fifth = foot switches. Dotted line = lack of normal heel switch activity. Squares = additional switch action. Length of solid line indicates the duration of foot switch activity.

Terminal stance and pre-swing. With heel rise, the medial metatarsal heads become the primary source of support in the valgus foot. Isolated floor contact by just this area, however, is unusual because of the demands of balance. Consequently, support is provided by the whole forefoot (Mt 1-5), but the center of pressure is medial.

During pre-swing, floor contact normally involves just the first metatarsal (Mt 1). Hence, this is not a diagnostic phase for valgus. Generally the great toe also is involved.

Causes of Coronal Plane Deviations

Excessive inversion and eversion generally relate to abnormal muscular control, with static deformities a secondary development. More proximal limb control causing torsion during stance can also have an affect. Because all the muscles controlling the ankle cross the subtalar as they insert on the foot, inversion and eversion abnormalities commonly occur in combination with ankle dysfunction.

In general terms, varus tends to be the dominant foot dysfunction in *spastic*

Table 11.2

Dynamic Varus Muscle Patterns

Muscle	Stance					Swing		
	IC	LR	MS	TS	PSw	ISw	MSw	TSw
ANTERIOR								
Tibialis Anterior				X	X	X		
Toe Extensors	o	o				o	o	o
POSTERIOR								
Soleus	X	X						X
Tibialis Posterior						X	X	X
FHL	X	X				X	X	X
FDL	X	X				X	X	X

Key:　X = phases of inappropriate activity contributing to varus　　PSw = pre-swing
　　　　0 = inactivity contributing to varus　　　　　　　　　　　　ISw = initial swing
　　　　IC = initial contact　　　　　　　　　　　　　　　　　　　MSw = mid swing
　　　　LR = loading response　　　　　　　　　　　　　　　　　TSw = terminal swing
　　　　MS = mid stance　　　　　　　　　　　　　　　　　　　　FHL = flexor hallucis longus
　　　　TS = terminal stance　　　　　　　　　　　　　　　　　　FDL = flexor digitorum longus

patients. Conversely flaccid paralysis tends to lead to valgus.

Causes of Excessive Varus

Dynamic Varus. Five muscles cross the subtalar joint on the medial side. All are aligned to invert the foot (Table 11.2). Four of the muscles (all but the anterior tibialis) also are plantar flexors. Hence, equinovarus is a common pathological finding when these muscles are overly active. Gait deviations generally result from the muscles being active at a time they normally are relaxed. The most common timing errors are premature or prolonged action. Occasionally there is a reversal of phasing (i.e., stance instead of swing or vice versa). Muscles that have significantly different levels of normal activity (e.g., soleus) also introduce gait deviation by an increase in intensity. Intramuscular contracture can have

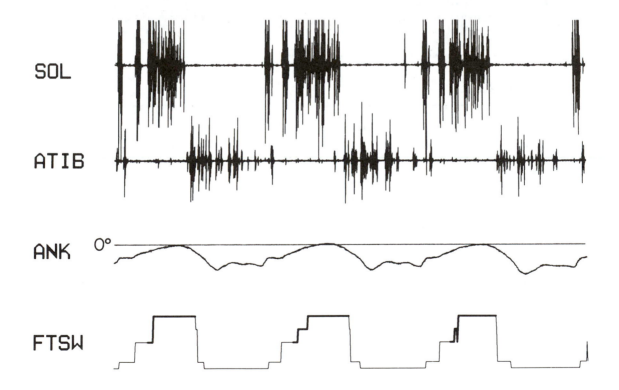

Figure 11.26 Tibialis anterior (ATIB) primitive pattern action. EMG starts at onset of swing and decreases to a nonsignificant intensity in terminal swing. Loading response action is lacking (single weak clonic beat). Soleus (SOL) action begins prematurely with clonic beats at onset of stance. ANK = ankle electrogoniometer. 0° = neutral. Stance dorsiflexion just to zero and plantar flexion in swing indicate a contracture that the moderately active ATIB could not oppose. FTSW = Foot switch of reference limb. Stance pattern indicates initial contact with Mt5, progression to H-5, H-5-1, and prolonged 5-1 (heel-off). Baseline is swing interval.

the same effect as excessive or ill-timed activity. A third cause of varus is the inactivity of a normal synergist. The primary cause of equinovarus is soleus overactivity or contracture.

Tibialis anterior and toe extensors. Swing varus with good ankle dorsiflexion is evidence of strong tibialis anterior action without toe extensors participation. This is the common deviation in spastic patients. Inversion of the forefoot at initial contact may either persist into the loading phase or cease. In *spastic* patients, the tibialis anterior (TA) action in swing is often part of the flexor pattern, but not the toe extensors. This causes swing phase foot inversion (varus). When the patient's limb control is dominated by the primitive locomotor patterns, the TA ceases to contract with the onset of the extensor pattern in stance (Figure 11.26). As a result, the varus in swing may abruptly reverse to neutral or even valgus. The gait pattern in stance will be determined by the actions of the other subtalar musculature.

Prolonged varus into mid and terminal stance may include stance action of

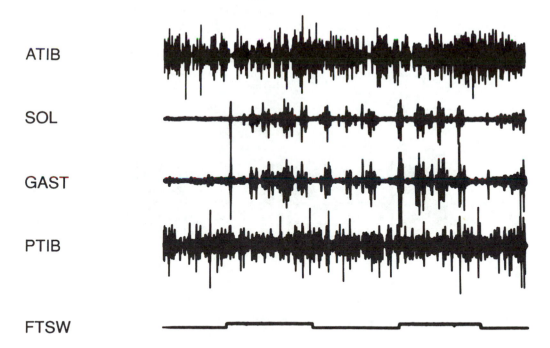

Figure 11.27 Tibialis anterior (ATIB) action prolonged in stance. EMG shows continuous activity. Soleus (SOL) and gastrocnemius (GAST) action is clonic and continues into swing. Tibialis posterior (PTIB) also continuous. Hence, there are three dynamic sources of varus. Foot switch (FTSW = Mt5) shows an equinovarus foot support pattern.

the tibialis anterior as well as the other inversion forces (Figure 11.27). Most commonly, the patient has an equinovarus. This accounts for 75% of the pathological varus in cerebral palsy[7] and probably a much higher percentage in stroke patients.[6]

Swing varus with good ankle dorsiflexion is evidence of strong tibialis anterior action without toe extensors participation. This is the common deviation in spastic patients.

Equinovarus in swing has three causes. As the natural ankle alignment is slightly oblique, passive plantar flexion (drop foot) includes a small amount of varus. Weak unassisted tibialis anterior action is capable of inverting the foot but lacks the strength to accomplish full dorsiflexion. Generally there also is some degree of posteriormedial contracture. Out-of-phase action by a posterior inverter, such as the posterior tibialis or a spastic soleus, is a dynamic cause of swing phase equinovarus.

Tibialis posterior. While normal gait involves the tibialis posterior, the activity of this muscle in patients is very inconsistent. The tibialis posterior also markedly varies its intensity as well as timing. Hence, one cannot assume a patient's varus is related to excessive or premature (Figure 11.28) tibialis posterior action. It may be totally quiescent (Figure 11.29). When active, however, it is a significant source of subtalar varus, as it has the longest leverage among the five inverting muscles (Figure 4.22). Phase reversal to swing action occurs in about 11% of cerebral palsy patients (Figure 11.30).[2]

Soleus. While primarily positioned for plantar flexion, the soleus also has good inversion leverage at the subtalar joint. This becomes significant because

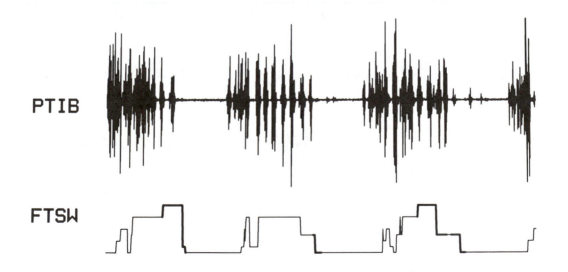

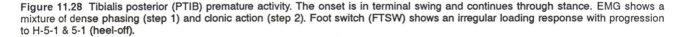

Figure 11.28 Tibialis posterior (PTIB) premature activity. The onset is in terminal swing and continues through stance. EMG shows a mixture of dense phasing (step 1) and clonic action (step 2). Foot switch (FTSW) shows an irregular loading response with progression to H-5-1 & 5-1 (heel-off).

Varus

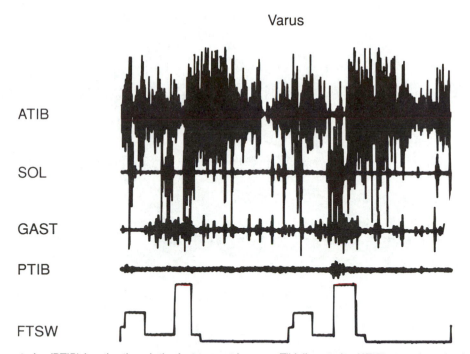

Figure 11.29 Tibialis posterior (PTIB) inactive though the foot support is varus. Tibialis anterior (ATIB) strongly active in stance as well as swing. Soleus (SOL) action is clonic and intermittent. Gastrocnemius (GAST) action is of low intensity with intermittent low spikes in swing. Foot switch (FTSW) pattern displays an unstable varus foot support pattern: H-5, Mt5 and 5- 1.

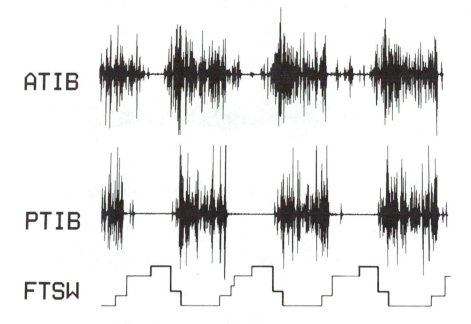

Figure 11.30 Tibialis posterior (PTIB) out of phase. EMG shows the onset in pre-swing, action through swing and cessation in early loading response. This timing is very similar to the anterior tibialis (ATIB). Foot switches (FTSW) display a slightly inconsistent normal sequence pattern (H, H-5-1, 5-1).

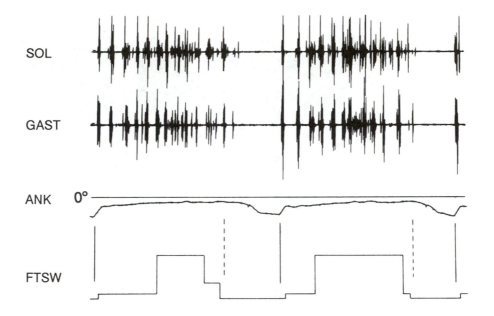

Figure 11.31 Soleus (SOL) and gastrocnemius (GAST) premature action. A clonic pattern of EMG begins with initial contact and persists through stance. Ankle motion (ANK) is continual equinus (below 0°). Foot switch (FTSW) indicates varus (Mt5 initial contact) progressing to equinus (prolonged Mt5-1).

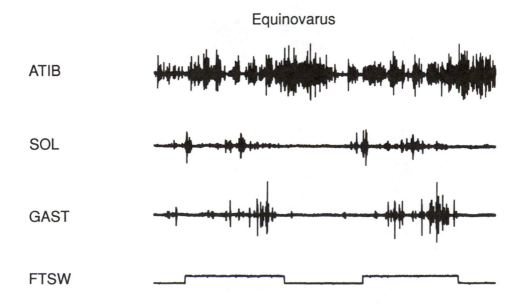

Figure 11.32 Soleus (SOL) activity reduced by contracture. EMG sparse and of low intensity, also gastrocnemius (GAST). Tibialis virtually continuously active. This would cause varus but no equinus. Foot switch (FTSW) shows Mt5 contact only.

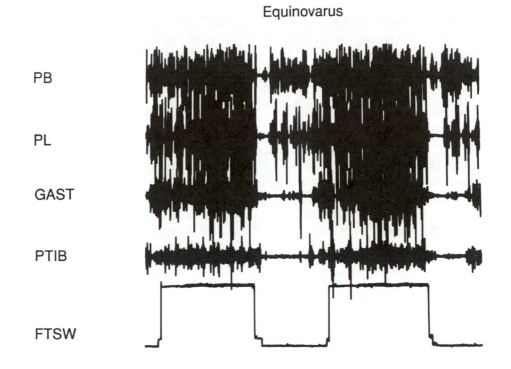

Figure 11.33 Peroneus longus (PL) and peroneus brevis (PB) with strong activity in a varus foot. (Provides lateral stability for weight bearing.) Gastrocnemius (GAST) and tibialis posterior (PTIB) also active through stance. Foot switch (FTSW) shows forefoot support (5-1) with Mt5 at start and end of stance.

of the muscle's size (five times the size of the tibialis posterior). Two abnormalities in soleus action lead to its contribution to inversion. Premature onset in terminal swing as part of the primitive extensor synergy prepositions the foot into varus and then maintains this undesirable posture throughout stance (Figure 11.31). The primitive control pattern also activates the soleus at a higher intensity during the loading response and mid stance than is normally needed before the terminal stance heel rise. As this is greater than the demand presented by the body vector, equinovarus results. Spasticity commonly increases the intensity of the soleus response. Conversely, a plantar flexion contracture can reduce the level of soleus action by diverting the stretch force (Figure 11.32).

Flexor hallucis longus and flexor digitorum. These commonly are included in the primitive extensor pattern and are thus prematurely activated in terminal swing. In addition, spasticity is frequently present in these muscles. As was described for the soleus, this leads to increased intensity of muscle action as well as premature timing. Both factors contribute to varus. Such overactivity is implied by the toe clawing seen in stance.

Peroneus longus and peroneus brevis. Patients who are able to walk with either varus or equinovarus display strong peroneal action by EMG testing. Generally, both peroneals are active, but either may dominate. Gastrocnemius activity also may be strong in equinovarus. Thus, insufficient evertor muscle action is not a component of varus gait (Figure 11.33).

Conversely, when inadequate peroneal muscle action is a cause of the varus, the foot is unstable and incapable of accepting body weight. The foot and ankle twist severely, and generally there is pain as the lateral tissues are strained.

Dynamic Valgus. Excessive eversion (valgus) during stance most commonly results from total weakness of the inverters, whether the primary pathology is flaccid or spastic paralysis, rather than excessive peroneal action (Figure 11.34). With soleus weakness there also is prolonged heel contact. Whether the arch collapses or persists depends on its structural integrity (ligamentous laxity).

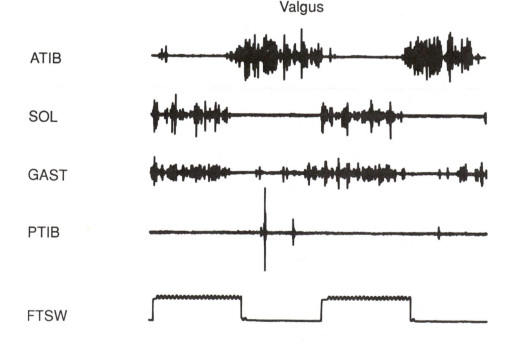

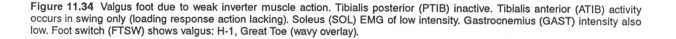

Figure 11.34 Valgus foot due to weak inverter muscle action. Tibialis posterior (PTIB) inactive. Tibialis anterior (ATIB) activity occurs in swing only (loading response action lacking). Soleus (SOL) EMG of low intensity. Gastrocnemius (GAST) intensity also low. Foot switch (FTSW) shows valgus: H-1, Great Toe (wavy overlay).

Valgus

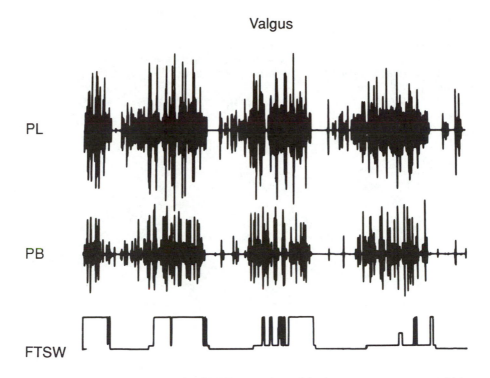

Figure 11.35 Peroneus longus (PL) and peroneus brevis (PB) excessive activity. Intense premature onset, high amplitude and dense EMG. Foot switch (FTSW) shows valgus: H-1.

Very infrequently, the cause of stance phase valgus is premature, strong peroneal muscle action accentuating the elevation of the lateral foot (Figure 11.35). With weakness of the other plantar flexors, occasionally peroneal muscle action can lead to a calcaneovalgus ankle/foot posture.

Eversion in swing always is abnormal, as the natural imbalance in the dorsiflexor muscles tends toward varus. Patients disabled by flaccid and spastic paralysis present different everting mechanisms. Flaccid, incomplete dorsiflexor paralysis, such as occurs in poliomyelitis, may create eversion in swing.

Strong toe extensor and peroneus tertius muscles can suspend the lateral side of the foot, while a weak or absent tibialis anterior muscle allows the medial side to drop. Floor clearance is less complete, and the foot is everted. This posture persists through all three gait phases.

References

1. Arsenault AB, Winter DA, Marteniuk RG: Bilateralism of EMG profiles in human locomotion. *American Journal of Physical Medicine* 65(1):1-16, 1986.
2. Barto PS, Supinski RS, Skinner SR: Dynamic EMG findings in varus hindfoot deformity and spastic cerebral palsy. *Dev Med Child Neurol* 26(1):88-93, 1984.
3. Eyring EJ, Murray WR: The effect of joint position on the pressure of intra-articular

effusion. *J Bone Joint Surg* 46A(6):1235-1241, 1964.
4. Kinney CL, Jaweed MM, Herbison GJ, Ditunno JF: Overwork effect on partially denervated rat soleus muscle. *Arch Phys Med Rehabil* 67:286-289, 1986.
5. Perry J, Mulroy SJ, Renwick S: The relationship between lower extremity strength and stride characteristics in patients with post-polio syndrome. *Arch Phys Med Rehabil* 71:1990.
6. Perry J, Waters RL, Perrin T: Electromyographic analysis of equinovarus following stroke. *Clin Orthop* 131:47-53, 1978.
7. Wills CA, Hoffer MM, Perry J: A comparison of foot- switch and EMG analysis of varus deformities of the feet of children with cerebral palsy. *Dev Med Child Neurol* 30:227-231, 1988.

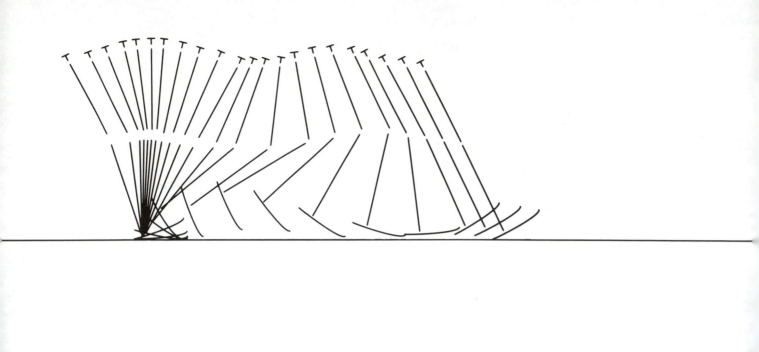

Chapter 12

Knee
Abnormal Gait

The most common types of knee dysfunction occur in the sagittal plane. Inappropriate arcs of motion result in excessive or inadequate flexion or extension. Less frequent are the deviations in the coronal plane (excessive valgus or varus). Excessive transverse plane rotation within the knee is reported, but the findings vary with the method of measurement. This results in a major inconsistency between laboratories, though each facility has confidence in its technic.[1]

Sagittal Plane Deviations

To accommodate clinical custom and reinforce the functional significance of both increased and reduced ranges of knee flexion or extension, the gait errors at the knee have been identified by four descriptors. *Inadequate flexion* defines the failure to accomplish the normal amount of flexion, with the resulting being limited or absent motion. *Excessive flexion* is more than the normal range. *Inadequate extension* relates to persistent flexion at a time the knee normally extends. *Excessive extension* indicates motion beyond neutral. The timing of these gait deviations relates to the normal incidence of the basic motions (Figure 12.1, Table 12.1).

Inadequate Flexion

In the four gait phases where flexion is a normal event, the loss of this motion carries functional significance. These phases are loading response, pre-swing, initial swing and mid swing.

The pathologies contributing to a lack of flexion in stance and swing differ markedly. Each situation also leads to very different substitutions.

Loading Response. During this weight accepting phase, limited knee flexion is evidence of intrinsic pathology. Absent knee flexion generally is a substitutive action.

Inadequate knee flexion reduces the limbs shock absorption quality. Failure to flex the knee more than 5 or 10 presents a relatively rigid limb. Loading impact transfers body weight directly from the femur to the tibia without muscular cushioning (Figure 12.2). If the patient is a slow walker, peak loading will not exceed body weight, because no significant acceleration will be added. Patients capable of a rapid gait may experience damaging microtrauma.

Full knee extension has the advantage of being the most stable weight-bearing position as the body vector is anterior to (or overlying) the joint axis. Consequently, absent knee flexion in the loading period is a desirable gait

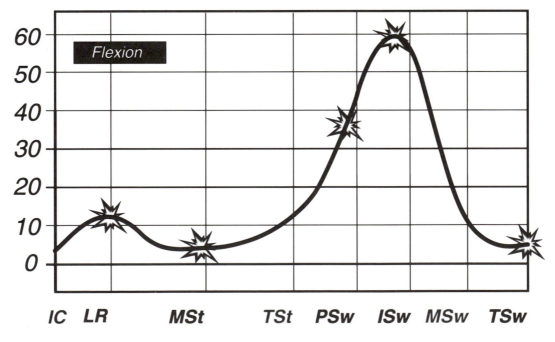

Figure 12.1 Gait phases where abnormal knee function is most significant.

Table 12.1

Phasing of the Gait Deviations at the Knee

	LR	MS	TS	PSw	ISw	MSw	TSw
Inadequate Flexion	X			X	X	X	
Excessive Extension							
Extensor Thrust		X					
Hyperextension		X	X	X			
Excessive Flexion	X			X	X	X	
Inadequate Extension		X	X				X
Coronal Gait Deviations							
Varus	X	X	X				
Valgus	X	X	X				

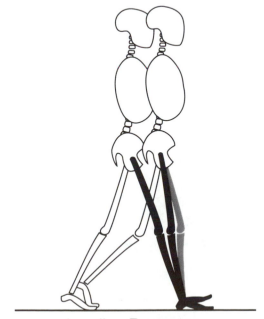

Loading Response

Figure 12.2 Inadequate knee flexion in loading response. Normal shock-absorbing flexion is lost.

deviation when the quadriceps muscle is too weak to repeatedly restrain a flexing knee.

Pre-Swing. Failure to adequately flex the knee in pre-swing makes toe-off more difficult. The transition between stance and swing is lost (Figure 12.3). A greater hip flexor or specific knee flexion effort will be required to lift the foot at the onset of initial swing.

There are no available substitutions until forward swing of the limb is initiated, because pre-swing still is a period of weight bearing.

Initial Swing. The lack of adequate knee flexion in initial swing causes toe drag with a corresponding inability to advance the limb (Figure 12.4). This difficulty results from the trailing posture tilting the foot downward. Without knee flexion the functional length of the limb between the hip and the toe (that area of the foot closest to the floor) is longer than that of the stance limb because its point of floor contact is the heel. After the toe has moved forward of the other limb, there is less need for knee flexion.

A more subtle display of inadequate knee flexion in initial swing is delay of peak knee flexion until mid swing. Toe drag is shorter. Insufficient pre-swing action is the usual cause. Lack of hip flexion is the other cause.

Mid Swing. Inadequate knee flexion in mid swing does not occur independently. It reflects either a lack of hip flexion or a continuation of the pathology in initial swing.

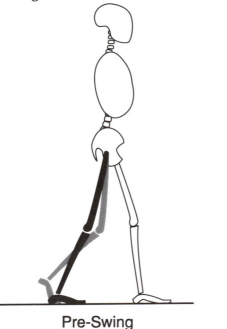

Pre-Swing

Figure 12.3 Inadequate knee flexion in pre-swing. Knee flexion is absent, ankle excessively dorsiflexed and heel contact prolonged.

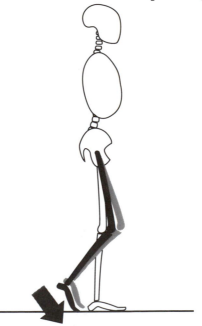

Initial Swing

Figure 12.4 Inadequate knee flexion in initial swing. Toe drag occurs as the leg and foot are not lifted sufficiently.

Excessive Extension

The generic term *excessive extension* has been replaced with two clinical phrases: extensor thrust and hyperextension. These two actions differ both in their arc of knee motion and in the vigor of the extensor action.

Extensor thrust is a term chosen to define the effect of an excessive extensor force when the knee lacks a hyperextension range. It is a dynamic, rapid action that causes the knee to move toward a posterior angle, but the range is not available (Figure 12.5).

Hyperextension occurs when the knee has the mobility to angulate backward (recurvatum). It may be slow and passive or actively abrupt. The onset of hyperextension can occur in any of the weight-bearing phases (Figure 12.6).

An extensor thrust often is the first reaction to limb loading. Hyperextension is a later development either as a reaction to the added stimulus of single limb support or advancement of the body (and thigh) over a stationary tibia. It can develop in either mid stance or terminal stance, and this posture, then, is continued into pre-swing. Timing varies with the severity of the contributing pathology.

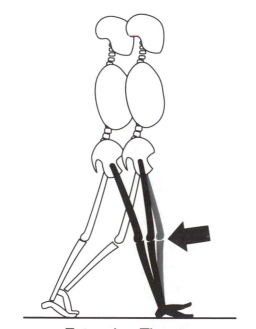

Extension Thrust

Figure 12.5 Extensor thrust inhibits knee flexion. It is accompanied by premature ankle plantar flexion and decreased hip flexion.

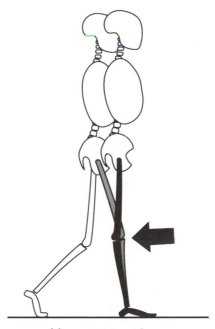

Hyperextension

Figure 12.6 Knee hyperextension. Dynamic retraction of the tibia (by the soleus) or retraction of the femur (by the gluteus maximus) pulls the knee into hyperextension if that range is available.

Causes of Inadequate Knee Flexion and Excessive Extension

Because the normal pattern of knee motion in stance flows from flexion to extension, the same pathology can influence both motions (Table 12.2). In stance, pathology that causes inadequate flexion (loading response or pre-swing) also commonly leads into excessive extension (mid or terminal stance). Swing phase dysfunctions more often have separate causes. An additional complexity is the sensitivity of knee function to the control and mobility at the ankle and hip.

Quadriceps Weakness

The function of the quadriceps is to support a flexed knee. When there is insufficient quadriceps strength to meet this demand a variety of substitutions are used to preserve weight-bearing stability. This pattern of action is the most common cause of absent loading response knee flexion and excessive extension during the other stance phases in persons with normal motor control (polio, femoral nerve injury, secondary disuse weakness). The deliberate actions used to prepare the limb for safe stance begin in terminal swing and continue through pre-swing.

Terminal Swing. Pass/retract action at the hip will extend the knee in the absence of a quadriceps. Quick hip flexion advances both femur and tibia. Then, rapid hip extension by the gluteus maximus retracts the femur while inertia holds the tibia. Generally, a neutral knee position is attained. More vigorous action by the gluteus maximus and an overly mobile joint may result in knee hyperextension.

Loading Response. Knee flexion is avoided as a deliberate action to protect a weak quadriceps (grade 4 to 3+) from the strain of decelerating a rapidly flexing knee. Patients use this substitution to preserve a good walking speed and endurance. The same mechanics are used to preserve weight-bearing stability when the quadriceps is incapable of controlling a flexing knee (grades 0-3).

Two actions prevent loading response knee flexion (Figure 12.7). Hip extension by the gluteus maximus (and adductor magnus) retracts the thigh. Premature ankle plantar flexion, initiated by the soleus, blocks tibial advancement so initial contact by the heel does not stimulate the normal rocker action.

Mid Stance and Terminal Stance. Hyperextension is used when an adequate passive range is available. This provides greater stability for an, otherwise, uncontrollable knee during weight bearing. The anterior body weight vector serves as a knee extensor force (Figure 12.8). Subtle balance between soleus muscle action, and the anterior vector maintains knee hyperextension throughout mid and terminal stance, while allowing the ankle to gradually dorsiflex at a slower than normal rate. There also is prolonged heel contact through terminal stance for optimum foot support.

Table 12.2

Causes of Knee Gait Deviations

Stance

	Inadequate Flexion	Excessive Extensor Thrust	Extension Hyper-Extension	Excessive Flexion	Inadequate Extension
Quadriceps Weakness	X	X	X		
Ankle PF Contracture	X	X	X		
Spasticity	X	X	X		
Hamstring Spasticity				X	X
Knee Flexion Contracture				X	X
Ankle PF Weakness					X

Swing

	Inadequate Flexion	Excessive Flexion	Inadequate Extension	Excessive Extension
Quadriceps Spasticity	X			
Hip Flexion Weakness	X			
Ankle DF Weakness		X		
Spasticity		X		
Hamstring Contracture			X	
Spasticity Primitive Pattern			X	
Quadriceps Weakness				X

Coronal Knee Gait Deviations

	Varus (Stance)	Valgus (Stance)
Osteoarthritis	X	
Rheumatoid Arthritis		X
Congenital	X	X
Trauma	X	X

The same actions are used to preserve knee extensor stability when there is no hyperextension range. These include prolonged gluteus maximus and soleus action and slight forward trunk lean to create an anterior vector.

Both substitutions can lead to long-term penalties. Disabling fatigue of the stabilizing muscles may develop. Also, chronic strain can cause degeneration of the ligaments supporting the hyperextended knee.

Pre-swing. Failure to flex the knee at the end of stance relates to combined muscle weakness at the knee and ankle. Quadriceps weakness necessitates the patient keeping the knee extended until it is fully unloaded by the transfer of body weight to the other limb. Activity of the weak quadriceps or the substitution musculature is continued into pre-swing. The knee is maintained in full extension (or hyperextension) until initial swing begins. This obstructs the passive freedom needed for knee flexion. Occasionally a momentary toe drag results. When hyperextension is the source of knee stability, the possible delay in toe clearance becomes greater.

Pain

Rapid motion of a knee with intrinsic joint pathology increases tissue tension and, therefore, pain. This leads to limited knee flexion in the three phases: loading response, pre-swing and initial swing.

Loading Response. Knee flexion is avoided by the same mechanisms used for quadriceps weakness. The purpose is to escape the shear force that accompanies joint motion. A second objective is to reduce the compressive force from a contracting quadriceps. Articular surface damage from arthritis or gross instability or scarring following multi-ligamentous injury are the common causes.

Pre-swing. Limitation of knee flexion also is a mechanism to escape the associated shear forces. This action is less complete, as weight bearing is rapidly reduced.

Initial Swing. Failure to move the knee rapidly results in an inadequate arc of flexion during walking. There may be sufficient passive range by clinical examination. The effect is a stiff-legged gait that may carry into mid swing.

Quadriceps Spasticity

Excessive muscular action is stimulated by a stretch reaction to rapid passive knee flexion. Loading response and initial swing are the sensitive phases of gait.

Loading Response. Knee flexion through the heel rocker action induces a rapid stretch of the quadriceps. An excessive response by the vasti inhibits the full flexion range. Premature knee extension results (Figure 12.9).

Throughout the rest of stance, continuation of a primitive extensor pattern

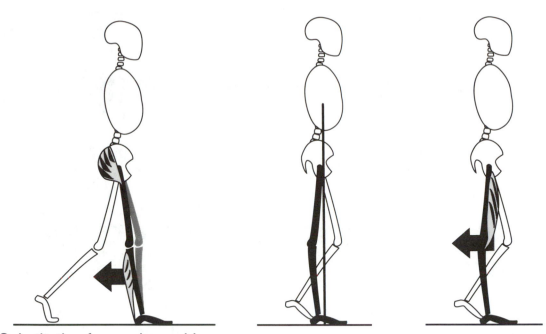

Substitution for weak quadriceps

Figure 12.7 Avoidance of loading response knee flexion by dynamic retraction of the tibia (by the soleus) and retraction of the femur (by the gluteus maximus).

Figure 12.8 Knee hyperextension substitution for a weak quadriceps. Vector is anterior to knee, providing an extensor torque.

Figure 12.9 Quadriceps overactivity (Vasti) can inhibit loading response knee flexion and create hyperextension.

accentuates the knee's position. A false impression of hyperextension may be created by a forward lean of the trunk, proximally combined with ankle plantar flexion distally, when the knee joint actually lacks the backward range. Sustained quadriceps action into pre-swing obstructs the passive freedom needed for knee flexion.

Initial Swing. Knee flexion can be inhibited by several patterns of quadriceps spasticity. All or part of this muscle group may be involved. The patterns of muscle action can not be differentiated by motion analysis or palpation. Dynamic EMG is required.

Rectus femoris activity obstructs initial swing knee flexion when the muscle's intensity is excessive and the action is prolonged (Figure 12.10). An underlying cause may be a gait velocity too slow to require rectus femoris restraint at the knee. The stimulus for inappropriate rectus femoris action is its primitive role as a hip flexor. Surgical release or transfer can significantly improve knee flexion.

Persistent vastus intermedius activity into (or through) swing is a second pattern of obstructive quadriceps action. It is not uncommon to see both rectus femoris (RF) and vastus intermedius (VI) action. The VI can be sacrificed by surgical release when there is appropriate stance phase action by the other vasti (Figure 12.11).

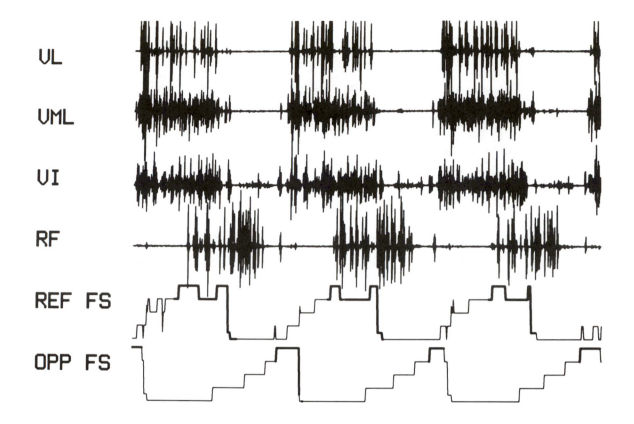

VL

VML

VI

RF

REF FS

OPP FS

Figure 12.10 Rectus femoris (RF) inhibition of knee flexion. RF onset is premature, prolonged and the intensity is excessive. Vasti (VL, VML VI) prolonged stance action inhibits pre-swing knee flexion. Reference limb foot switches (REF FS) shows inconsistent progression with heel off (5-1) and foot flat (H-5-1) alternating. The opposite foot switch pattern (OPP FS) is normal. Overlap of OPP FS with end of REF FS identifies the pre-swing phase.

The third pattern of quadriceps obstruction to initial swing knee flexion is prolonged action of all the vasti into a major portion of swing. If all or most of the vasti continued their activity until toe-off, the effectiveness of an RF release or transfer is reduced because pre-swing knee flexion is inhibited (Figure 12.12). Prolongation of the vasti through initial swing presents an uncorrectable situation, as the the vastus lateralis (VL), vastus medialis longus (VML) vastus medialis oblique (VMO) are not expendable.

Excessive Ankle Plantar Flexion

This is the primary cause of knee hyperextension. It can initiate the problem any time within stance, depending on the severity and etiology of the patient's plantar flexion (Figure 12.13).

Loading Response. Knee flexion can be inhibited from the moment of initial contact by two mechanisms. The heel rocker is reduced, and advancement of

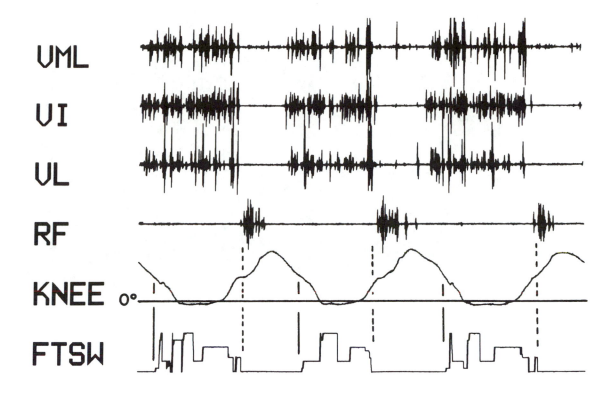

Figure 12.11 Rectus femoris (RF) delay of initial swing knee flexion. RF action is overly intense and prolonged.Vasti (VML, VL, VI) also prolonged. Knee motion (KNEE) shows premature stance knee extension and hyperextension. Initial swing flexion partially inhibited. Peak swing flexion follows relaxation of RF. Foot switches (FTSW) indicate an unstable stance.

the tibia is inhibited. There are three pathological situations that commonly produce the reduced knee flexion: deliberate tibial control, a planter flexion contracture or soleus muscle spasticity (Figures 12.13a and 12.13b).

Mid Stance and Terminal Stance. Onset of knee hyperextension relates to less severe forms of ankle plantar flexion contracture or spasticity. The excessive knee posture develops as the femur attempts to advance beyond the range of tibial motion (Figure 12.13c). An ankle with dorsiflexion to neutral will not cause hyperextension until the last half of mid stance. In terminal stance, excessive ankle plantar flexion may also lead to a late heel rise, creating a further postural strain at the knee due to the forward alignment of body weight. This may persist through pre-swing until the limb is unloaded.

Hip Flexor Weakness

Knee flexion is lost in initial swing when inadequate hip flexion deprives the patient of the momentum normally used to flex the knee. This problem is accentuated by inadequate pre-swing function. The range still is incomplete and the initiation delayed (Figure 12.14). Slow walkers also need increased hip

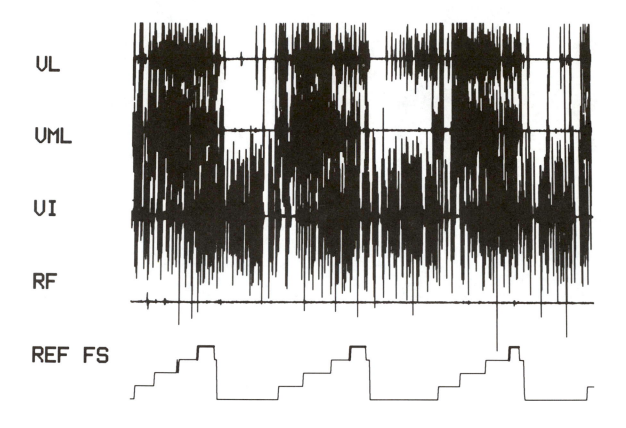

Figure 12.12 Quadriceps inhibition of knee flexion by overactivity of the vasti. (a) Vastus lateralis (VL) and vastus medialis longus (VML) show intense, prolonged action through stance. Vastus intermedius (VI) has continuous activity. Rectus femoris (RF) is inactive. Foot switches of reference limb (REF FS) show a normal sequence with slight irregularity in the first two steps.

flexor effort to bend the knee. They rely on femoral advancement and tibial inertia for knee flexion. With weak hip flexors, the thigh stays vertical and the knee relatively extended. Patients with a strong short head of the biceps substitute moderately well.

Extension Contractures

The knee flexion needed for swing may be lost through two mechanisms. There may be insufficient passive range from capsular scarring or quadriceps contracture (i.e., less than 60°). More commonly, the passive range obtained by clinical examination is sufficient, but the tissues cannot yield rapidly enough to meet the motion demands of initial swing. The functional requirement of 60° knee flexion within 0.2 seconds (pre-swing and initial swing combined) has exceeded the plasticity of scar tissue. Consequently a knee that bends adequately under slow passive teasing still may display severe limitations during walking.

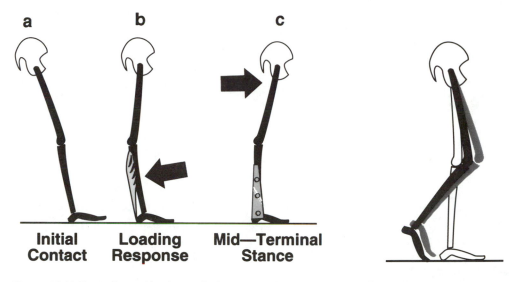

a   **b**   **c**

Initial Contact   **Loading Response**   **Mid—Terminal Stance**

Figure 12.13 Excessive ankle plantar flexion causes knee hyperextension by inhibiting tibial advancement. (a) Initial contact ankle PF reduces heel rocker. (b) Premature soleus muscle action retracts tibia. (c) Ankle PF contracture restrains tibia. Knee hyperextended as body momentum (arrow) advances femur.

Figure 12.14 Hip flexor weakness causes inadequate knee flexion in initial swing (black limb). Thigh advancement is inadequate. (Gray limb indicates normal function.)

Excessive Knee Flexion

Excessive flexion is seen in two phases of gait: loading response and mid swing. Each represents very different pathology.

Loading Response. Excessive knee flexion during early stance relates to a knee posture greater than 25 (Figure 12.15). Most of this flexion arc develops in loading response, but a few more degrees of knee flexion actually follow the added thrust of single limb support at the onset of mid stance. This timing presents slight confusion in the phasic interpretation of knee dysfunction. To differentiate the major purpose of mid stance (progressive knee extension), the term *excessive flexion* has been identified with the loading response phase.

Mid Swing. Excessive knee flexion at this time generally represents the secondary effect of increased hip flexion and gravity drawing the tibia to a vertical posture (Figure 12.16). It is not a clinical concern.

Inadequate Extension

Inability to fully extend the knee is a common gait error that may occur in either stance or swing. The three gait phases where inadequate extension may be a problem are mid stance, terminal stance and terminal swing.

Mid Stance and Terminal Stance. During mid stance, the knee fails to move toward extension. In terminal stance the knee does not extend within 10° of neutral (Figure 12.17). Generally, these gait errors represent a continuation of the excessive flexion displayed in loading response.

Terminal Swing. Recovery of knee extension following peak flexion earlier in swing is incomplete. Consequently, the limb is not fully prepared for stance (Figure 12.18).

Causes of Excessive Flexion and Inadequate Extension

There are four major causes of excessive knee flexion or inadequate knee extension. A flexion contracture or inappropriate hamstring muscle activity influences knee motion in both swing and stance. Soleus (and gastrocnemius) weakness only disrupts stance. Quadriceps weakness can reduce knee extension in terminal swing.

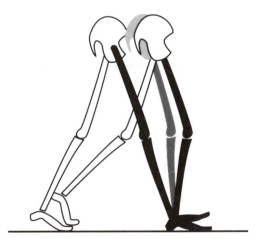

Excessive Knee Flexion—Loading Response

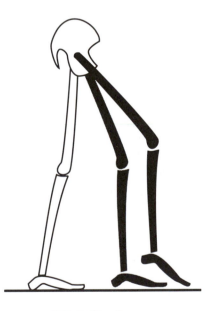

Mid Swing

Figure 12.15 Excessive knee flexion in loading response (black limb). The ankle is excessively dorsiflexed. Dark gray limb = initial contact. Light gray limb = normal loading response motion.

Figure 12.16 Excessive knee flexion in mid swing to compensate for excessive ankle plantar flexion. Without compensation the toe drags. Increased hip flexion to lift a plantar flexed foot for clearance also increases knee flexion.

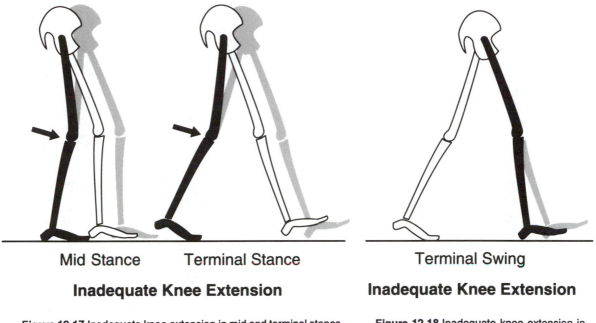

Mid Stance	Terminal Stance		Terminal Swing

Inadequate Knee Extension   **Inadequate Knee Extension**

Figure 12.17 Inadequate knee extension in mid and terminal stance. Both phases also show excessive ankle dorsiflexion. Gray images show loss of body advancement by the pathologically restrained thigh position (black limb).

Figure 12.18 Inadequate knee extension in terminal swing (black limb). Loss of terminal reach displayed by gray limb.

Inappropriate Hamstring Activity

Patients with upper motor neuron lesions commonly display overactivity of the hamstrings. This generally is attributed to spasticity. Recent experience with selective dorsal rhizotomy, which surgically divides the sensory fibers that stimulate spasticity, does not eliminate the hamstring overactivity.[2] Thus, it is logical to assume that inappropriate hamstring activity also is a common part of the primitive mass extensor muscle synergy in diplegic cerebral palsy. A second functional error in hamstring timing is voluntary use of these muscles to supplement or replace gluteus maximus insufficiency. Excessive hamstring activity may be premature or prolonged.

Hamstring Spasticity. Primitive pattern activation of these muscles generally begins in early mid swing and continues through mid stance or longer. Seldom are the hamstrings active in initial swing (Figure 12.19). This contrasts markedly with the precision of normal function (Figure 12.20).

Mid Swing and Terminal Swing. Stretch of spastic hamstrings by flexor momentum results in premature onset of muscle action and greater intensity than is displayed by normal function. The passive knee extension that normally occurs in mid swing is inhibited. Further stretch occurs as the quadriceps begin

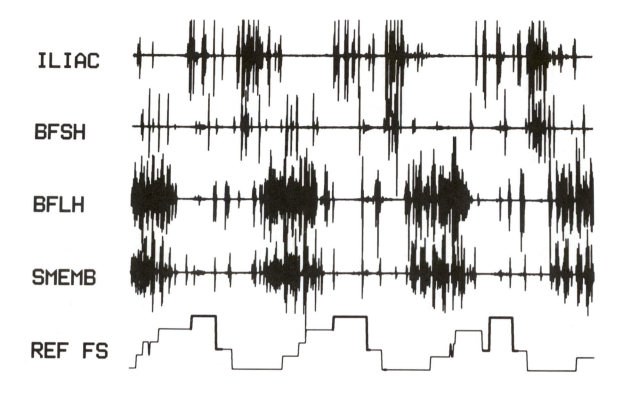

Figure 12.19a Hamstring spasticity causing inadequate knee extension in stance. Biceps femoris long head (BFLH) shows sustained high intensity action through mid stance. Brief clonic response to pre-swing stretch. Semimembranosis (SMEMB) pattern similar. Biceps femoris short head (BFSH) dominant activity is in initial swing. Iliacus (ILIAC) dominant action is initial swing, semi-clonic activity in terminal stance suggests a spastic response to stretch. Footswitches (REF FS) show an inconsistent, normal sequence.

active knee extension in terminal swing. Failure of the knee to extend implies that the hamstrings have a mechanical advantage over the quadriceps.

Loading Response. Knee flexion is increased by the effect of floor contact being added to the continuing hamstring pull. Weight-bearing stability is preserved by strong quadriceps action to support the flexed knee, with further stimulus of the primitive extensor pattern.

Mid Stance and Terminal Stance. knee flexion action during these phases may represent continued participation of the hamstrings in the primitive extensor pattern or a response to forward trunk lean. The patient's forward posture to accommodate inadequate ankle dorsiflexion increases the need for hip extensor support. While out of the normal timing, this would be appropriate hamstring response to a functional demand (Figure 12.20).

Selective substitution of the hamstrings for weakness of the gluteus maximus (and adductor magnus) leads to a mild loss of knee extension in stance because of the muscles' insertion on the tibia. From loading response through terminal stance, the knee remains flexed approximately 15° if forward lean of the trunk

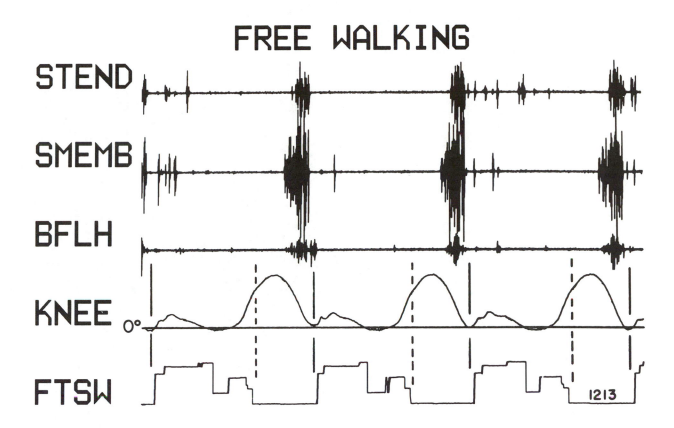

Figure 12.19b Normal hamstring EMG: There is vigorous activity during terminal swing and prompt cessation during early loading response.

is used to keep the body vector anterior to the knee, as a substitution for a weak quadriceps. Knee stability is precarious as the secondary flexion of the knee by the hamstrings also increases the need for a forward lean.

Knee Flexion Contracture

As the resting position for a swollen knee is about 30°, this is not an uncommon posture for a contracture (Figure 10.7). Numerous pathologies may lead to this deformity, of which major trauma, arthritis, and knee surgery are the most likely causes. Flexion contractures introduce a constant limitation to extension. With a 30° flexion contracture, all phases of the gait cycle will be abnormal except initial swing.

Partial recovery of the passive range to a 15° contracture will allow loading response and pre-swing also to have normal posturing. Knee extension in terminal swing, initial contact, and mid and terminal stance will still be inadequate.

While the difference between 15° and 30° may not be obvious during the

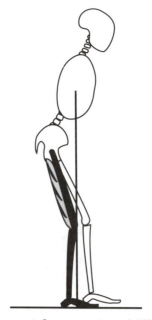

Figure 12.20 Prolonged hamstring activity in mid stance. Hip extension support of flexed trunk also causes excessive knee flexion.

Hamstrings extend Hip,

flex Knee

loading response, inadequate extension in the single limb support phases will be really apparent. The penalty for loss of extension in terminal swing is shortening of step length. Inability to appropriately extend the knee in mid and terminal stance increases the demand on the quadriceps. Active control will have to substitute for the loss of passive positioning.

Soleus Weakness

Inability of the soleus to effectively control the tibia is an obscure yet major cause of inadequate knee extension in mid and terminal stance. The lack of sufficient plantar flexor muscle strength allows the tibia to fall forward as body vector advances. As a result, the tibia advances faster than the femur, causing continued knee flexion (Figure 11.5). The quadriceps, despite having adequate strength to support the flexed knee, cannot reestablish knee extension because the base from which it pulls (the tibia) is unstable. As the quadriceps acts to draw the femur forward for knee extension, it also advances the body mass resting on the hip. This moves the body vector forward and increases the demand torque at the ankle, which the weak soleus cannot resist. Hence the whole limb advances rather than just the femur, and knee extension remains inadequate.

Mid Stance and Terminal Stance. Knee motion is a continuation of the flexion attained during the loading response. Associated with this is excessive ankle dorsiflexion. In addition, there will be sustained heel contact as an additional sign of soleus weakness.

Excessive Ankle Plantar Flexion

The distance between the hip joint and toe is increased by ankle plantar flexion. Whenever the swing limb must pass the stance limb, this relative lengthening must be accommodated by knee flexion if there is no anatomical shortening.

Mid Swing. Advancement of the limb will be obstructed by an ankle plantar flexion contracture or dorsiflexor paralysis. To assure foot clearance of the floor, the limb is lifted (Figure 12.21). Hip flexion is the basic action, while gravity, which holds the tibia vertical, flexes the knee. The visibility of the knee makes excessive knee flexion appear to be the obvious substitution, but this is only accomplished through the added hip flexion.

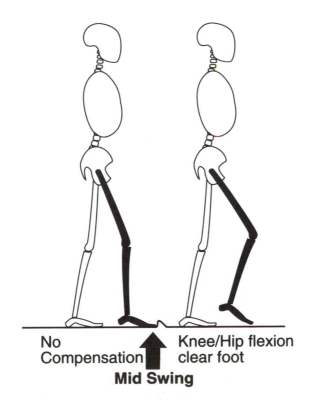

No Compensation

Knee/Hip flexion clear foot

Mid Swing

Figure 12.21 Mid swing excessive hip flexion as a compensatory action for a drop foot. (a) Toe drag without compensation. (b) Floor clearance by excessive hip flexion lifting limb.

Wobble

This term was adopted to identify small, alternating arcs of flexion and extension occurring during stance. It may represent a search for stability in a joint with impaired proprioception. Spastic clonus is a second cause.

Coronal Plane Gait Deviations

The terms *abduction* (valgus) and *adduction* (varus) refer to lateral and medial angulations of the tibia at the knee in the coronal plan. A false impression of knee joint distortion can be gained when knee flexion and limb rotation are combined. This faulty interpretation is very likely with observational analysis, unless the presence of the confounding motions has been screened. Misinterpretation of knee angulation can also occur in single camera filming (or video). As both rotation and flexion occur in swing, the presence of coronal plane malalignment should only be diagnosed during the stance period of the gait cycle.

Excessive abduction (valgus) refers to excessive lateral deviation of the distal tibia from the center of the knee (Figure 12.22). The normal abduction of approximately 10° represents an angulation within the femur while the tibia is vertical. Pathological abduction at the knee causes the tibia to tilt laterally with corresponding lateral displacement of the foot. This clinically is called a valgus deformity or *knock-knee.* During quiet standing, the distance between the feet will be greater than at the knees. Combined internal hip rotation and knee flexion can give a false impression of abduction during either stance or swing.

Excessive adduction (varus) of the knee is displayed by a medial tilt of the tibia and medial displacement of the foot relative to the knee (Figure 12.23). Femoral alignment is also altered as the hip abducts to accommodate the foot displacement. Rather than the deforming, medial angulation within the knee causing the foot to cross the midline for stance, the entire limb is moved laterally by hip abduction. This also widens the distance between the knees. Clinically this deformity is called varus or *bowleg.* Quiet standing now shows the knees to be farther apart than the feet. A false impression of knee varus may result from the combination of flexion and external rotation.

Causes of Coronal Plane Gait Deviations

Both varus and valgus can result from static or dynamic influences. Static deformities will be present on manual examination. Dynamic angulations represent the effects of altered body position and ligament laxity. Patients often display a mixture of the two mechanisms.

Static Factors

Intrinsic congenital or developmental deformities are childhood mechanisms. Trauma can induce a static malalignment of the knee at any age.

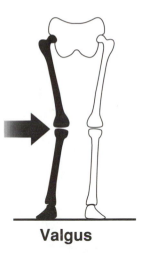

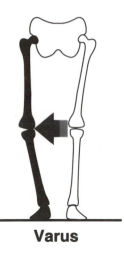

Valgus **Varus**

Figure 12.22 Knee valgus (excessive abduction). Knee is displaced medially from the line between hip and ankle because tibia is tilted laterally.

Figure 12.23 Knee varus (excessive adduction). Knee is displaced laterally from the line between hip and ankle because tibia is tilted medially.

Dynamic Deviations

The position of the knee at rest is increased by the dynamics of walking.

Osteoarthrosis allows the knee to yield to the persistent medial alignment of the body weight vector throughout stance. This creates a greater load on the medial tibial plateau. The osteoarthritic knee reacts to the unequal loads with degenerative changes and increasing knee deformity. Progressive malalignment toward varus results. Patients can partially unload the medial knee by lateral trunk sway.[3]

Rheumatoid arthritis tends to produce knee valgus. The causative mechanisms may be the lateral trunk lean used to unload the painful hip or a valgus foot deformity.

Paralytic gait may also induce coronal malalignment at the knee. Valgus is the more common abnormality. The mechanism is the lateral trunk lean to stabilize the hip when the abductor muscles are weak (the gluteus medius limp). This can be sufficient to deform the knee. Posturing into knee varus may occur in patients with a contralateral pelvic drop. Knee deformity is a rare consequence, however.

References

1. Biden E, et al.: Comparison of gait data from multiple labs. *Transactions of the Orthopaedic Research Society* 12:504, 1987.
2. Cahan LD, et al.: Instrumented gait analysis after selective dorsal rhizotomy. *Dev Med Child Neurol* 32(12):1037-1043, 1990.
3. Prodromos C, Andriacchi T, Galante J: A relationship between gait and clinical changes following high tibial osteotomy. *J Bone Joint Surg* 67A:1188-1193, 1985.

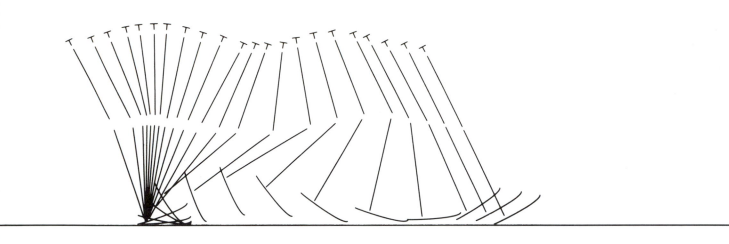

Chapter 13

Hip Gait Deviations

The multidirectional mobility of the hip makes this joint sensitive to dysfunction in all three planes. A further complexity to assessing the effects of hip pathology is its role as the junction between the lower limb and trunk. Abnormal hip function may be displayed by malalignment of either the thigh or pelvis (and indirectly the trunk). Pelvic motion may either accompany the displacement of the thigh, remain stationary, or move in the opposite direction, depending on the mobility of its articulation with the trunk. Thus, in the assessment of walking, thigh motion analysis should be separated from that of the pelvis. The functional patterns of both segments, however, are influenced by the interplay between postural demand and hip joint mechanics (mobility and the actions of its controlling muscles).

The potential gait errors in the sagittal plane include inadequate extension and excessive or inadequate flexion (Figure 13.1). Deviations in the other planes are excessive adduction, abduction and transverse rotation (internal or external).

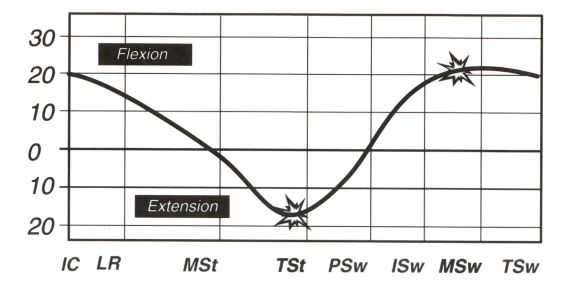

Figure 13.1 The phasing of the most significant gait deviations: terminal stance extension and mid swing flexion.

Inadequate Extension

The lack of hip extension threatens the person's weight-bearing stability. It also impedes progression. Failure to move the thigh toward neutral alignment in mid stance or attain hyperextension in terminal stance are the common errors.

Mid Stance

Limited hip extension can modify the alignments of either the pelvis or thigh. This introduces three postural errors in adjacent body segments: forward trunk lean, lumbar spine lordosis and a flexed knee (Figure 13.2).

Forward tilt of the pelvis is the sign of inadequate hip extension when the supporting limb advances to a vertical position over an extended knee in mid stance, that is, the thigh is vertical (Figure 13.2a). Without postural compensation, the trunk also will be forward, placing the body weight vector anterior to the hip joint. This increases the demand on the hip extensor muscles.

The least stressful means of reducing the resulting flexor leverage is lumbar lordosis (Figure 13.2b). Hip flexion of 15 is easily accommodated by the spine, unless it is abnormally stiff (Figure 13.3). Greater loss of hip extension begins to tax spine mobility. Each degree of anterior pelvic tilt (symphysis down) moves the base of the lumbar spine (lumbosacral joint) proportionally more anterior to the hip joint (Figure 13.4). To realign the body vector over the hip joint, the spine must arch further to carry the trunk mass back an equivalent distance. In general, children develop more lordosis than adults, since spinal growth

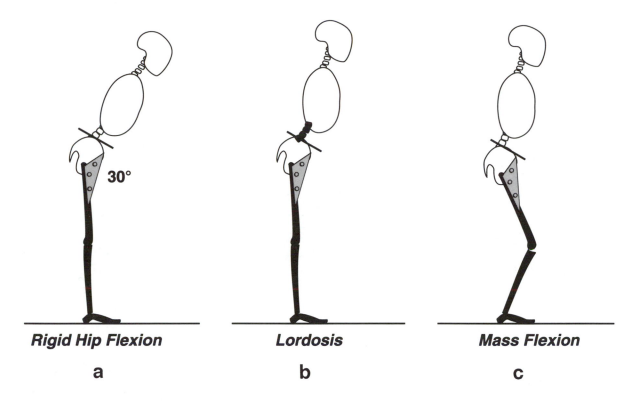

Rigid Hip Flexion

a

Lordosis

b

Mass Flexion

c

Figure 13.2 Inadequate hip extension in mid stance. (a) Without compensation the pelvis and trunk are tilted forward. Bolted plate indicates a rigid contracture. (b) Lumbar lordosis can restore an erect trunk. (c) Knee flexion equal to the fixed hip flexion can right both the pelvis and trunk.

absorbs the postural stresses (Wolff's Law, Figure 13.4). Failure to provide sufficient lumbar lordosis leaves the body vector anterior to the hip joint, and a corresponding degree of extensor muscle action (hip and back) is required.

Flexing the knee tilts the thigh back and allows the pelvis to retain its normal alignment, despite fixed hip flexion (Figure 13.2c). Hence, a crouch posture is an alternate means of accommodating to inadequate hip extension in mid stance. This is very inefficient, as the flexed knee must be stabilized by increased quadriceps control. Also, excessive ankle dorsiflexion or heel rise onto forefoot support is required. This mode of substitution for inadequate hip extension also significantly reduces body progression.

Terminal Stance

The added demands for hyperextension of the hip at the end of the single limb support period magnify the functional limitations of inadequate hip extension. Now the patient generally exhibits two functional deficits: anterior pelvic tilt and loss of a trailing thigh (Figure 13.5). Tilting of the pelvis

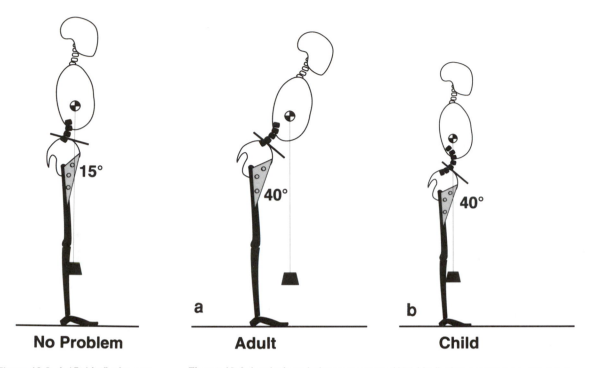

No Problem   **Adult**   **Child**

a   b

Figure 13.3 A 15° hip flexion contracture is readily compensated by lumbar lordosis to place the body vector over the supporting foot.

Figure 13.4 Lordosis to balance a severe (40°) hip flexion contracture. (a) Adults lack the spine mobility to fully compensate. C/G remains anterior to area of foot support. (b) Children's growth malleability allows the spine to develop the necessary lordosis for postural compensation.

(symphysis down) with its associated lumbar lordosis is the first change.

As the limits of spine mobility are challenged, the thigh assumes a less trailing position. Knee flexion may be increased to reduce the extensor strain on a hip with inadequate range. The lack of hip extension shortens the step of the other limb.

Excessive Flexion

As the thigh normally flexes 20° during swing (30° hip joint flexion), excessive flexion, generally, represents a major change in limb posture. The one exception is pre-swing, at which time the hip needs only to exceed neutral alignment to be excessively flexed.

Pre-Swing and Initial Swing

Excessive hip flexion during pre-swing most commonly represents a continuation of inadequate hip extension in the previous stance phases. Occasionally there is a rapid advancement of the thigh when weight transfer to the other foot unlocks the limb and releases flexors that previously had been held under tension. In either situation, hip flexion for swing is initiated prematurely and may continue into initial swing.

Mid Swing

An increase in hip joint angle due to intrinsic pathology most often is reflected by greater pelvic tilt than altered thigh position. Excessive elevation of the thigh in mid swing, however, is a common substitution for excessive ankle plantar flexion (Figure 13.6).

Causes of Inadequate Extension and Excessive Hip Flexion

There are five common pathologies that restrict the mobility of the anterior hip joint tissues (Table 13.1). Each can cause inadequate hip extension or excessive hip flexion. These are a flexion contracture, anterior iliotibial band

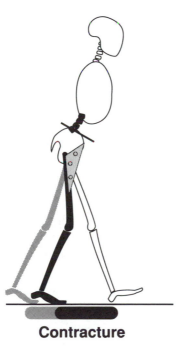

Contracture

Figure 13.5 Inadequate hip extension in terminal stance prevents a trailing thigh (black limb). Body advancement and step length are shortened. Gray limb displays normal alignment for comparison.

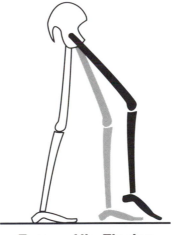

Excess Hip Flexion

Figure 13.6 Excessive hip flexion is used voluntarily in mid swing to provide floor clearance by a plantar flexed ankle.

Table 13.1

Causes of Gait Deviations at the Hip

	Inadequate Extension	Excessive Flexion	Inadequate Flexion	Excessive Extension
Flexion Contracture		X	X	
IT Band Contracture		X	X	
Flexor Spasticity		X	X	
Arthrodesis	X	X	X	X
Pain		X	X	
Voluntary	X	X	X	

	Excessive Adduction	Excessive Abduction	Excessive Rotation
Abduction Weakness	I	C	
Adduction Contracture Spasticity	I	C	
Scoliotic Pelvic Obliquity	I/C	I/C	
Abduction Contracture	C	I	
Iliotibial Band Contracture	C	I	
Arthrodesis	X	X	X
Voluntary		I	X
Muscle Overactivity			X
Hip Anteversion			X

Key: C = Contralateral
        I = Ipsilateral
        I/C = Ipsilateral and Contralateral
        X = Not side-oriented

contracture, spasticity of the hip flexors, pain, and hip joint arthrodesis. Voluntary posturing is an additional cause of excessive flexion. Often differentiating the cause of the limited motion depends on dynamic electromyography rather than motion analysis.

Hip Flexion Contracture

Anterior fibrous tissues, shortening of the joint capsule or flexor muscles is the most common limitation of full hip extension (Figures 13.2 and 13.5). As the contracture introduces a fixed hip position, its functional significance varies with the normal angle used during walking.

Iliotibial Band Contracture

A variant of a hip flexion contracture, is a tight iliotibial band (Figure 13.7). During walking the patient exhibits a greater limitation of hip extension than when lying supine. The difference is the relative adduction that occurs with weight-bearing. This increases iliotibial band tension and introduces an equivalent forward tilt of the pelvis.

The clinical finding in a supine lying test of full passive extension, with the hip widely abducted and fixed flexion when the hip is neutrally aligned, localizes the contracture to the iliotibial band (Figure 13.8).

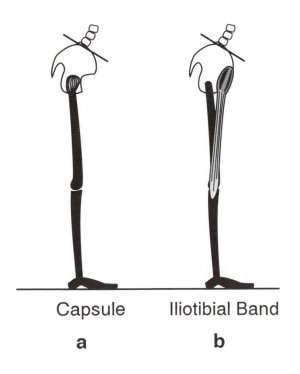

Capsule   Iliotibial Band

a   **b**

Figure 13.7 Iliotibial band contracture can mimic a rigid joint contracture.

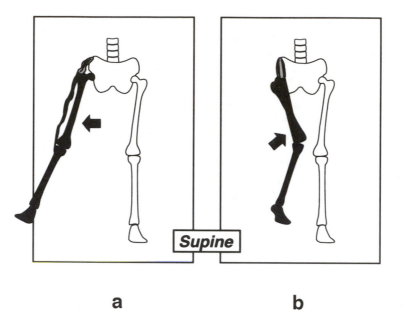

a   b

Figure 13.8 Iliotibial (IT) band contracture limitation of hip extension. (a) With limb abducted, IT band is slack and hip extends fully. (b) With thigh adduction, IT band is tightened and the hip flexes.

Hip Flexor Spasticity

Stretch stimulates spastic muscles to contract. During walking the spastic hip flexors react when the muscle's free range is exceeded. As eight muscles cross the hip anteriorly and any or all may be spastic, the timing and magnitude of hip extension limitation varies with the individual. There also is much overlap of associated adduction, abduction and rotation. Dynamic electromyography is the only means of identifying the offending muscles (Figure 13.9).

Similarly, stretch caused by the dangling limb can stimulate a spastic response during the swing phases of walking in patients with upper motor neuron lesions. This would be superimposed on the voluntary action (selective or primitive patterning). Flexion in excess of 40°, however, is unusual unless there is an associated contracture.

Pain

Arthritis and other joint pathology that cause swelling within the hip joint introduce a flexed posture. Intra-articular pressures are least when the hip is flexed 30° to 40° (Figure 10.8).[1] Hence, this position is assumed reflexly. The actual degree of flexion varies with the intensity of the joint pathology. Single limb support is reduced as progression increases the tension on the joint capsule, leading to greater pain.

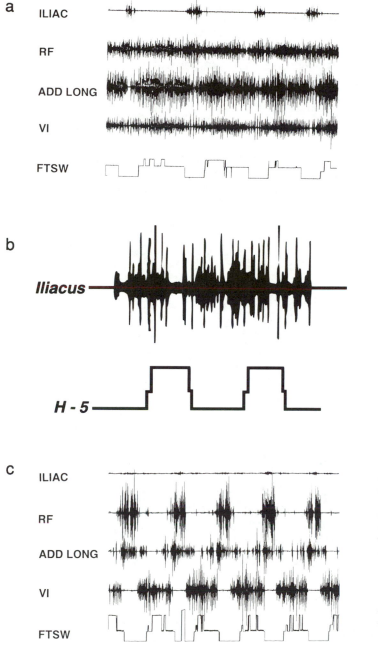

Figure 13.9 Spastic hip flexors limit hip extension in stance. (a) Rectus femoris (RF) and adductor longus (ADD LONG) show continuous EMG while iliacus (ILIAC) timing is normal. (b) Continuous activity of a spastic iliacus. (c) Useful swing phasing of rectus (RF) and adductor longus (ADD LONG) as a substitution for the inactive iliacus (ILIAC). Vastus intermedius (VI) has extended action through stance. Foot switches (FTSW) shows stance instability.

Arthrodesis

Loss of joint motion from either surgical arthrodesis or spontaneous ankylosis denies the patient the hip extension used during walking. Customarily, the hip is fixed in a position of flexion between 20° and 45°, as a compromise between the needs of walking and sitting. The times within the gait cycle when this limitation occurs depend on the position of joint fixation.

Hence, the hip fused at 20° flexion results in inadequate extension, while flexion is excessive only in pre-swing. The more severe posture (45°) presents excessive swing phase flexion also.

Voluntary Flexion

Deliberate flexion of the hip above 30° in mid swing gains floor clearance when the foot is plantar flexed (Figure 13.6). The added flexion might carry over into terminal swing but would not persist as the limb approached the floor.

Pass-Retract

In terminal swing, the hip is aggressively flexed and then rapidly reversed into extension (Figure 13.10). There are two subtle variations of this action. Mid swing may be a period of excessive hip flexion, with the terminal swing extension returning the thigh to the normal 30° posture. Flexion may not exceed the normal range, and the subsequent extension in terminal swing results in a reduced posture for initial contact.

Pass-retract hip motion is used by persons with paralyzed quadriceps and normal neural control (poliomyelitis) to extend the knee. Rapid hip flexion advances both thigh and tibia. Quick, active retraction of the femur allows inertia to continue advancing the tibia. In this way, the limb is prepared for initial contact. The action may be overt or very subtle.

Dominance of the primitive patterns in spastic patients also can introduce a pass-retract motion pattern. In mid swing the flexor pattern provides limb advancement and floor clearance. Preparation for stance in terminal swing initiates the extensor pattern. This may cause hip extension as the knee is straightened. Now, the retraction of a previously flexed hip represents inability to mix hip flexion and knee extension.

Inadequate Hip Flexion

The need for hip flexion begins in initial swing, continues through the other phases of swing and into initial contact. Evidence of inadequate hip flexion may arise in any of these phases.

Initial Swing

Failure to flex the hip 15° in initial swing reduces limb advancement (Figure 12.4). A secondary effect is limited knee flexion since the thigh momentum needed to initiate this action is lacking. This, in turn, contributes to toe drag and

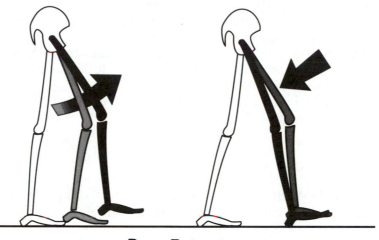

Pass-Retract

Figure 13.10 Voluntary excessive hip flexion and its release in terminal swing to rapidly advance and retract the thigh to extend the flaccid knee. The *pass-retract* maneuver.

ankle plantar flexion. As a dragging toe can also inhibit hip flexion, function of the knee and ankle in other gait phases is used to elucidate the cause of the observed limitation at the hip.

Mid Swing

Inadequate hip flexion in mid swing generally is a continuation of limited initial swing action. Little additional flexor muscle action is available.

Terminal Swing, Initial Contact and Loading Response

Hip position during these phases reflects the limitations experienced in mid swing, as no additional flexion normally occurs in any of these phases. The result is a shortened step length.

Causes of Inadequate Hip Flexion

The lack of adequate hip flexion generally relates to the nonavailability of active muscle control. Loss of hip joint mobility is an infrequent cause.

Hip Flexor Insufficiency

Weakness or inability to activate the hip flexor muscles may be displayed by a loss of speed or inadequate range. Failure of these muscles to meet the functional demand indicates a major physical impairment since walking requires little of the flexor muscles. With normal motor control grade 2+ (poor plus), muscle strength is sufficient for an average gait.

Upper motor neuron lesions commonly make the patient dependent on the mass flexor pattern for limb advancement. Normal initial swing acceleration is lacking. Hence, the limb flexes slowly in initial swing, resulting in an inadequate range. Patients dependent on primitive patterned control reach their maximum hip flexion in late mid swing.

Hip Joint Arthrodesis

Flexion of the hip during swing is dictated by the fixed position of the joint. Seldom is this a cause of inadequate hip flexion. Only if the hip were fused in a position less than 20° flexion would a swing phase have inadequate posturing. Initiating thigh advancement in pre-swing is delayed until the limb is unloaded. The strength of the abdominals, combined with back mobility, determines the rate the limb moves forward in initial swing.

Substitutive Actions

Several substitutions are possible for advancing the limb when primary hip flexion is inadequate. They generally begin in initial swing. Posterior tilt of the pelvis (symphysis up) uses the abdominal muscles to advance the thigh (Figure 13.11). Circumduction is common. This includes hiking and forward rotation of the pelvis and abduction of the hip. Advancing the limb in this manner utilizes considerable energy because so much trunk mass must be moved.

Voluntary excessive knee flexion is an indirect means of flexing the hip (Figure 13.12). The posterior alignment of shank and foot weight introduces passive thigh advancement to balance total limb weight under the point of suspension (the hip joint). A modest but useful amount of hip flexion results.

Additional substitutions used to assure floor clearance by an unflexed limb include contralateral vaulting and lateral lean of the trunk to the opposite side.

Excessive Coronal Plane Motion

Deviation of the thigh from its normal alignment may be either lateral or medial. In observational gait analysis, it is common practice to merely designate the gait deviations as *abduction* or *adduction*. With instrumented analysis, the requirements are more stringent. The normal alignment of the thigh is adducted relative to vertical. Also, quantitated motion analysis has identified minor arcs of normal motion beyond the neutral alignment. Functionally significant gait

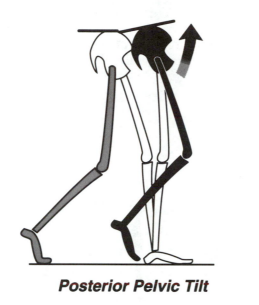

Posterior Pelvic Tilt

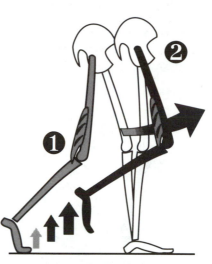

**Rapid Knee Flexion
Causing Hip Flexion**

Figure 13.11 Voluntary posterior pelvic tilt to advance the thigh when hip flexion is inadequate.

Figure 13.12 Voluntary excessive knee flexion to flex the flaccid (or contracted) hip (arrow) by changing the limb's C/G.

deviations represent excessive arcs. To accommodate these different situations, the terms *excessive adduction* and *excessive abduction* will be used.

Excessive Adduction

In stance, there are two patterns of excessive adduction of the hip. The thigh may have an excessive medial angle (coxa vera), with a corresponding increase in the valgus alignment of the knee. This will persist throughout the weight-bearing period.

A contralateral drop of the pelvis also increases hip adduction during the weight-bearing period of walking. While this posture is assumed during loading response and persists through single limb support, it corrects in pre-swing as body weight is transferred to the opposite limb.

In swing, excessive hip adduction relates to medial alignment of the whole limb. This begins in initial swing, as the hip is flexed, and progresses during swing (Figure 13.13). When it is sufficiently severe to cause the swing limb to cross the stance limb, the patient is said to have a *scissor gait*. The result of excessive adduction in swing is a narrow base of support. With a severe scissor gait, progression can be blocked. Floor contact with the foot on the opposite side of the midline obstructs forward swing of the other limb. In initial swing the foot can catch on the stance limb, and advancement is obstructed.

Excessive adduction is often confused with combined internal rotation and knee flexion (pseudo adduction, Figure 13.14). This combination of limb postures directs the knee inward, even to the extent of overlap with the other limb. The two situations are differentiated by the relative closeness of the feet. With pseudo adduction the feet are separated. Conversely, they approximate each other when true adduction exists.

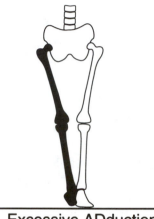

Excessive ADduction

Figure 13.13 Excessive hip adduction in swing limb causing a *scissor gait*. Whole limb moves medially (thigh and foot).

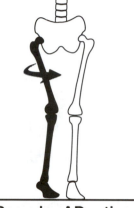

Pseudo ADuction

Figure 13.14 Pseudo adduction. Combined hip flexion and internal rotation excessively adducts the thigh (knee), but the foot is lateral.

Causes of Excessive Adduction

The dynamic causes of coronal plane deviations relate to muscle weakness, spasticity or voluntary substitutions. Static malalignment can also result in an inappropriate hip position during gait. Because obliquity of the pelvis causes excessive adduction of one hip and excessive abduction of the other hip, mobility and muscular control of both sides must be considered in seeking the cause of coronal plane deviations.

Ipsilateral Pathology

Abductor Weakness. Lifting the one foot for swing removes the support for that side of the pelvis while body weight is medial to the supporting hip. This creates a strong adduction torque that must be stabilized by the hip abductors. Hip abductor muscles (gluteus medius primarily) with grade 3 strength or less cannot prevent the pelvis and trunk falling to the opposite side (contralateral drop) (Figure 13.15). This lateral fall begins with the rapid transfer of body weight onto the stance limb in loading response. The pelvic drop continues through the weight-bearing period because there is no mechanism to raise it until the other foot again contacts the floor in pre-swing.

Adduction Contracture or Spasticity. Static posturing of the hip by either fibrous tissue or bony fixation causes a continuous deviation throughout the gait cycle (Figure 13.16). Very commonly, an adduction contracture is associated with internal rotation and flexion. Spasticity can mimic contracture when the patient is standing, but be mild or absent with the patient supine.

Adductors as Hip Flexors. Substitution of the adductor muscles (longus, brevis or gracilis) for a weak or absent iliacus muscle (the primary hip flexor) leads to medial displacement of the thigh (excessive adduction) in swing (Figure 13.17). Spasticity activation of the adductor muscles by stretch of the dangling limb creates the same situation.

If the hip is fully extended at the onset of adductor muscle action, advancement of the thigh will be accompanied by external rotation. Having a flexed position at the start of the adductor muscle action introduces internal rotation.

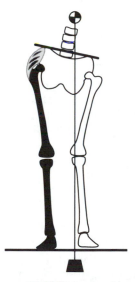 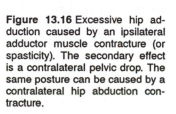 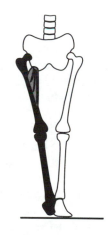

Figure 13.15 Excessive hip adduction caused by weak hip abductors (gluteus medius) allowing a contralateral pelvic drop as the swing limb is lifted.

Figure 13.16 Excessive hip adduction caused by an ipsilateral adductor muscle contracture (or spasticity). The secondary effect is a contralateral pelvic drop. The same posture can be caused by a contralateral hip abduction contracture.

Figure 13.17 Excessive hip adduction caused by these muscles serving as the primary hip flexors (voluntary or spastic overuse).

Contralateral Pathology

Contralateral Hip Abduction Contracture. Tightness of the lateral musculature of the other hip draws the pelvis down toward the femur. This results in an contralateral pelvic tilt (drop) for the reference limb and relative adduction of that hip (Figure 13.16). The passive posture of the reference limb is the same as that created by its own adduction contracture. During swing this can create an apparent scissor gait, but the fault is on the other side. As the pelvis falls (abduction of the contralateral stance hip) it draws the swinging reference limb closer to the midline.

Excessive Abduction

Lateral displacement of the thigh during stance presents a wide based gait. The form of excessive hip abduction increases stance stability, but also requires greater effort during walking to move the body from one limb to the other. In swing, floor clearance is made easier.

Causes of Excessive Abduction

Ipsilateral Pathology

Abduction Contracture. Shortening of the abductor musculature or capsule displaces the femur laterally. The patient's gait generally is a mixture of wide base (foot to the side) and an ipsilateral pelvic drop (Figure 13.18). This relatively lengthens the leg, making the initiation of swing difficult. Abductor spasticity could create the same situation, but this is infrequent. Conversely, grossly inadequate adductor tone can result in an excessively abducted limb.

A tight iliotibial band causes hip abduction with extension, but neutral alignment is possible when the hip is flexed (Figure 13.8) Hence, patients generally show a mixture of excessive flexion, abduction and pelvic tilt.

Short Leg. The ipsilateral pelvic tilt used to accommodate the lack of leg length puts the hip into excessive abduction. This is not a significant finding unless the leg length discrepancy is severe.

Voluntary Abduction. Patients with good control of their trunk muscles commonly substitute abduction for the lack of adequate hip flexion as the means of advancing the limb in swing (Figure 13.19). Generally hip abduction is combined with pelvic rotation and hiking to complete the motion complex commonly called *circumduction.* Ipsilateral abduction as part of a trunk lean is also used to help the other limb clear the floor.

Abduction in stance is used to widen the base of support. This is a frequent substitution for impaired balance.

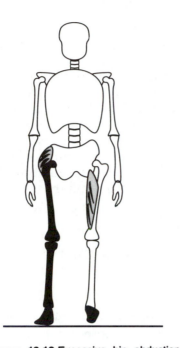

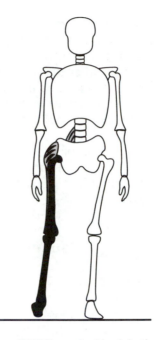

Figure 13.18 Excessive hip abduction caused by an abduction contracture. The limb is displaced laterally (wide-based gait). An ipsilateral pelvic drop partially accommodates. The same posture can be caused by a contralateral adduction contracture pulling the pelvis toward the femur medially.

Figure 13.19 Excessive hip abduction by voluntary displacement to provide floor clearance in swing as a substitution for inadequate knee flexion.

Contralateral Pathology

Contralateral Hip Adduction Contracture. As the contracted limb assumes a vertical alignment for weight bearing, the pelvis is tilted down. This creates an ipsilateral pelvic rise for the reference limb that also results in relative lengthening (Figure 13.18). If there is adequate quadriceps and hip extensor control, the patient substitutes with knee flexion to shorten the limb.

Scoliosis with Pelvic Obliquity

Pelvic obliquity secondary to scoliosis leads to excessive abduction in the hip on the low side. Conversely, the hip on the high side will be in excessive adduction. The oblique pelvis can also represent an accommodation to fixed abduction or adduction within the hip joint.

Excessive Transverse Rotation

Any visible transverse rotation of the limb represents excessive motion as the normal arc of 5 (10 total displacement) is obscured by the anterio-posterior changes in limb alignment.

While the arcs of transverse hip rotation in normal gait are too small to be apparent by observational analysis, the terms *excessive internal* and *excessive external* are necessary to accommodate instrumented motion analysis. The magnitude of rotation that is significant of pathology varies with the measurement system.

Excessive rotation of the limb can arise within the hip joint or be secondary to rotation of the pelvis or within trunk. Hence, the originating site of the excessive rotation must be determined as well as the magnitude of the limb displacement.[2]

Causes of Excessive Rotation

External Rotation

Gluteus Maximus Overactivity. Terminal swing use of the gluteus maximus as the prime source of hip extension causes rapid external rotation. The small external rotator muscles can have the same effect as they attempt to substitute for the larger hip extensors.

Excessive Ankle Plantar Flexion. External rotation in mid stance commonly accompanies persistent foot flat floor contact from a rigid ankle equinus. This appears to be a useful means of circumventing the barrier to progression that the lack of ankle dorsiflexion imposes.

In terminal stance, excessive external rotation may accompany marked equiovarus if the natural obliquity of the metatarsal head axis provides asymmetrical forefoot support.

Internal Rotation

Medial Hamstring Overactivity. The semimembranosus and semitendinosus lie both posterior and medial to the hip joint, making these muscles natural internal rotators. Overactivity as a result of spasticity or strong involvement in a primitive pattern would accentuate the rotatory effect of these muscles. Because the hamstring muscles are flexors at one joint (knee) and extensors at the other (hip), their action can accompany either the flexor or extensor primitive locomotor patterns.

Adductor Overactivity. Flexion of the hip by the adductors is accompanied by internal rotation if the hip's resting position included some flexion. Internal, rather than the expected external, rotation occurs because the flexed position displaces the femur forward of the functional limb lever between the hip and foot.

Anterior Abductor Overactivity. The tensor fascia lata and anterior portion of the gluteus medius produce internal rotation. Use of these muscles to assist hip flexion will result in excessive rotation of the hip.

Quadriceps Weakness. Internal rotation of the thigh utilizes the lateral knee ligament and iliotibial band to resist the sagittal thrust of limb loading that, otherwise, would flex the knee. This is a voluntary substitution for a very weak (or absent) quadriceps when there is no available hyperextension at the knee.

References

1. Eyring EJ, Murray WR: The effect of joint position on the pressure of intra-articular effusion. *J Bone Joint Surg* 46A(6):1235-1241, 1964.
2. Tylkowski CM, Simon SR, Mansour JM: Internal rotation gait in spastic cerebral palsy. In Nelson JP (Ed): *The Hip.* St Louis, The C.V. Mosby Company, 1982, pp. 89-125.

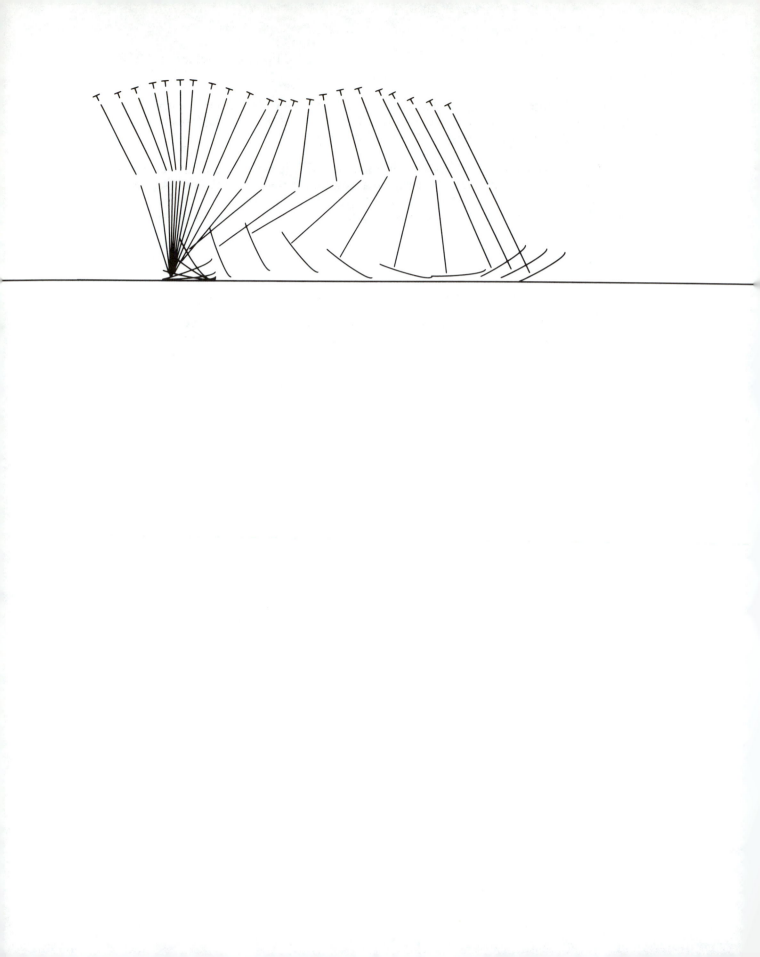

Chapter 14

Pelvis and Trunk Pathological Gait

As the average change in the position of the pelvis is 5° or less and the trunk normally maintains a neutrally aligned erect posture, visible deviations of the pelvis or trunk from neutral represent abnormal function. Instrumented analysis would have similarly small margins for normal function.

Pelvis

Abnormal pelvic motion is displayed as excessive action. Any of the three planes of motion may be altered. Inadequate pelvic motion is seen as stiffness.

Sagittal Plane

Gait errors in this plane are identified as forms of pelvic tilt. The direction of the motion has been described by two, commonly used, sets of terms: *anterior* and *posterior* or *upward* and *downward*. Definition of these terms has varied according to the anatomical site selected as the apex of the motion, that is, the symphysis or the sacrum. To circumvent this confusion, the more obvious terms of *symphysis up* and *symphysis down* have been substituted. As these phrases are euphemistically awkward, their best use may be to clarify the definitions of anterior tilt (symphysis down) and posterior tilt (symphysis up).

Anterior Tilt (Symphysis Down). The normal 10° anterior angulation of the sagittal pelvic axis (a plane through the posterior and anterior superior iliac spines) increases.[1] A tilt of 30° is not uncommon. Phasic timing of the abnormal posturing varies with the cause (Figure 14.1).

Causes of Anterior Pelvic Tilt

Weak Hip Extensors. In loading response, the symphysis moves down as a reaction to the anterior alignment of the C/G relative to the hip joint when the extensor muscles lack the strength to restrain the pelvis. This posture may continue throughout stance or revert to neutral when the limb assumes a trailing position in terminal stance. Surgical release or lengthening of spastic hamstrings to relieve a crouch gait is a common cause of hip extensor weakness, especially when there is also spasticity of the hip flexors.

Hip Flexion Contracture or Spasticity. The pelvis may be drawn into an anterior tilt in any of the stance phases depending on its severity. With

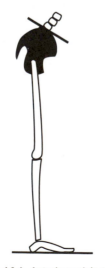

Figure 14.1 Anterior pelvic tilt (symphysis down). Hip is flexed, trunk is forward.

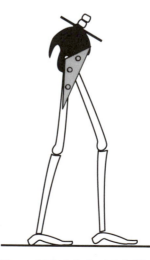

Figure 14.2 Anterior pelvic tilt resulting from a hip flexion contracture (or spasticity).

contractures of 30°, the postural change starts in mid stance as the limb becomes vertical and increases in terminal stance and pre-swing when the thigh assumes a trailing posture (Figure 14.2). Lesser deformities start later. Contractures that exceed 40° may introduce a symphysis down posture at initial contact and become prominent by loading response. Spasticity can be partially differentiated from contracture by supine clinical testing. During gait, dynamic electromyography is needed. This distinction assists in surgical planning and prediction of long term outcome.

Posterior Tilt (Symphysis Up). Raising the pelvic axis above the horizontal for a posterior tilt must be differentiated from correction of a previous anterior tilt. Return to neutral is not a gait error. Tilting the pelvis posteriorly to create a symphysis up posture is an infrequent event. It generally is a deliberate action, occurring in swing (Figure 14.3). The purpose is to advance the limb in the absence of effective hip flexors.

Coronal Plane

Two clinical terms are used to define abnormal pelvic motion in the coronal plane: *hip hike* and *pelvic drop*. Hip hike (more correctly called pelvic hike) indicates lateral elevation of the pelvis above the neutral axis. Pelvic drop, conversely, implies descent of the pelvis. This is differentiated into contralateral drop and ipsilateral drop. For both deviations, it is important to isolate a primary motion error from correction of prior malpositioning.

Pelvic Hike. The clinical term *pelvic hike* refers to excessive elevation of the ipsilateral side of the pelvis. This is a swing phase event (Figure 14.4). It is a deliberate action that begins in initial swing, continues through mid swing, and then corrects in terminal swing. The purpose is to assist foot clearance when either hip or knee flexion are inadequate. The presence of excessive ankle plantar flexion is a common cause of pelvic hiking.

Mild (5°) ipsilateral elevation of the pelvis in stance is a normal recording with instrumented gait analysis since the middle of the pelvis is the point of reference and it drops at the onset of limb loading.

Contralateral pelvic hike occurs as the other limb experiences the same functions.

Contralateral Drop. Descent of the opposite side of the pelvis occurs in stance. It begins as body weight is dropped onto the limb in loading response and persists through terminal stance (Figure 14.5). With instrumented motion analysis, contralateral pelvic drop is identified as ipsilateral pelvic elevation. This occurs because the midline reference point drops while the stance limb's hip joint maintains its height.

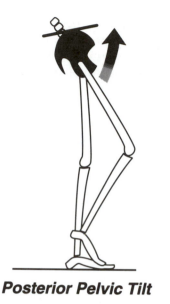

Posterior Pelvic Tilt

Figure 14.3 Posterior pelvic tilt (symphysis up). Trunk leans back. Thigh is advanced if hip remains at neutral (swing limb). With thigh vertical, hip is hyperextended (stance limb).

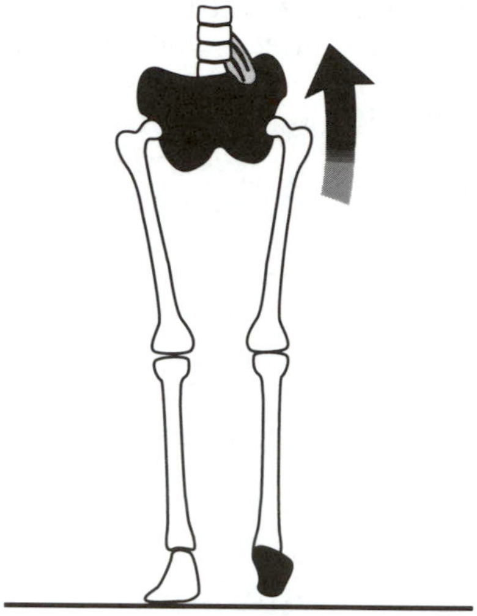

Pelvic Hike

Figure 14.4 Ipsilateral pelvic hike. Reference side of pelvis is elevated. This is a voluntary coordination with the swing limb.

Causes of Contralateral Pelvic Drop

Weak Hip Abductor Muscles. Abductor muscle strength less than grade 3+ creates an unstable pelvis in stance. Unloading the opposite limb in preparation for swing removes the support for that side of the pelvis. As body weight is medial to the supporting hip joint, the pelvis falls (Figure 14.6a). This action begins in loading response because of the rapid transfer of body weight to the stance limb. With greater incompetency of the abductors, the contralateral pelvic drop is accompanied by an ipsilateral trunk lean to preserve stance stability (Figure 14.6b). Weakness of the hip abductor muscles can be masked by a tight iliotibial band.

Hip Adductor Contracture or Spasticity. During mid stance, the pelvis is drawn down as the femur assumes a relatively vertical posture (Figure 14.7). Generally, there is associated hip flexion and internal rotation.

Contralateral Hip Abductor Contracture. The same pattern of pelvic obliquity seen with tight hip adductors can be created by excessive abduction in the opposite hip (Figure 14.7). This makes the ipsilateral limb relatively short.

Ipsilateral Drop. Dropping of the ipsilateral side of the pelvis occurs in swing (Figure 14.8). Often it reflects contralateral pathology.

Causes of Ipsilateral Pelvic Drop

Contralateral Hip Abductor Weakness. The pelvis drops with the onset of initial swing and persists through terminal swing (Figure 14.8). Lifting the limb removes the support for that side of the pelvis, and the hip abductor muscles of the stance limb lack stabilizing strength.

Short Ipsilateral Limb. Preparation for loading a short leg may induce an ipsilateral pelvic drop in terminal swing. This occurs when other substitutions are lacking. Alignment of the pelvis after initial contact varies with the way the patient accommodates the difference in limb length. The ipsilateral drop may persist, or the pelvis may become level.

Calf Muscle Weakness. Insufficient calf muscle strength for weight-bearing heel rise in terminal stance results in an ipsilateral pelvic drop. The lack of heel rise relatively shortens the limb as it assumes a trailing position. Limb length is

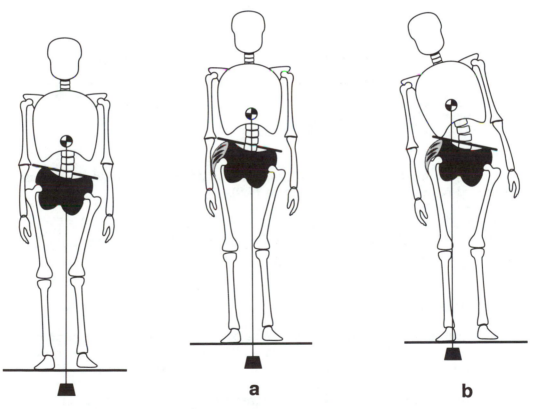

a   **b**

Figure 14.5 Contralateral pelvic drop. Side opposite the reference limb drops as swing limb is lifted. C/G is displaced laterally.

Figure 14.6 Contralateral pelvic drop resulting from weak ipsilateral hip abductors. (a) Body center of gravity (C/G) displaced away from stance limb. (b) Compensating trunk lean with a change in pelvic posture. C/G moves toward stance limb.

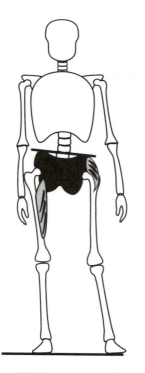

Figure 14.7 Contralateral pelvic drop resulting from ipsilateral adductor contracture (spasticity) or contralateral abduction contracture (spasticity).

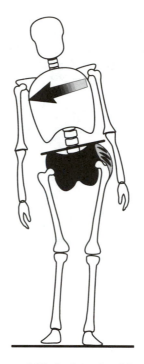

Figure 14.8 Ipsilateral pelvic drop accompanies swing limb when contralateral hip abductors are weak.

gained by dropping the pelvis on that side. This is accompanied by excessive backward rotation of the pelvis (Figure 14.9).

Scoliosis. Deformity in the spine presents static malalignment of the pelvis as either contralateral or ipsilateral drop. Deviations of the pelvis may be oblique, as well as lie in the coronal plane (Figure 14.10).

Transverse Plane

Rotation of the pelvis may be excessive or lacking. Also, the direction of the gait error may be forward or backward. Whenever rotation of the pelvis is visible, it is excessive. By instrumentation this would be greater than 5°.

Excessive Forward Rotation. The pelvis may have a fixed forward alignment or move in company with the swing limb. Rapid pelvic forward rotation in initial swing and continuing into mid swing is a means of advancing the limb when the hip flexors are incompetent.

Excessive Backward Rotation. Again, the pelvis may have a fixed backward alignment. Dynamic backward rotation occurs in terminal stance. It is a fairly abrupt motion that accompanies persistent heel contact in a person who has a moderately good gait velocity. The cause is calf muscle weakness (Figure 14.9). The lack of heel rise makes the limb relatively short. Length is gained by a combined backward and downward rotation of the pelvis.

Lack of Pelvic Rotation (Forward or Backward). Insufficient pelvic motion is seen in patients with spastic rigidity of the spine. Surgical fusion is a less frequent cause. Visually the patients appear stiff.

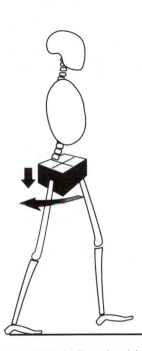

Figure 14.9 Ipsilateral pelvic drop and posterior pelvic rotation. The cause is a weak soleus on the stance limb ipsilateral leading to a loss of heel rise and relative lengthening of limb.

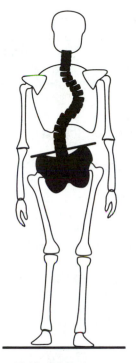

Figure 14.10 Pelvic drop as part of the scoliosis curve.

Trunk

A direct correlation between trunk (spine or abdominal) muscle strength and posture has not been recorded. Clinical experience, however, indicates there is no significant deviation from normal until the muscle weakness is marked, generally less than grade 3 (fair). This is consistent with the small amounts of muscular activity needed to control the minor postural deviations induced by the mechanics of walking. When muscle strength is insufficient, the postural deviation is constant. This also is true for spastic muscle imbalance or skeletal abnormalities causing scoliosis, kyphosis, lordosis or pelvic tilt. The phasic changes in trunk or pelvic alignment recorded during walking represent postural adaptations to inadequate mobility or faulty muscle control at the hip, knee or ankle.

Deviations in trunk alignment from the neutral upright posture are classified as a trunk lean. The direction may be backward, forward, ipsilateral or contra-lateral. Also, the trunk may rotate toward or away from the reference limb.

Backward Lean

Displacement of the trunk posterior to the vertical axis uses the weight of the trunk as a substitution for inadequate hip muscle strength. Different types of limb control deficits initiate a backward lean in stance and swing. There are two elements to the backward lean posture: posterior displacement of the upper trunk with normal lumbar alignment and increased lumbar lordosis (Figure 14.11).

Causes of Backward Lean

Weak Hip Extensors. In stance, a backward lean of the trunk substitutes for weak hip extensors by placing the body vector behind the hip joint axis (Figure 14.11). The need for such a substitution begins with loading response and continues throughout stance, ending in pre-swing. In anticipation, patients commonly assume the posture at initial contact. Patients with bilateral hip extensor weakness maintain a backward lean of the trunk during the entire stride.

The severity of lumbar lordosis associated with the backward lean is related to the degree of hip flexion contracture present (Figure 14.12). This displaces the base of the spine (lumbosacral joint) anterior to the hip joints, thereby, necessitating greater backward lean of the thoracic trunk segment. The head maintains a vertical posture.

Inadequate Hip Flexion. During swing, a backward lean of the trunk may be used to assist limb advancement when hip flexor range or muscle control is inadequate. As upward rotation of the pelvis (posterior tilt) is a more direct substitution, using the trunk implies a need for further force to substitute for the inadequate hip function (Figure 14.13). The cause for involving the trunk could either be lumbar spine immobility or poor control of the abdominal muscles. In the latter instance, backward lean of the trunk uses the abdominal muscle mass as a passive strap. Backward lean of the trunk in swing can also indicate contralateral hip extensor weakness when there is bilateral pathology.

Forward Lean

Positioning the trunk forward of the vertical moves the body vector anteriorly (Figure 14.14). The basic indications are to preserve weight-bearing balance and to stabilize the knee. Pathology at the ankle, knee or hip most

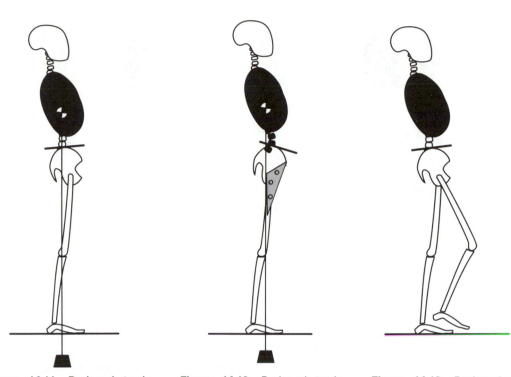

Figure 14.11 Backward trunk lean. Displacement of C/G behind hip joint will substitute for weak hip extensors. Hip hyperextension and ankle dorsiflexion are needed to maintain C/G over foot support area.

Figure 14.12 Backward trunk lean as a voluntary use of lordosis to accommodate a rigid hip flexion contracture. Pelvis is tilted anteriorly.

Figure 14.13 Backward trunk lean as a voluntary effort will assist a posterior tilt to advance the thigh in swing.

commonly creates the need for anterior displacement of the vector by forward lean of the trunk. Other possible causes are a lack of spine mobility or abdominal muscle weakness. The cause of forward trunk lean changes with the gait phase. Defining the different mechanisms is accomplished by relating the actions at the other joints.

Ankle plantar flexion persisting into mid stance, terminal stance or pre-swing, combined with continued heel contact, requires forward lean of the trunk to place the body weight vector over the area of foot support (Figure 14.15). The cause may be a contracture or spasticity of the soleus/gastrocnemius musculature.

Quadriceps weakness at the knee stimulates a forward trunk lean as a substitute. This posture provides a passive knee extensor force by placing the body vector anterior to the knee (Figure 14.16). Forward lean begins in loading response and persists through the rest of stance, until body weight is transferred to the other limb in pre-swing. This substitutive posture can be very

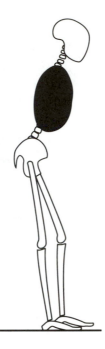

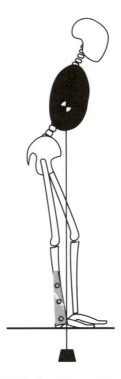

Figure 14.14 Trunk forward lean. Lumbar lordosis keeps the trunk erect while the mass is forward.

Figure 14.15 Trunk forward lean compensates for a rigid ankle plantar flexion contracture, positioning the stance limb posteriorly. C/G remains over supporting foot.

subtle if an insufficient quadriceps is the only impairment. Forward trunk lean is increased if there is an associated knee flexion contracture.

Hip extensor weakness of a moderate degree initiates forward trunk lean in loading response and early mid stance. As body weight is dropped onto the limb, the weak extensors allow the pelvis to fall forward, and the trunk follows when either spine mobility or control is insufficient to provide compensatory lumbar lordosis. Postural lengthening of the muscle fibers provides the strength needed to stabilize this forward position. This represents an extensor lag of the hip muscles. As the limb advances beyond vertical in late mid stance, passive extension removes the stimulus for a forward lean.

Hip flexion contractures without compensatory lordosis result in a forward lean of the trunk during mid stance, terminal stance and pre-swing (Figure 14.17).

Phasing of Forward Lean

Loading response has two causes for a forward trunk lean. The most common stimulus is quadriceps muscle inadequacy of any magnitude, as this is a phase of high demand. Deliberate reduction of quadriceps action to protect the anterior cruciate ligament is more subtle use of a forward trunk lean. Mild hip extensor weakness will create an extensor lag that is reflected as a forward lean at this time.

Mid Stance and Terminal Stance. Ankle plantar flexion becomes a third potential cause in addition to the continuation of the loading response mechanisms. Residuals from hip or knee extensor weakness should have decreased, though a few patients fail to assume the optimally efficient posture. With the onset of pre-swing, the transfer of body weight to the other limb terminates the mechanisms, inducing forward trunk lean. Consequently, unless there are similar problems in the contralateral limb, the trunk resumes its upright posture.

Lateral Lean

The trunk may fall or be deliberately displaced toward the same (ipsilateral) or opposite (contralateral) side. One also may refer to the direction of trunk

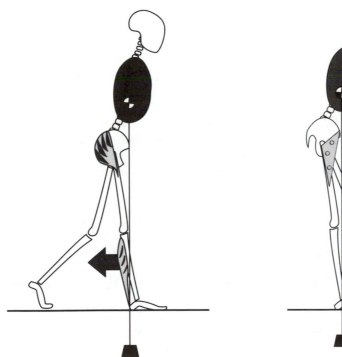

Figure 14.16 Trunk forward lean compensates for quadriceps weakness by moving vector anterior to knee. Tibia is actively retracted (arrow) by soleus.

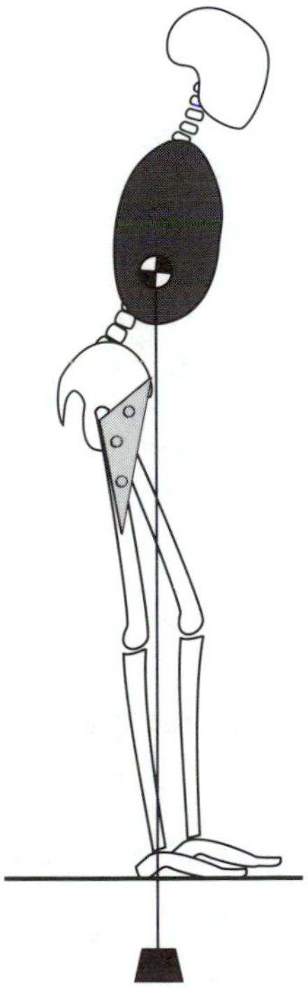

Figure 14.17 Trunk forward lean follows the anterior pelvic tilt created by a rigid hip flexion contracture. Ankle plantar flexion allows C/G to remain over the foot.

displacement as right and left, but this is not recommended, since the functional significance is obscured. Lateral deviation of the trunk in either direction may also occur in either stance or swing, though most causes relate to standing stability.

Causes of Lateral Trunk Lean

Ipsilateral Trunk Lean. Moving the trunk toward the stance limb is a deliberate action. In contrast, ipsilateral trunk lean in swing is incompatible with stability. Thus, it occurs only with the attempted first step. Lateral fall of the trunk toward the limb being lifted for swing represents failure to accommodate for the lack of limb support.

Causes of Ipsilateral Trunk Lean

Weak Hip Abductors. Shifting the trunk toward the supporting limb in stance to restore balance is a useful substitute for inadequate hip abductors. This is a deliberate action that reduces the adduction torque created by the trunk mass (Figure 14.18). Body weight is moved toward the center of the hip joint. Substitutive ipsilateral trunk lean begins with the loading response and persists through terminal stance. The amount of lateral lean varies with the weakness of the hip musculature.

Contracture. Two types of contractures can cause ipsilateral trunk lean. Adductor muscle contracture has the same effect as weak hip abductors. By pulling the pelvis down, the tight adductors move the body C/G away from the stance limb. To correct this imbalance, the trunk leans toward the stance limb (Figure 14.19).

Contracture of the lateral hip structures, most commonly a tight iliotibial band (ITB), move the stance limb away from the midline. Now the trunk leans to that side to place the C/G closer to the area of support. As the ITB also has a flexor component, the resulting trunk posture tends to be a mixture of forward and lateral lean (Figure 14.20).

Short Limb. Inadequate leg length by itself is seldom a cause of lateral trunk lean, unless it is marked, that is, $1^1/2$ inches or greater. The influence of a short limb becomes more severe when accompanied by a lateral contracture.

Scoliosis. Spinal curves that displace the upper trunk lateral to the midline create a static form of lateral trunk lean.

Impaired Body Image. In swing, fall of the trunk toward the limb being lifted (Figure 14.21) can occur when the patient is indifferent to not having that half of his body supported. Hemiplegic patients with an impaired body image are unaware of the location of their body weight line. Having no sense of instability, they fail to make any postural adaptations. The resulting imbalance is incompatible with walking.

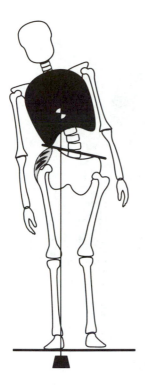

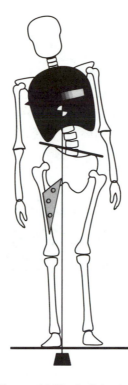

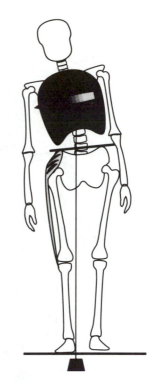

Figure 14.18 Ipsilateral trunk lean moves C/G close to stance limb to reduce the demand on weak hip abductors.

Figure 14.19 Ipsilateral trunk lean to preserve C/G alignment when a hip adduction contracture causes a contralateral pelvic tilt.

Figure 14.20 Ipsilateral trunk lean to move C/G closer to area of support when a hip abduction contracture or tight iliotibial band displaces the foot laterally (wide stance base).

Contralateral Trunk Lean. In stance, contralateral trunk lean represents failure to compensate for a situation that threatens balance. Contralateral trunk lean in swing is a deliberate substitutive action.

Inadequate Hip Flexion for swing stimulates leaning to the opposite side as a means of raising the foot to clear the floor (Figure 14.22). The cause can be either a lack of joint mobility or hip flexor muscle weakness. Both situations would cause the lateral trunk lean to begin in initial swing and persist through mid swing. Inadequate joint mobility also introduces abnormal trunk posturing in terminal stance, while hip flexor weakness does not require a substitutive action until the onset of swing.

Excessive Trunk Rotation

Excessive and out-of-phase rotation of the trunk are identifiable gait errors, but have little functional significance other than an increase in energy cost. Most commonly, the deficit is dynamic. Rotatory scoliosis is a static cause of transverse plane malalignment of the trunk.

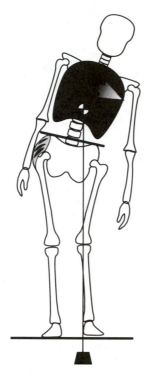

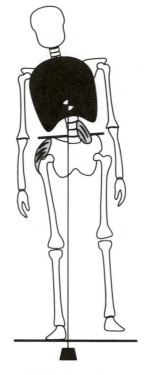

Figure 14.21 Contralateral trunk lean in stance. Trunk falls away from stance limb because the impaired body image fails to identify an unsupported swing side. This is incompatible with walking.

Figure 14.22 Contralateral trunk lean in swing as a voluntary act to assist pelvic hiking for foot clearance.

Dynamic Causes of Excessive Trunk Rotation

Synergy With the Pelvis. The trunk may accompany the pelvis as it follows the swing limb, rather than providing the normal counterbalance in the opposite direction. This results in excessive (and out-of-phase) forward rotation of the ipsilateral side of the trunk during mid and terminal swing. If the response is bilateral during stance, the trunk will move into excessive backward rotation by terminal stance.

Walking Aid Synergy. Trunk rotation may accompany the walking aid. In persons relying on a single walking aid, the trunk may follow the crutch or cane. The pattern of rotation varies depending on the location of the walking aid. When the support is ipsilateral, as for a painful knee, the cane (or crutch) follows the limb. This results in contrary phasing with excessive forward rotation at initial contact and peak backward rotation in pre-swing. Contralateral use of the walking aid, as is the practice with hip pathology, results in normal phasing of the rotation but with an increased range. Now, at initial contact the trunk displays excessive backward rotation. By terminal stance, there is excessive forward rotation.

Arm Swing Synergy. Normal phasing of trunk rotation occurs, but it can become excessive as exaggerated arm motion is used to assist balance. The pattern of motion is similar to that of single contralateral cane use.

Reference

1. Mundale MO, Hislop HJ, Robideau RJ, Kottke FS: Evaluation of extension of the hip. *Arch Phys Med Rehabil* 37(2):75-80, 1956.

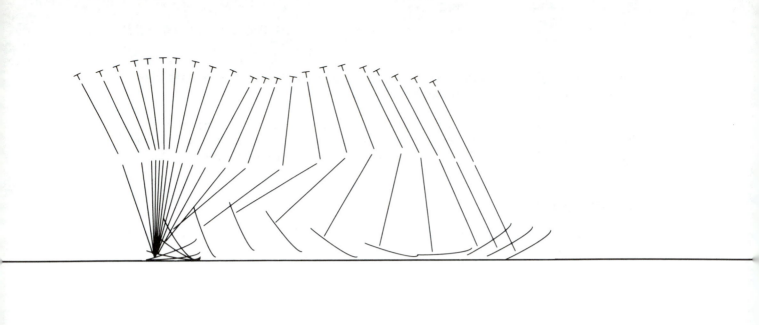

Chapter 15

Clinical Examples

In the first sections of this book, diagrams were used to illustrate the events that occur during normal and pathological gait for the purpose of isolating and emphasizing the action of the numerous joints and muscles. The purpose of this third section is to provide a clinical bridge with the diagrammatic information by presenting a series of characteristic examples. While representative situations have been selected, the reader must be fully aware that each patient has a unique mixture of pathology, normalcy and substitutive capability. The examples are not models from which one can make general conclusions for all patients with that particular diagnosis. Instead, these clinical examples should be used as guidelines for interpreting the abnormal actions identified by the gait analysis. As the basic clinical technic is observational analysis, the gait patterns are described first by this technic. Then, as available, laboratory data are used to clarify and quantitate the gait deviations seen. Varying with the complexity of the problem, motion has been recorded either with electrogoniometers or an automated, Vicon™, multiple video camera system. Muscle action was documented by dynamic electromyography, using wire electrodes.

Contracture

The primary functional impairment imposed by the loss of joint mobility from contractures is restraint of progression. During stance, patients either are delayed or inhibited from advancing over the supporting foot. In swing, inhibition of floor clearance or reach is the deterrent to normal progression. When patients are neurologically intact, as is true of the examples selected, they have both the proprioceptive feedback and the selective control to substitute.

Ankle Plantar Flexion (Trauma)

Contracture of the fibrous tissue in the muscles or capsule that cross the ankle posteriorly is common in patients subjected to a lengthy period of non-weight bearing (bed, chair or plaster cast). Accompanying most disability is a significant interval of inactivity. Failure to mobilize the tissues leads to contracture. At the ankle, this occurs in about 15° plantar flexion, because that is the joint's natural resting position.

During normal walking, 10° dorsiflexion is used to roll over one's forefoot for a full stride in terminal stance. The difference between normal mobility and a 15° PF contracture is a 25° functional deficit. As a plantar flexion contracture seldom is an isolated event, the functional significance of the lost mobility is masked in most patients by their more prominent primary pathology of paralysis or arthritis.

Patient A. To demonstrate the effects on walking when an ankle lacks dorsiflexion above 15° PF a patient with no additional pathology has been selected (Figure 15.1). The diagnosis is delayed healing of a complicated tibial shaft fracture, which necessitated prolonged non-weight bearing immobilization in a cast. Most of his gait deviations occur during the stance phases. Throughout swing, only the mid swing phase is functionally significant.

Initial contact is made with a *low heel strike*. Despite the 15° PF ankle posture, the heel is the first portion of the foot to reach the floor, because the foot has been sufficiently tilted upward by the normal 30° hip flexion and full knee extension (Figure 15.1a). Without close observation (eye or instrument), this gait error would be overlooked. As the limb is loaded, there will be only a brief *heel-only* support period available, because the forefoot is close to the floor at the time of initial contact. This limits the heel rocker stimulus to flex the knee for shock absorption.

Progression across the supporting foot causes premature loading of the forefoot. At the onset of mid stance, the tibia is more posterior than normal, and tibial advancement is inhibited by the lack of ankle rocker mobility

(Figure 15.1b). Advancement of the body mass results in increased metatarsal head pressure against the floor. Guarding of the forefoot from excessive pressure is evidenced by the plantar flexed position of the clawed toes. In terminal stance, the excessive heel rise (Figure 15.1c) shows that this patient has the substitutive ability to roll up onto his forefoot because he is healthy, strong and vigorous. Rolling onto the forefoot without the usual ankle dorsiflexion range reflects considerable propulsive energy by the trunk and hip extensors. The high heel rise, while not a conspicuous deviation, is significant evidence of greater metatarsal head strain from prolonged weight bearing.

The natural toe down (equinus) posture of the foot in pre-swing and initial swing masks the patients contracture (Figure 15.1d). The potential delay in knee flexion has been overcome by selective action of the hip and knee flexor muscles. In mid swing, however, the vertical tibia exposes the fixed plantar flexion (Figure 15.1e). Toe drag is avoided by the substitution of excessive hip and knee flexion to lift the plantar flexed foot higher than normal.

Thus, there are three major functional penalties from an isolated ankle plantar flexion contracture. The heel rocker is reduced by the early forefoot floor contact. This decreases the momentum for progression and the knee flexion contribution to shock absorption. Premature loading of the forefoot and the early heel rise in mid stance increases the duration of pressure on the metatarsal heads with corresponding tissue strain. Forward progression over the foot is delayed, as the only fulcrum for tibial advancement becomes the metatarsal heads, instead of also using the ankle joint. Consequently, the body must be lifted as well as rotated forward over the forefoot rocker. This added resistance retards tibial advancement while the femur rolls forward at the knee, creating a relative hyperextension torque that locks the knee. The limb must be unloaded in the pre-swing double support period to unlock the knee for swing. As running does not have a double support period, this otherwise vigorous man cannot run. In swing, the increased demand is greater hip flexion to lift the foot. While most conspicuous, the mid swing gait deviation usually has little functional significance, since increasing hip flexion is an easy task for most patients.

Knee Flexion (Degenerative Arthritis)

As the joint surfaces and underlying bone deteriorate, deformities develop. Increasing angulation of the joint's weight-bearing alignment not only adds to the severity of the deforming forces but it also imposes greater demands on the supporting muscles.

Patient B. At the knee, the most common problems related to degenerative arthritis are varus and flexion. Weight bearing with a knee flexion deformity increases the demand on the quadriceps for stance stability.[2,9] Sagittal plane vector analysis shows that the patient uses a forward trunk lean to move the body vector anterior to the knee joint axis to decrease the necessary quadriceps action (and associated joint force) (Figure 15.2a). This posture, however,

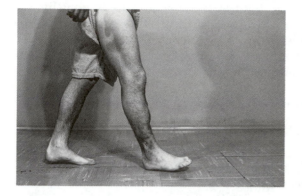

Figure 15.1 Patient A: Ankle plantar flexion contracture.
Figure 15.1a Initial contact with a low heel strike.

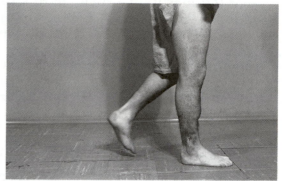

Figure 15.1b Mid stance posture showing excessive ankle plantar flexion.

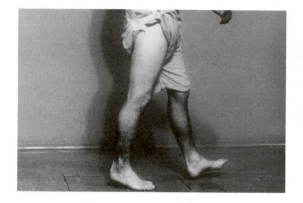

Figure 15.1c Terminal stance displays excessive heel rise.

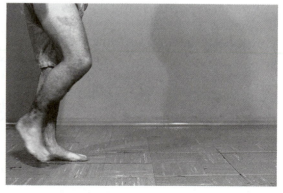

Figure 15.1d Initial swing limb alignment obscures the excessive ankle plantar flexion.

imposes a greater flexor torque at the ankle and hip. Consequently, the extensor muscles (soleus and gluteus maximus) have an increased load.

Coronal plane vector analysis demonstrates an excessive medial torque (Figure 15.2b). This creates a self-perpetuating deformity, as the progressive bone loss is greatest in the areas of maximum compression (i.e., the medial condyles). No substitution is used by this patient.

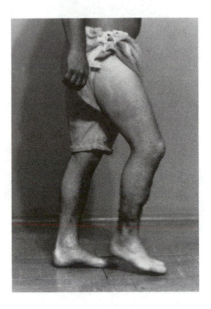

Figure 15.1e Mid swing use of excessive hip and knee flexion to avoid the toe drag from excessive ankle plantar flexion.

Hip Flexion (Burns)

Contractures at the hip severely limit the patient's progressional capability, even when there is normal neurological control. A secondary reaction is the development of knee flexion contractures due to the constant posturing of the femur. Step length is significantly shortened by the inability to extend the limbs in terminal stance and terminal swing. Weight-bearing muscular effort is also increased.

Patient C. A child, disabled by extensive burns on both lower extremities, is one example. The lengthy immobilization needed to regain adequate skin coverage led to fibrous rigidity. The 30° flexion contractures at the hips and knees reflect the natural resting positions of these joints (Figures 10.7, 10.8). Ankle dorsiflexion to approximately 5° has been preserved.

Advancement of the body over the foot in mid stance is severely restricted. While the tibia reaches a vertical position, fixed knee flexion restrains the thigh (Figure 15.3a). To accommodate the excessive knee flexion, the ankle would need to be excessively dorsiflexed. As this mobility is lacking, the junction of pelvis and thighs remains behind the supporting foot. Excessive hip flexion and forward lean of the trunk are required to place the body vector over the

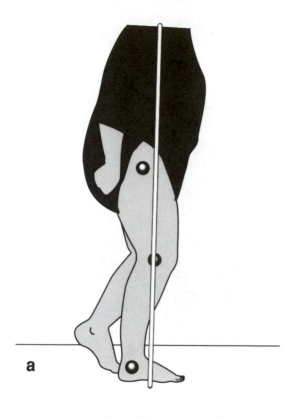

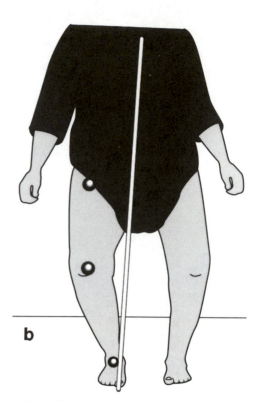

a

b

Figure 15.2 .Patient B: Knee deformity (Degenerative arthritis).
Figure 15.2a Forward trunk lean moves the vector anterior to the flexed knee, lessening the demand on the quadriceps.

Figure 15.2b Varus (excessive adduction) deformity with a marked medial vector.

supporting foot for weight-bearing balance. The flexed knee posture also increases the demand on the quadriceps.

Inability to extend the hip and knee in terminal stance prevents effective advancement of the body weight ahead of the supporting foot (Figure 15.3b). The flexed hip does not allow the limb to assume a trailing position. Step length is severely shortened by the inability to advance the pelvis beyond the supporting foot. In terminal swing, the patient lacks knee extension for a significant forward reach of the limb (Figure 15.3b, left leg).

Having a bilateral disability, the patient has minimal ability to substitute. Consequently, the residual deformities have severely limited the patient's walking ability. Shortened stride lengths necessitate a corresponding increase in step rate to accomplish the desired distance.

Weakness

Loss of muscle strength limits both progression and weight-bearing stability. The ability to substitute is dependent on the balance of muscle strength within the

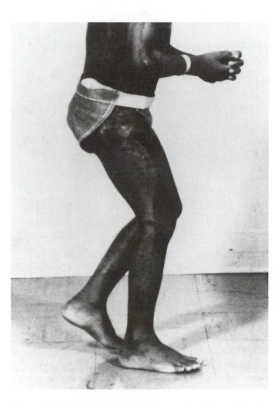 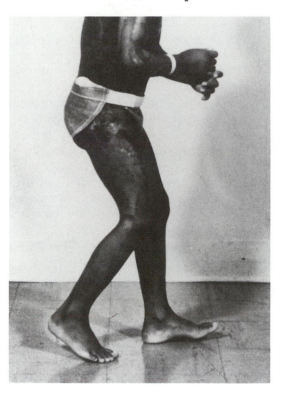

Figure 15.3 Patient C:Hip flexion contractures (Burn).
Figure 15.3a Hip and knee flexion deformities have placed pelvis behind the supporting foot as excessive ankle dorsiflexion is not available.

Figure 15.3b Trailing limb posture is lost. Step length is markedly shortened.

limb and between the two limbs. Thus, bilateral impairment significantly reduces the patient's function, as the opportunity to substitute is reduced.

Muscle weakness can result from lower motor paralysis, muscle degeneration or through the inhibition of muscle action by pain.

Quadriceps Insufficiency (Poliomyelitis)

Partial or complete paralysis of the quadriceps muscle mass impairs weight-bearing stability during stance. Loading response is the phase of maximum challenge as the normal heel rocker gait pattern initiates an arc of knee flexion that requires direct quadriceps control. Effective substitutions are developed by patients with inadequate quadriceps strength and/or endurance when they also have normal selective control and proprioception. The gait mechanics of patients disabled by poliomyelitis provide clear examples how joint motion and muscle use are altered.

Poliomyelitis has no characteristic pattern of paralysis, though involvement of the quadriceps is a typical disability. The residual impairment may be minimal or complete. While the virus initially invades 95% of the motor cells, the effect is highly varied, with a recovery rate that ranges from 12% to

91%.[1] Among 2371 muscles in 203 affected limbs, Sharrad found that the residual impairment after 3 years was about equal for the 16 major muscles (5% to 7% of the total) but the ratio of paresis to paralysis differed significantly, 3.7 to 0.5.[10] For example, the quadriceps and hip abductors were most often involved, but weakness rather than complete paralysis was the more likely result. Conversely, tibialis anterior involvement was a little less frequent but generally led to complete paralysis. Major contractures occur only in the severe, totally neglected limbs. Having normal control, normal proprioception and good mobility, post-poliomyelitis patients soon learned to minimize their disability with highly selective substitutions.

Today there are two gait patterns for post-poliomyelitis quadriceps paralysis (early and late onset disability). Early, complete quadriceps paralysis most commonly was followed by the development of excessive knee hyperextension. Residual hip extensor and calf musculature are used to control the limb so the body vector remains anterior to the knee during stance (Figure 15.4). While this assures stance stability, as the knee deformity increases, there is an ever greater extensor (stretching) torque on the knee's posterior structures, as well as greater compression on the anterior margins of the joint. Pain and instability may become significant.

Recently, a late development of additional muscle weakness after years of effective function has become evident. This post-polio syndrome, as it often is called, displays more subtle gait deviations.

Patient D. This patient had early, complete quadriceps paralysis that persisted, while the gluteus maximus and soleus muscles retained useful strength (grades 3+ to 4). The knee also had a mild knee hyperextension range initially. Prolonged substitution for the absent quadriceps has resulted in excessive knee hyperextension.

Loading response knee stability is gained by the substitution of knee

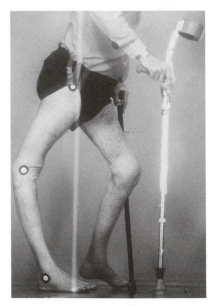

Figure 15.4 Quadriceps paralysis substitution (Poliomyelitis). Knee hyperextension for stance stability. Anterior alignment of the body vector stabilizes the knee.

hypertension for the absent quadriceps (Figure 15.5a). The flexor thrust of a heel rocker is avoided by immediate foot flat as the ankle drops into plantar flexion. Hip flexion is limited by retraction of the femur to assist knee hyperextension.

During mid and terminal stance, knee stability is maintained by a clever interplay of knee hyperextension and decreasing ankle plantar flexion while the body advances over the support foot (Figure 15.5b). The tibia is allowed to move forward by slow relative ankle dorsiflexion, which decreases the prior plantar flexion. Hip hyperextension allows the trunk to remain upright. Heel contact is maintained throughout terminal stance to preserve the hyperextension knee lock (delayed heel off). The lack of a forefoot rocker limits progression. Continuation of the same crutch position, from loading response through terminal stance, indicates the knee no longer tolerates the full body-weight requirement of single limb support.

Pre-swing double limb support with full foot contact, knee hyperextension and hip hyperextension bilaterally provides the stance stability needed for advancement of the crutches (Figure 15.5c). Heel rise (delayed heel off) and knee flexion begin only after the crutches have been advanced and body weight is on the other limb (Figure 15.5d).

Knee flexion for swing is a very deliberate act involving rapid and excessive hip flexion (Figure 15.5e). Momentum for adequate knee flexion is gained from the excessive hip flexion. In terminal swing, the lack of a functioning quadriceps prevents the patient from attaining full knee extension, despite some hip retraction (Figure 15.5f). Deceleration of the femur (with minimal loss of hip flexion) and progression of the body over the other foot have allowed tibial inertia to extend the knee. Hence, step length is preserved. The only terminal swing preparation for loading of the limb with an absent quadriceps is premature ankle plantar flexion. A comparison of the terminal swing and loading response postures (Figures 15.5b and 15.5f) shows the use of rapid thigh retraction to gain a stable hyperextended knee for weight acceptance.

Patient E. The late development of functionally significant quadriceps weakness in a knee lacking hyperextension mobility displays only a loss of the loading response flexion. Anterior joint pain is the patient's disability. Dynamically, the same mechanics to preserve knee stability are used, that is, relative hyperextension as a substitution for quadriceps weakness. The potential heel rocker is reduced, the thigh is retracted and tibial advancement is delayed.

Initial contact is made with a fully extended knee and slight ankle plantar flexion (Figure 15.6a). While floor contact is by the heel, closeness of the forefoot to the floor minimizes the potential for any heel rocker action. Loading response lacks tibial advancement. This results in the loss of all knee flexion (Figure 15.6b). In mid stance, as the limb rolls across the supporting foot, tibial advancement is slower than the femur (Figure 15.6c) to maintain full knee extension without placing a demand on the weak quadriceps. With the femur ahead of the tibia and adequate ankle stability, the knee is sufficiently locked by passive alignment for the patient to tolerate a heel rise at the end of terminal stance (Figure 15.6d). Momentum from the velocity of the opposite limb rolls body weight onto the forefoot, despite the lack of dorsiflexion beyond neutral. The resulting forefoot rocker action in

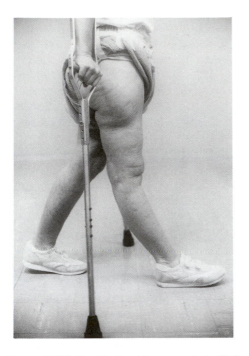

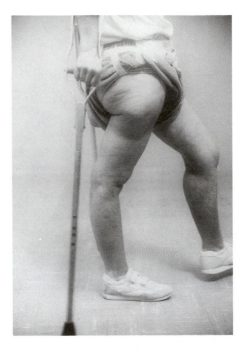

Figure 15.5 Patient D: Quadriceps paralysis (Poliomyelitis).
Figure 15.5a Loading response stance stability gained by thigh retraction, excessive plantar flexion and avoidance of a heel rocker.

Figure 15.5b Mid and terminal stance progression gained by reducing ankle plantar flexion.

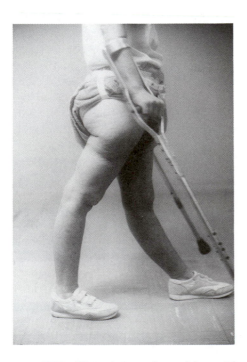

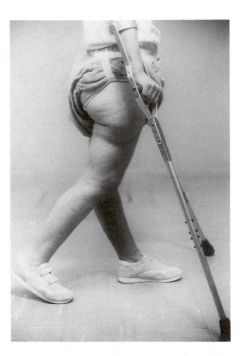

Figure 15.5c Bilateral stance is used for crutch progression. Heel contact is maintained to preserve knee hyperextension.

Figure 15.5d Pre-swing knee flexion is limited.

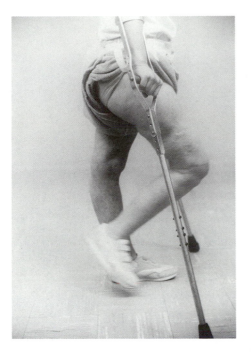 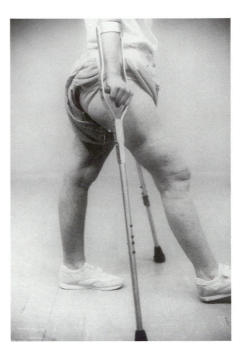

Figure 15.5e Initial swing uses excessive hip flexion to gain knee flexion for toe clearance of the floor.

Figure 15.5f Terminal swing knee extension is incomplete.

terminal stance preserves a significant portion of the patient's stride length. The postural knee lock, however, does not prepare the limb for pre-swing. Consequently, knee flexion is lacking at this time (Figure 15.6e). This is overcome in initial swing by rapid, active knee flexion for floor clearance (Figure 15.6f). The dynamic nature of this knee flexion is implied by the arc of knee motion that is much greater than that at the hip. Advancement of the limb through the rest of swing is normal (Figure 15.6g). Floor clearance in mid swing is assured by ankle dorsiflexion.

The substitutive motions identified by observation of the patient's gait are confirmed by the electrogoniometer recordings of the knee and ankle (Figure 15.6h). Ankle plantar flexion (10°) begins at the onset of terminal swing, once the mid swing need of dorsiflexion for floor clearance has passed, and is maintained through loading response. In mid and terminal stance, dorsiflexion for progression occurs slowly, not reaching neutral until the middle of the single stance period. The maximum ankle position in terminal stance is less than 5° DF. Pre-swing plantar flexion and the subsequent recovery of neutral dorsiflexion in swing follow the normal pattern.

The knee is fully extended by the end of terminal swing, and this posture (0°) is maintained throughout stance. The minor amount of hyperextension (2° or 3°) during loading response indicates inadequate dynamic stability. Pre-swing knee flexion begins slowly as the limb is unloaded, resulting in only 20° before toe off. In initial swing, the knee very rapidly flexes to 60° for floor clearance by the toe.

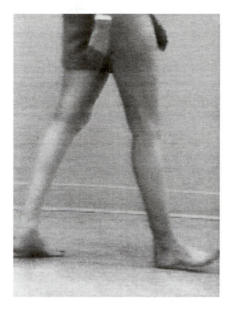

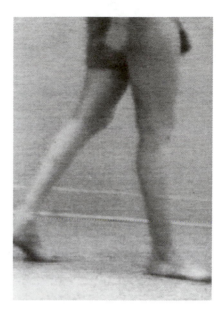

Figure 15.6 Patient E: Quadriceps weakness (Post polio).
Figure 15.6a Initial contact with a low heel strike.

Figure 15.6b Loading response with no knee flexion.

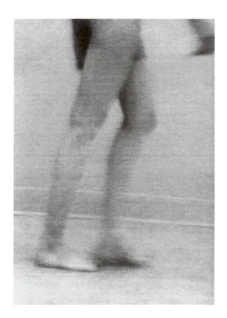

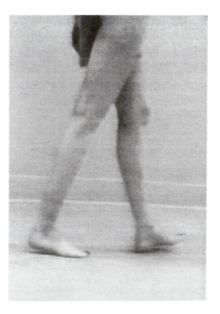

Figure 15.6c Mid stance with limited ankle dorsiflexion.

Figure 15.6d Terminal stance with a heel rise but limited ankle dorsiflexion.

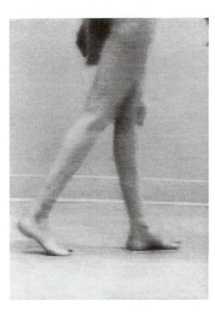

Figure 15.6e Pre-swing lacking knee flexion.

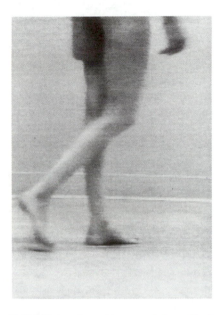

Figure 15.6f Initial swing with normal knee flexion but limited hip flexion.

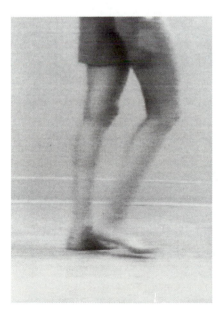

Figure 15.6g Mid swing with delayed knee extension.

Following a delay in mid swing, the knee quickly extends to neutral (0°) in terminal swing.

The foot switch record shows a normal floor contact sequence, though the time spent in each foot support mode varied among the steps. This variation is consistent with there being some joint control insecurity.

Dynamic electromyographic recordings confirm that the patient accomplishes this effective gait without relying on her easily fatigued quadriceps (Figure 15.6i). To do so, the patient significantly modifies the activity of her other limb muscles.

In terminal swing, preparation of the limb for stance begins by a premature burst of gluteus maximus action to retract the femur, so that tibial momentum extends the knee rather than the quadriceps. Assistance in limb retraction is provided by a strong burst of biceps femoris long head (BFLH) action (Figure 15.6j). This muscle, then, promptly ceases its activity with floor contact, so there will be no destabilizing knee flexor pull. At the same time, the larger semimembranosus shows only minimal activity.

For initial contact and loading response, continuing gluteus maximus action stabilizes the knee by restraining the femur. At the same time, premature and intense soleus action to restrain the tibia becomes the primary source of knee extensor stability (Figure 15.6i). This strong soleus muscle action continues through terminal stance. Assistance by gastrocnemius action is delayed until mid stance, when there is a passive extensor alignment to oppose the knee flexion potential of this muscle (Figure 15.6j). Pre-swing is a period of muscular silence. Initial swing knee flexion begins with a strong burst of out-of-phase semimembranosus action. This timing of the semimembranosus indicates that direct knee flexion for toe clearance is more critical than the loss of hip flexion for limb advancement, due to the muscle's extensor action at the hip. Slight shortening of step length is the result. Activity of the biceps femoris, short head (BFSH) assists in maintaining peak knee flexion (Figure 15.6j). With the need to start extending the knee in mid swing, BFSH ceases and there is a marked reduction in semimembranosus intensity. Joined by BFLH, the two hamstrings begin hip deceleration in preparation for stance. As identified earlier, the gluteus maximus augments this function by becoming prematurely active in terminal swing.

Thus, stance knee stability was attained without quadriceps participation by premature (really out-of-phase) gluteus maximus action, modification of the BFLH intensity pattern, premature and overly strong action of the soleus, and modified gastrocnemius intensity. Knee flexion for swing was accomplished by a phase reversal of the semimembranosus and normal BFSH action.

Hip and Knee Extensor Weakness (Muscular Dystrophy)

This combination of muscle loss limits the patient's ability to supplement the weakness with a passive stabilizing vector, as the optimum alignment for one joint contradicts the need at the other. Spontaneous primary impairment of these two muscle groups is a characteristic finding in lower limb muscular dystrophy.

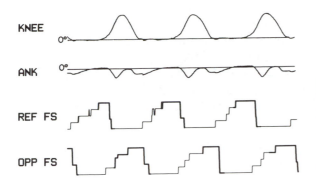

Figure 15.6h Electrogoniometric recording of knee and ankle. ANK = ankle; REF FS = foot switch trace for the reference limb; OPP FS = Foot switch trace for the opposite limb; baseline = swing; elevated segments = stance. Height of foot switch steps indicates area of contact, length of step identifies duration of that mode of contact.

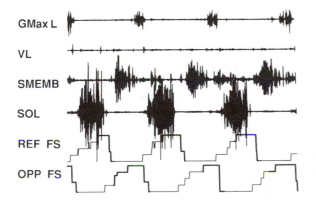

Figure 15.6i Dynamic Electromyography (raw data). GMAX L = gluteus maximus, lower; VL = vastus lateralis; SMEMB = semimembranosus; SOL = soleus.

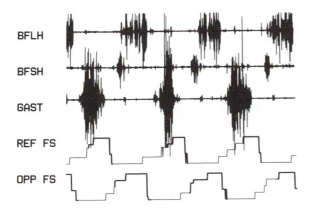

Figure 15.6j Dynamic Electromyography (raw data). BFLH = biceps femoris, long head; BFSH = biceps femoris short head; GAST = gastrocnemius.

The Duchenne type of muscular dystrophy is the most common form of this progressive muscle disease, occurring in about 85% of the patients. Characteristically, the muscle loss in the lower limbs begins at the hips and progresses to include the quadriceps and ankle dorsiflexes (tibialis anterior), and lastly, all the muscles.[7,8] As the muscle fibers degenerate, there is fibro-fatty replacement. The resulting pathology is progressive weakness and contracture formation. While some contractures provide substitutive stability, others obstruct efficient limb posturing. Foot and knee stability are helped by the fibrotic replacement of lost muscle, but there also is a strong tendency to develop excessive ankle plantar flexion, foot inversion, and flexion contractures at the hips and knees. The patient's gait reflects the functional balance between weakness and contractures. At the onset of the dysfunction, the gait changes are subtle,[11] but become very characteristic as the pathology progresses.

Patient F. Initial contact is made by the forefoot, as a result of the combination of ankle plantar flexion and mild knee flexion (Figure 15.7a). The effect of these deformities is minimized by continued good hip flexion for step length.

Loading response is characterized by a rapid reduction in hip flexion, as weakness of the hip extensor muscle does not allow weight acceptance on a flexed limb (Figure 15.7b). Hence, the loading posture shows a nearly vertical thigh (inadequate hip flexion). There also is a loss of the normal knee flexion during the loading response, as a result of the extensor thrust created by the plantar flexed ankle. This inhibition of tibial advancement protects the weak quadriceps.[11] EMG studies show premature calf muscle activity in some patients, indicating that the tibial control can be dynamic, but it doesn't occur in all.[7] Early hypertrophy of the gastrosoleus muscle group is a common finding on biopsy.[6] With further muscle loss and increased fibrosis, the resulting plantar flexion contracture becomes the more significant stabilizing mechanism.

Hyperextension of the knee is obstructed by the knee flexion contracture. The reason for this contracture has not been specifically identified by EMG analysis, but there are three possible mechanisms. Weakness of the quadriceps could lead to incomplete knee extension since twice the force is required to extend the knee to zero (0°) as is used to attain the 15° flexed position.[9] Use of the hamstrings as hip extensors to supplement the weak gluteus maximus would also cause slight flexion at the knee. Gastrocnemius contracture or its premature activity could create a knee flexion torque as the muscle is stretched at the ankle.

In mid stance, advancement of the body over the supporting foot reduces the ankle plantar flexion by stretching the elastic element of the contracture (Figure 15.7c). Continued soleus action assures the amount of tibial restraint needed to preserve knee extension.[7] Once the contracture's elasticity is exceeded, the heel rises prematurely. Hip extension stability requires an erect trunk to align the vector posterior to the joint.[11]

The terminal stance forefoot rocker available with the heel rise allows the body to roll forward and continue hip extension (Figure 15.7d). To gain a trailing posture for good step length in terminal stance, despite the presence of a slight hip flexion contracture, the pelvis is drawn into a slight anterior tilt. The continued slight knee flexion indicates a contracture or, as mentioned earlier, gastrocnemius tightness. This protects the knee from passive hyperextension. Flexibility of the posterior ankle tissues is indicated by the move toward dorsiflexion, as the forward position of body weight creates a strong stretching force. Ankle stability (and indirectly, knee stability) continues to be provided by the contracture, augmented by calf muscle action.

Limited pre-swing knee flexion is gained as a result of several factors. Passively, there is momentum to roll over the forefoot rocker, and the knee already is unlocked by its flexion contracture. Action by the gastrocnemius (visible muscle bulge) increases both ankle plantar flexion and knee flexion (Figure 15.7e). Initial swing knee flexion appears normal, though there might be a 5° increase in knee flexion to assure floor clearance with such a plantar flexed ankle (Figure 15.7f). Because of the trailing posture of the limb, the excessive ankle plantar flexion has only minimal functional significance in initial swing.

Mid swing clearly displays the excessive ankle plantar flexion. Increased hip flexion is used to gain floor clearance (Figure 15.7g). Two factors contribute to the equinus foot posture: tibialis anterior weakness and a plantar flexion contracture. Now there is no passive force to stretch the tight fibrous tissues as was present in mid stance. The relative elasticity of the contracture is readily demonstrated during quiet standing (Figure 15.7h).

Soleus and Hip Extensor Weakness (Myelodysplasia)

As a congenital form of spinal cord injury, the myelodysplastic patient's paralysis is complicated by sensory loss in addition to the muscle weakness. A high potential for contractures is another complication, for the disability is present at birth. Myelodysplasia also subjects the joints to abnormal weight-bearing postures from the onset of walking. These multiple factors significantly reduce the patient's ability to substitute.

The severity of the gait deviations increases with each higher level of paralysis. Sequentially, impaired control of the limb involves the foot musculature, hip extensors, knee extensors (quadriceps) and hip flexors.

Patient G. A major functional division is the strength of the quadriceps. Patients with a low lumbar lesion (L_4 intact) retain a strong quadriceps. This provides weight-bearing stability at the knee, but function is seriously compromised by the lack of ankle plantar flexor, hip extensor and hip abductor musculature. This paralytic pattern has a very characteristic gait.

Initial contact is made with a flexed knee and flat foot for several biomechanical reasons (Figure 15.8a). Hip flexion is excessive because of the inability of weak (or absent) hamstrings to adequately restrain the thigh in terminal swing. Lack of a forefoot rocker on the other limb has inadequately advanced the body mass. It is necessary to keep the foot within a weight-accepting range. To meet these limitations the patient is voluntarily relying on his strong quadriceps. The lack of dorsiflexor musculature allows the foot to drop into mild plantar flexion. Hence, preparation for weight acceptance is a compromise.

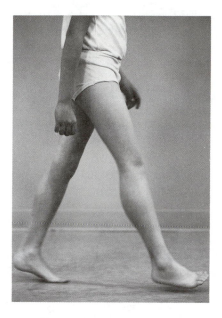

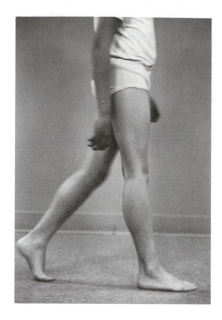

Figure 15.7 Patient F: Hip extensor weakness (Muscular dystrophy).
Figure 15.7a Initial floor contact with the forefoot.

Figure 15.7b Loading response characterized by limb retraction (reduced hip flexion, extended knee, plantar flexed ankle).

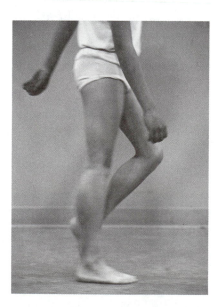

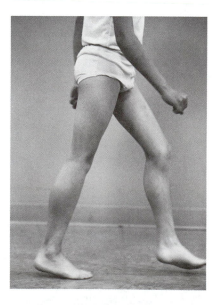

Figure 15.7c Mid stance ankle rocker limited to elasticity of the plantar flexion contracture.

Figure 15.7d Terminal stance ankle plantar flexor stability allows a forefoot rocker. This, in turn, stabilizes the knee and hip.

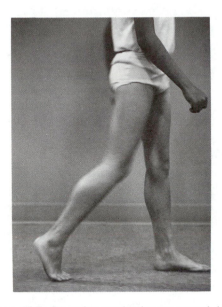

Figure 15.7e Pre-swing mechanics are normal. Knee flexion may be slightly reduced.

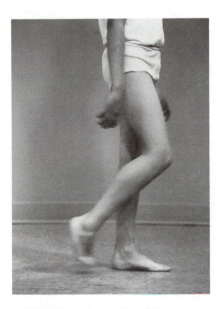

Figure 15.7f Initial swing trailing tibia posture masks the excessive ankle plantar flexion. Floor clearance is accomplished by the knee flexion.

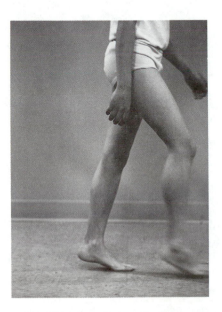

Figure 15.7g Mid swing displays the excessive ankle plantar flexion because the tibia is vertical. Toe clearance gained by excessive hip and knee flexion.

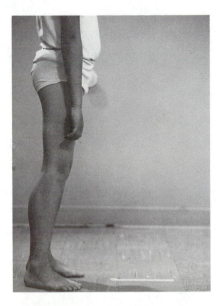

Figure 15.7h Standing posture is well balanced because the ankle plantar flexion contracture is stretched by the dorsiflexion body weight vector.

Loading the limb increases both knee and hip flexion, while ankle plantar flexion only slightly decreases (Figure 15.8b). This limb posture represents slight collapse, because the paralyzed gluteus maximus cannot stabilize the femur. Any substitutive hip extensor action by the hamstrings merely adds to the knee flexion. The markedly flexed posture at the knee presents a very strong demand on the quadriceps to preserve weight-bearing stability.

Mid stance advancement of the body onto the supporting limb leads to excessive ankle dorsiflexion and persistent knee flexion (Figure 15.8c). The lack of tibial control at the ankle moves the knee joint more anterior to the body vector, increasing the demand on the quadriceps. The patient cannot reduce this strain by leaning forward, since this would increase both the dorsiflexion demand at the ankle and introduce a flexor torque at the hip and spine. Increased action by the quadriceps is the only source of knee stability, because it is the sole weight-bearing muscle group. Terminal stance involves further advancement of body weight over the foot, while the trunk remains erect to provide passive hip extensor stability (Figure 15.8d). Ankle dorsiflexion becomes extreme and knee flexion increases. Thus, postural relief for the quadriceps by moving the vector anteriorly is not available to this patient. Stride length is gained by using total body rotation to add pelvic width to the distance between the two feet (Figure 15.8e). During pre-swing, heel contact continues until the limb is lifted for swing. In mid swing, excessive hip flexion

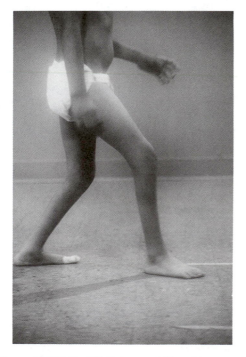

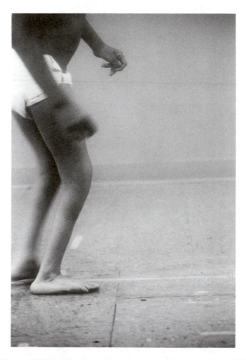

Figure 15.8 Patient G: Soleus and hip extensor weakness (L$_4$ Myelodysplasia).
Figure 15.8a Initial contact by the forefoot with excessive knee and hip flexion.

Figure 15.8b Loading response showing increased hip and knee flexion, the ankle is slightly less plantar flexed.

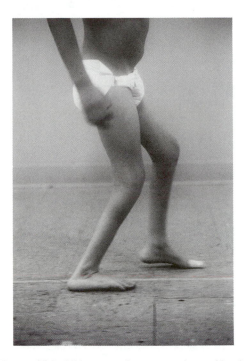

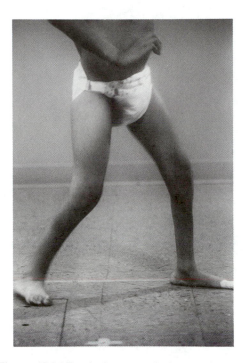

Figure 15.8c Mid stance has excessive ankle dorsiflexion and continued knee flexion.

Figure 15.8d Terminal stance displays extreme dorsiflexion and additional knee flexion as the body approaches the anterior margin of the supporting foot.

is required both to accommodate the drop foot and the lower pelvic position created by the contralateral knee flexion (Figure 15.8f).

Soleus Weakness (Rheumatoid Arthritis)

Loss of muscle strength is much greater in rheumatoid arthritis than degenerative arthritis. A major factor is the pain induced by the inflammatory nature of the rheumatoid pathology. Pain is an inhibitor of muscle action. The inhibition reflex relieves pain by reducing the muscle force crossing the joint. Motion also is decreased. The secondary effect of this enforced inactivity is the development of significant disuse muscle weakness. During gait, the postural strain imposed on the muscles can be visualized by vector analysis.

Patient H. An obscure but very significant factor that limits the walking ability of persons disabled by rheumatoid arthritis is calf muscle weakness. This patient also has a mild (10°) knee flexion contracture.

Loading the limb with the knee flexed induces a challenging torque to a quadriceps with only borderline (grade 3+) strength. The flexion places the body weight vector posterior to the knee joint axis (Figure 15.9a). The patient is able to meet the resulting flexor demand through two mechanisms. As the flexion contracture is less than 15°, the quadriceps has a favorable moment arm

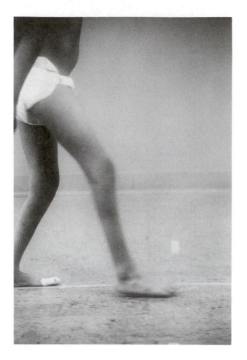

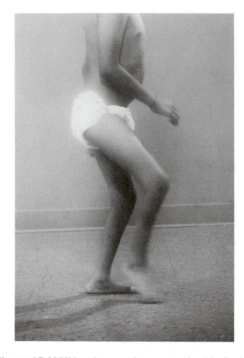

Figure 15.8e Pre-swing double limb support displays the amount of total body rotation use to gain step length.

Figure 15.8f Mid swing requires excessive hip flexion to lift the plantar flexed foot clear of the floor.

that makes this demand no greater than would be experienced with a 5° position.[9] Also, dynamic flexion at the knee is minimized by the short step, which allows almost vertical loading of the limb and flat foot contact. There is no heel rocker to accelerate knee flexion. Vertical leg alignment also allows the weak calf muscles to stabilize the tibia for optimum quadriceps action without the challenge of a dorsiflexion torque.

Progression of the body over the supporting foot in mid stance increases both ankle dorsiflexion and knee flexion (Figure 15.9b). The cause is inability of the weak plantar flexor muscle mass (grade 2) to oppose the resulting dorsiflexion torque. Soleus and gastrocnemius activity has been inhibited by metatarsal joint arthritis, which makes the forefoot intolerant of full weight bearing. Persistent quadriceps action provides the necessary knee stability. In terminal stance, further advancement of the body vector to the midfoot reduces knee flexion with a minimal increase in ankle dorsiflexion (Figure 15.9c). The newly acquired tibial stability reflects passive tension of the gastrosoleus as the ankle reaches the limit of its dorsiflexion range. Relative extension of the knee occurs as the femur advances more than the tibia. This moves the vector closer to the knee and reduces the demand on the quadriceps. The patient, however, has insufficient strength to roll onto the metatarsal head for a forefoot rocker. Advancing the vector to the forefoot would lengthen the dorsiflexion lever arm beyond that which the weak calf muscles could control. Continued foot flat

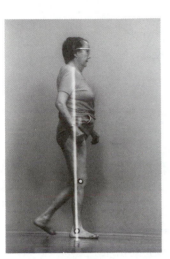

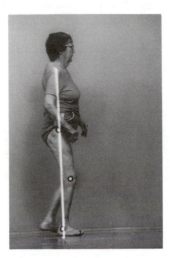

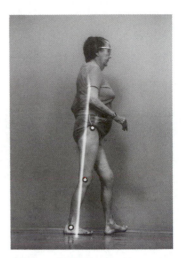

Figure 15.9 Patient H: Soleus weakness (Rheumatoid Arthritis). **Figure 15.9a** Loading response with the vector posterior to the flexed knee and at the axis of ankle. Vertical line = the body weight vector.

Figure 15.9b Early mid stance showing increased knee flexion displaces the joint axis more anterior to the vector. Vertical line = the body weight vector.

Figure 15.9c Terminal stance with the base of the vector at mid foot, anterior to the dorsiflexed ankle and slightly posterior to the knee. Vertical line = the body weight vector.

contact also reduces the weight applied to the painful metatarsal heads. Pre-swing knee flexion is lacking, because there is no forefoot rocker to advance the tibia ahead of the vector (Figure 15.9d). Instead, heel rise is delayed until most of body weight has been transferred to the other limb. The sum of these factors is a very short step.

Initial swing knee flexion is a deliberate act that lifts the tibia more than the hip flexes (Figure 15.9e). Ankle dorsiflexion to neutral assists floor clearance. Mid swing advancement of the limb also is aided by the early ankle dorsiflexion while the hip flexors pull the femur forward (Figure 15.9f).

Tibialis Anterior Weakness (Spinal Cord Injury, Cauda Equina)

Fractures within the lumbar vertebrae are below the spinal cord per se, but may involve the mass of roots lying within the spinal canal called the cauda equina. Injuries to these roots cause lower motor neuron (flaccid) paralysis. The functional impairment varies among patients according to the completeness of the root damage.

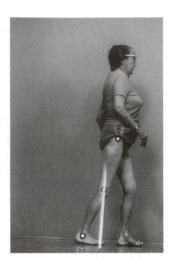

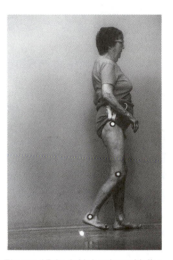

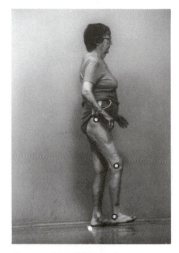

Figure 15.9d Pre-swing includes a limited heel rise with the ankle dorsiflexed and inadequate knee flexion. The low level of the vector indicates only partial weight bearing. Vertical line = the body weight vector.

Figure 15.9e Initial swing with limited knee flexion and excessive ankle dorsiflexion.

Figure 15.9f Mid swing with excessive ankle dorsiflexion limiting the amount of hip and knee flexion needed for floor clearance.

While similar, the impairment seen in cauda equina spinal cord injury (SCI) patients differs from that occurring with myelodysplasia, as there is less anatomical consistency in the lesions. The SCI disability also differs from poliomyelitis by the presence of sensory, particularly, proprioceptive impairment in patients. This varies markedly among patients. Often the residual sensation does not correlate with the level of motor impairment, as the anterior location of the vertebral fracture may spare the posterior rami.

Patient I. A mid lumbar neurological lesion has caused complete paralysis of the tibialis anterior and other ankle muscles as well as the knee flexors, hip extensors and abductors. The quadriceps muscle group has grade 3+ strength. Sensation is intact at the knees, but impaired at the feet.

Terminal swing preparation of the limb for stance is incomplete because there is marked ankle plantar flexion (Figure 15.10a). Initial contact will be made with the forefoot. The dorsiflexion advancement of the tibia in mid and terminal stance reveals the passive nature of the terminal swing equinus, that is, tibialis anterior paralysis rather than a contracture (Figure 15.10b). There is however, a useful degree of ankle plantar flexion contracture to provide weight-bearing limb stability by slight knee hyperextension. Passive tension on the contracture restrains the tibia at 5° DF while the femur rolls forward and hyperextends the knee. Alignment of the body weight line (trunk center to mid foot) provides an extensor torque to supplement the weak quadriceps. There is continual weight bearing on the arms as a substitution for the paralyzed hip extensor and abductor muscles. A functional compromise between progression and stability is gained by the plantar flexion contracture stretching to 5° dorsiflexion with the advancement of the body vector.

Initial swing is delayed by a passive drop foot (absent tibialis anterior) and the lack of active knee flexion (Figure 15.10c). Preparing the limb for swing is a deliberate process that includes transferring a major portion of body weight onto the crutches through the arms. Elevation of the shoulders is a sign of intense weight bearing. Advancement of the limb for swing depends on direct hip flexor action. Mid swing floor clearance requires excessive hip flexion to accommodate the passive drop foot (Figure 15.10b, left leg).

Hip Abductor Weakness

Gluteus medius muscle weakness occurs in many types of pathology. Ipsilateral lateral trunk lean in the coronal plane is used to stabilize the hip. The mobility developed by patients who experienced their acute poliomyelitis in childhood allows the greatest freedom to use this substitution. Complete abductor muscle paralysis can be fully accommodated by shifting the trunk laterally until the body vector lies over the hip joint (Figure 15.11). A secondary effect of that posture is valgus of the knee as a result of the laterally displaced weight line.

Adult onset hip abductor incompetence, such as occurs with rheumatoid arthritis, allows lesser degrees of lateral trunk lean. Again, the knee experiences a valgus thrust (Figure 15.12).

Below Knee Amputation

Amputations cause a loss of limb length, normal joint mobility, direct muscular control and local proprioception, particularly, the precise awareness of foot contact on the floor. Modern prosthetic design has made major strides in replacing these deficits, yet the gait of the amputee still is less than normal.

Patient J. A below knee prosthesis has the potential for optimum function, as the patient has retained normal hip and knee control, and there is adequate prosthetic length to incorporate one of the new dynamic elastic response feet. These feet (of which there are several designs) provide controlled mobility at the ankle area. The experienced walker in Figure 15.13 is currently using a Quantum™ foot.

Initial contact is made by the heel with the limb normally postured (Figure 15.13a). Loading response displays excessive knee flexion, a vertical tibia and the ankle at neutral dorsiflexion. Hip flexion is maintained (Figure 15.13b). This loading pattern implies excessive heel rocker action. While prosthetic feet have

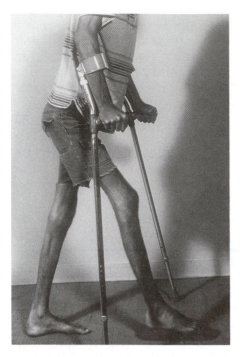

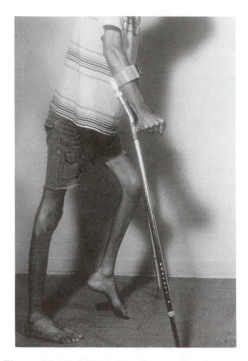

Figure 15.10 Patient I: Anterior tibialis paralysis (spinal cord injury, cauda equina).
Figure 15.10a Terminal swing with excessive ankle plantar flexion and inadequate knee extension.

Figure 15.10b Mid stance shows mild ankle plantar flexion and knee hyperextension.

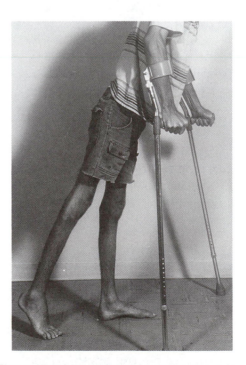

Figure 15.10c Pre-swing with a severe drop foot and no knee flexion to prepare for floor clearance.

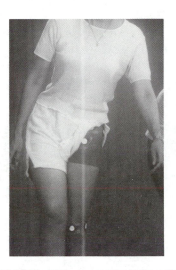

Figure 15.11 Hip abductor paralysis limp (Poliomyelitis). Lateral trunk lean for abductor muscle loss. The body vector passes through the hip joint. Vertical line = body weight vector.

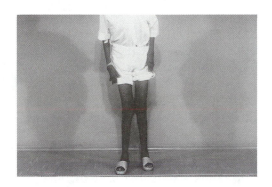

Figure 15.12 Hip abductor paralysis limp (Rheumatoid arthritis). Lateral trunk lean for gluteus medius inadequacy.

a cushioned heel to reduce loading impact, the one this patient is wearing appears not to have decreased the heel rocker by simulated ankle plantar flexion. The resulting knee flexion presents an increased demand on the quadriceps. In the middle of mid stance, the ankle is in slight dorsiflexion while both the knee and hip are minimally flexed (Figure 15.13c). The trunk is over the mid foot, and the other foot is slightly trailing. Terminal stance has a normal heel rise, further ankle dorsiflexion, full knee extension and a trailing thigh position (Figure 15.13d). Hence, there is good prosthetic tibial control to provide an extended knee. At the same time, the prosthetic ankle is yielding for optimum progression and step length. By the end of pre-swing, the knee has normal flexion, although the thigh has not advanced enough to attain a fully vertical position (Figure 15.13e). This implies direct knee flexor action as a supplement to a limited prosthetic forefoot rocker.

Motion analysis shows a relatively normal pattern at each joint (Figure 15.13f). The ankle, beginning in neutral alignment at initial contact, plantar flexes approximately 10° in loading response. From this position, the change toward dorsiflexion is initially abrupt, but then slows during mid stance, followed by accelerated dorsiflexion in terminal stance to 20°. Throughout swing, the ankle is at neutral (0°). The knee advances from full extension (0°) at initial contact to 20° flexion by 18% GC. This is followed by progressive extension, reaching 4° hyperextension at 40% GC. There then is a sharp reversal into flexion during the last portion of terminal stance, which continues through pre-swing and initial swing. The timing of peak knee flexion is normal (72% GC), but the magnitude is excessive (73°). Extension of the knee reaches 2° hyperextension just before initial contact (95% GC). The thigh has an early onset of progressive extension during the loading response, but does not exceed the 20° hyperextension in terminal stance. Subsequent thigh flexion follows the normal pattern, reaching 25° in mid swing.

Electromyographic recordings of his key muscles show an increase in intensity and some prolongation of action. At the hip, the gluteus maximus (GMax) intensity is prematurely high, as its activity accompanies a vigorous semimembranosus (SMEMB) (Figures 15.13g and 15.13h). Biceps femoris long head (BFLH) has prolonged action. This muscle pattern implies a strong thigh retraction effort that is consistent with the full knee extension in terminal swing and the early reduction of thigh flexion in loading response. Prolongation of strong quadriceps action (VL) is appropriate for the sustained knee flexion displayed in his motion graphs (Figure 15.13i). The brief period of rectus femoris action at the terminal stance/pre-swing junction is decelerating the overly rapid knee flexion that accompanies the accelerated ankle dorsiflexion and heel-off.

The patient's gait velocity is normal (93m/min). His foot switch pattern shows rapid progression from the heel (H), across a brief foot flat interval (H-5), onto sustained heel-off support (5-1). Thus, this physically fit man has attained a gait that closely mimics normal function by modifying his muscle action to compensate for the small abnormalities in prosthetic function.

Muscle Weakness Summary

The patients selected to illustrate the effects of muscle weakness represent the functional differences between the three major weight-bearing muscle groups.

In the poliomyelitis patients, quadriceps paralysis was the major impairment. Passive knee hyperextension or its equivalent mechanism provided good weight-bearing stability. Limb posturing depended on adequate hip extensor control of the femur and calf control of the tibia. Also, there were no impeding contractures.

The patient with myelodysplasia had the reverse impairment. The quadriceps was his strongest muscle. Protective posturing was not available. Hence, the quadriceps muscle of this patient is a prime candidate to wear out from overuse by early adulthood.

A less severe state of calf muscle insufficiency was presented by the patient with rheumatoid arthritis. Limited hip extensor musculature is still available to stabilize the thigh as means of reducing the increased quadriceps demand imposed by the weak gastrosoleus muscles.

Hip extensor and quadriceps weakness, knee flexion contracture and a strong ankle plantar flexor mass (muscle plus contracture) characterized the muscular dystrophy patient. As with the polio patient, quadriceps weakness was well accommodated by dynamic substitutions, but the knee flexion

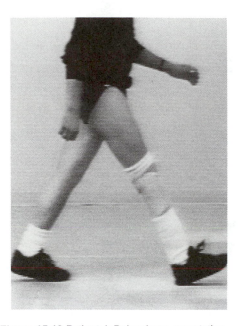

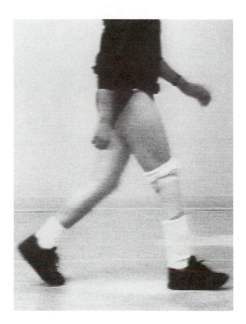

Figure 15.13 Patient J: Below knee amputation.
Figure 15.13a Initial contact with normal limb alignment.

Figure 15.13b Loading response with excessive knee flexion and excessive ankle dorsiflexion.

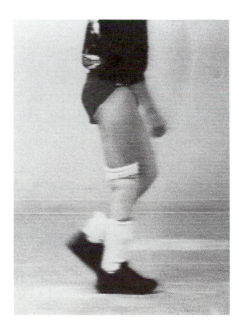

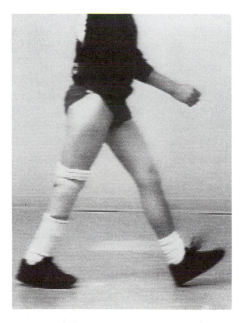

Figure 15.13c Mid stance with slight flexion at the knee and hip and ankle dorsiflexion.

Figure 15.13d Terminal stance with a low heel rise and excessive ankle dorsiflexion provide good progression.

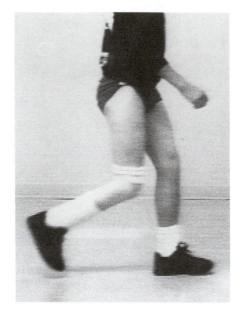

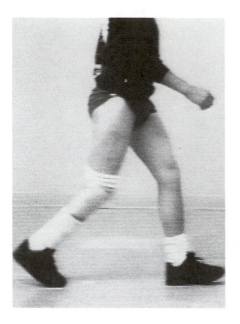

Figure 15.13e Pre-swing thigh advancement and ankle plantar flexion are less than normal, yet there is adequate knee flexion. This implies increased knee flexor muscle action.

Figure 15.13f Initial swing showing normal knee flexion but limited thigh advancement.

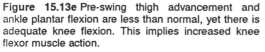

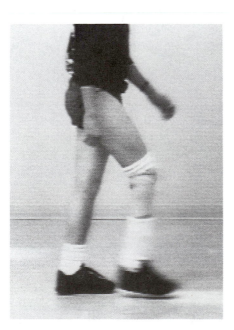

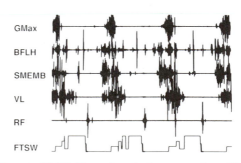

Figure 15.13h Dynamic electromyography. GMax = Gluteus maximus; BFLH = Biceps femoris long head; SMEMB = Semimembranosis; VL = Vastus longus (quadriceps); RF = rectus femoris; FTSW = foot switches.

Figure 15.13g Mid swing elevation of the foot is slightly excessive.

MOTION ANALYSIS
Pathokinesiology Service   Rancho Los Amigos Medical Center

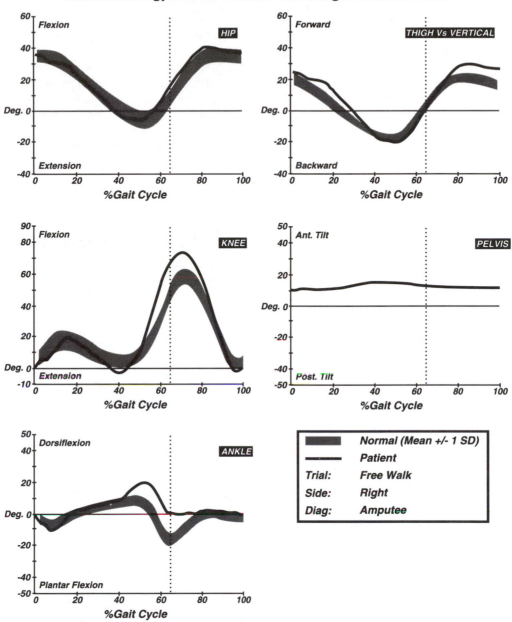

Figure 15.13i Motion analysis. The vertical axis is degrees of motion (flexion is positive). The horizontal axis is the percents of the gait cycle. The vertical dotted line divides stance and swing (toe-off). Gray areas indicate the 1 standard deviation band of normal function. Black line is patient data.

contracture limited the effectiveness of these secondary actions.

The amputee displayed a strong quadriceps, being capable of accepting the added loading torque imposed by the limited mobility of the prosthetic foot. During the rest of stance, however, the quadriceps was protected by the tibial stability offered by the dynamic elasticity of the prosthetic ankle.

Control Dysfunction

The control deficits resulting from a stroke, head trauma, high spinal cord injury or cerebral palsy may cause a variety of gait deviations. While all patients exhibit the increased reflexes of spastic paralysis, the severity may range from mild to severe. A more subtle, yet profound change with an upper motor neuron lesion is the limitation in muscle control. This, too, differs among individuals. Some patients merely display local weakness, which signifies impairment of selective control. For others, the dominant mode of limb control is through primitive patterns. In this situation, the loss of selective control is replaced by mass action of the flexor muscles for swing (hip flexor, tibialis anterior and perhaps a knee flexor) (Figure 15.14a). For stance, the extensor pattern is activated (quadriceps, gastrosoleus and gluteus maximus) (Figure 15.14b). Impaired proprioception prevents some patients from using their available motor control, because they lack positional feedback. A statistical study of gait measurement of cerebral palsy patients showed the severity of the control deficit (mild, moderate, severe) was more significant than its anatomical extent (i.e., hemiplegia, diplegia, quadriplegia).[13]

Adult Hemiplegia

Paralytic involvement of one side of the body can vary markedly in its severity. Within the mixture of individual disability, there are several characteristic patterns of dysfunction. These include a drop foot (excessive plantar flexion), equinovarus (excessive plantar flexion and inversion), genu recurvatum (excessive extension) and a *stiff-knee gait* (inadequate flexion). Hemiplegic patients have some ability to substitute through the good function in the other limb.

The influence of the primitive patterns is particularly prominent at the foot. This can confuse the diagnosis of ankle control. As the functional purposes of the swing phases change, muscle activation is abruptly modified. Mid swing is dominated by the flexor pattern to assure floor clearance. Flexion of the hip is accompanied by full ankle dorsiflexion (Figure 15.14c). Terminal swing begins the extensor pattern to prepare the limb for stance. This involves extension of the knee, accompanied by ankle plantar flexion (Figure 15.14d). The typical EMG pattern of the ankle muscles shows prematurely curtailed tibialis anterior action and premature onset of soleus muscle activity (Figure 11.26). The terminal swing and loading response phases of the tibialis anterior are lost as the ankle control of the flexor pattern shifts to the extensor pattern and soleus begins its action prematurely.

Drop Foot

Patient K. A simple drop foot may be the only visible gait deviation of the mildly hemiplegic stroke patient. The cause is impaired selective control (without primitive flexor synergy emergence), which results in inadequate

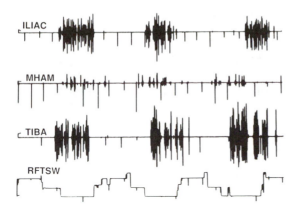

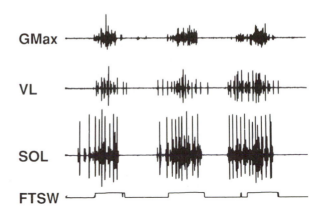

Figure 15.14 Primitive mass patterns during walking.

Figure 15.14a Dynamic EMG of the basic flexor muscles (wire electrodes). ILIAC = iliacus; M HAM = medial hamstring; TIB A = tibialis anterior; FTSW = right foot switch.(Perry J. Integrated Function of the Lower Extremity Including Gait Analysis. In Cruess RL, Rennie WR., Eds. *Adult Orthopedics.* New York: Churchill Livingstone, 1984; 1161-1207.)

Figure 15.14b Dynamic EMG of the basic extensor muscles (wire electrodes). GMax = gluteus maximus; VL = vastus lateralis; SOL = soleus; FTSW = right footswitch. (Perry J. Integrated Function of the Lower Extremity Including Gait Analysis. In Cruess RL, Rennie WR., eds. *Adult Orthopedics.* New York: Churchill Livingstone, 1984; 1161-1207.)

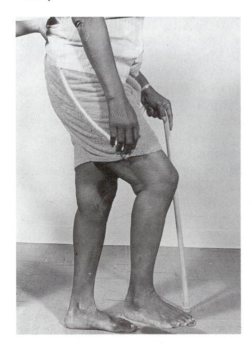

Figure 15.14c Mid swing use of the primitive mass pattern. Hip flexion is accompanied by knee flexion and ankle dorsiflexion.

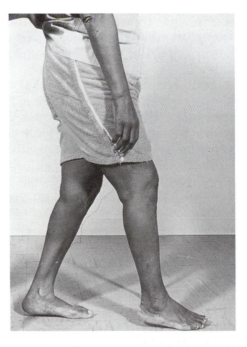

Figure 15.14d Terminal swing use of the primitive mass extensor pattern. Knee extension (incomplete) is accompanied by ankle plantar flexion and reduced hip flexion.

activation of the dorsiflexor muscles. The findings are selected phases of excessive plantar flexion with an otherwise normal gait.

Initial contact is made with a low heel strike (Figure 15.15a). While the ankle is in excessive plantar flexion, total limb alignment places the forefoot slightly above the heel.

Stance phase ankle dorsiflexion follows the normal pattern when dorsiflexor inactivity is the only deficit (Figure 15.15b). There may be minimal loss of tibial advancement due to the reduced heel rocker, but terminal stance and pre-swing heel rise are appropriate.

Mid swing is the phase where the disability becomes apparent (Figure 15.15c). The excessively plantar flexed ankle causes a toe drag, while hip and knee flexion are normal. This patient's failure to avoid the toe drag suggests an inability to voluntarily increase his hip flexion and the lack of a substitutive flexor synergy.

Dynamic Varus (Swing)

Patient L. The hemiplegic foot frequently displays varying degrees of varus during swing, stance or throughout the gait cycle. Spasticity and the primitive locomotor patterns are the dominant sources of muscle dysfunction. The effect on the knee varies with the activity of the hamstrings and severity of the equinus.

The mode of impaired foot control displayed by this patient results from hemiplegia following a ruptured aneurysm. Swing phase varus is the dominant deviation. The apparent cause is strong tibialis anterior muscle action as part of the flexor pattern, while the long toe extensors are far less active.

Initial contact is made with the lateral side of the foot (H5) while the knee is excessively flexed and there is normal hip flexion (Figure 15.16a). A prominent tibialis anterior tendon is evident. The immediate concern is having a stable foot posture for weight acceptance. Will the tibialis anterior continue its activity or relax as the extensor pattern takes over?

Loading response involves a rapid drop of the foot into a safe plantigrade support pattern (H,5,1) with the tibia vertical (Figure 15.16b). This signifies prompt tibialis anterior relaxation as the extensor muscle synergy takes over.

Persistence of the plantigrade foot alignment now depends on the intensity of the plantar flexor muscle action. Total foot contact in pre-swing implies adequate mediolateral balance (Figure 15.16c). It also signifies insufficient ankle dorsiflexion range to fully move body weight over the metatarsal heads to have achieved an earlier forefoot rocker. The absence of a forefoot rocker has also denied the patient pre-swing knee flexion.

Initial swing initiation of limb flexion in preparation for floor clearance stimulates foot inversion (Figure 15.16d). Close inspection of the anterior ankle provides a visible muscle test. A prominent anterior tibialis tendon indicates strong muscle action, while inconspicuous toe extensor tendon implies poor function of this lateral group. The latter also is confirmed by a lack of toe hyperextension at the metatarsophalangeal (MP) joints. Such

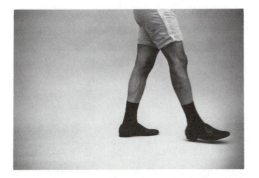

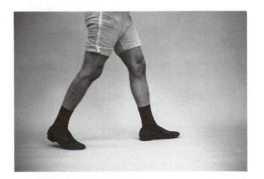

Figure 15.15 Patient K: Hemiplegia drop foot.
Figure 15.15a Terminal swing limb alignment for low heel contact. The cause is excessive ankle plantar flexion.

Figure 15.15b Terminal stance with a normal-appearing end of phase limb posture.

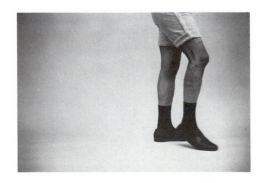

Figure 15.15c Mid swing toe drag resulting from excessive ankle plantar flexion with normal hip and knee flexion.

findings imply the tibialis anterior muscle is the dominant ankle dorsiflexor. Limited knee flexion results in an early toe drag.

In mid swing, strong tibialis anterior muscle action causes marked varus, yet the foot appears to be in slight equinus. There really are two patterns of foot dorsiflexion (Figure 15.16e). The medial side of the foot (first two rays) is at neutral. Laterally, however, the foot is slightly plantar flexed. Hence, the tibialis anterior has the strength to dorsiflex the ankle, but its tendon

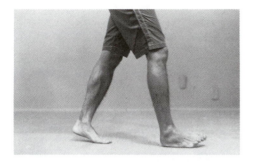

Figure 15.16 Patient L: Hemiplegic varus foot.
Figure 15.16a Initial contact with the heel and fifth metatarsal. There is excessive knee flexion. The tibialis anterior tendon is prominent.

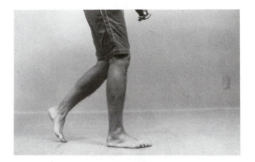

Figure 15.16b Loading response with total foot contact (heel, Mt5, Mt1). Tibia is vertical, knee and hip flexed.

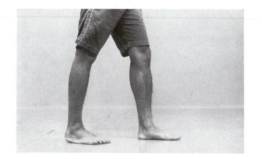

Figure 15.16c Pre-swing foot flat contact (H, Mt5, Mt1). Ankle mildly dorsiflexed, knee slightly hyperextended.

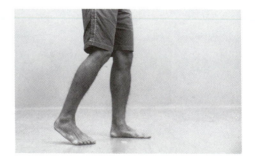

Figure 15.16d Initial swing foot inversion as flexor pattern is initiated. Knee incompletely flexed.

alignment first inverts the foot. The limited ability of even strong tibialis anterior action to raise the whole foot is most apparent from an anterior view of the foot (Figure 15.16f). Depression of the fifth ray is a potential source of foot drag if there is no substitutive action. This patient, lacking free knee flexion, must lift the whole limb by using contralateral vaulting as an alternate substitution (Figure 15.16e).

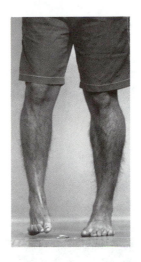

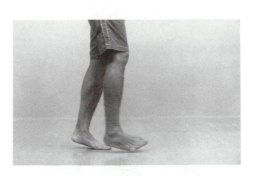

Figure 15.16e Mid swing with severe foot varus (inversion), prominent tibialis anterior tendon and drop of the lateral side of the foot. Knee flexion incomplete.

Figure 15.16f Anterior view of foot showing a drop of the lateral side. The tibialis anterior tendon is prominent but not the extensor digitorum longus and peroneus tertius. Toe clawing is by the short toe extensor tendons.

Stance Equinus and Stiff Knee Gait

Patient M. Two characteristic gait deviations dominate this patient's mode of walking. Equinus during stance inhibits the progression of this stroke patient. It also deprives the patient of shock-absorbing knee flexion. During swing, limb advancement is impeded by inappropriate quadriceps action.

Initial contact is made by the fifth metatarsal (Mt5) as a result of three contributing factors (Figure 15.17a). There is excessive ankle plantar flexion, combined with subtalar varus that drops the lateral side of the foot. The knee is slightly flexed and hip flexion is limited.

The loading response to the body weight being transferred onto the forefoot generates three actions. While the ankle maintains its plantar flexed position, the heel makes delayed contact with the floor (Figure 15.17b). This prevents tibial advancement and the loss of shock-absorbing knee flexion.

Mid stance progression of the body across the supporting foot creates a dorsiflexion torque that decreases the ankle plantar flexion slightly (Figure 15.17c). At the same time, advancement of the femur over the stationary tibia hyperextends the knee. The two deformities compensate each other sufficiently to allow a relatively vertical position of the limb with the hip aligned over the ankle. Unless the ankle yields, he will have no mechanism for unlocking the knee.

Pre-swing displays a very short contralateral step, indicating the weight-bearing limb has no further progressional mobility beyond that attained in mid stance (Figure 15.17d). The inadequate knee flexion reflects the tibial restraint caused by the relatively neutral posture of the ankle and the low heel rise. This deprives the patient of the mechanisms that smooth the transition from stance to swing.

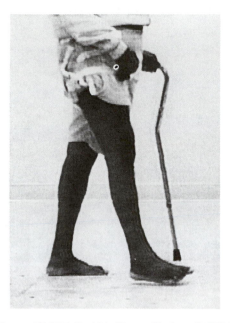

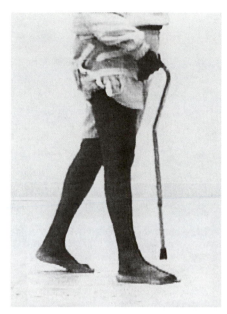

Figure 15.17 Patient M: Stance Equinus & Stiff Knee Gait (Hemiplegia).
Figure 15.17a Initial contact will be by the fifth metatarsal due to equinovarus of the foot combined with inadequate knee extension and hip flexion.

Figure 15.17b Loading response shows knee hyperextension, the ankle plantar flexed, flat foot contact and hip center over the foot.

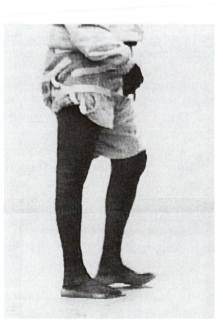

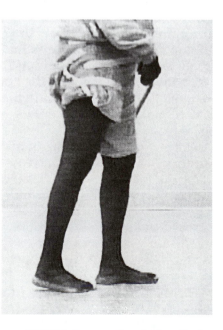

Figure 15.17c Mid stance has continuing knee hyperextension while the ankle is in less plantar flexion with flat foot contact. The hip remains over the foot.

Figure 15.17d Late pre-swing displays the knee fully extended while the ankle is at neutral and heel moderately elevated. The thigh has trailing posture.

While some body advancement was gained by knee hyperextension, the ankle plantar flexion proved to be a major obstruction. Even ankle dorsiflexion to neutral is insufficient to align the body vector over the forefoot. Also, the patient's slow gait velocity (19m/min, 22% normal) does not provide the momentum needed to roll onto the metatarsal heads. A further problem is the need for complete transfer of body weight to the other limb before the hip and knee can be unlocked to allow any flexion. Hence, the initiation of limb advancement is delayed until the end of pre-swing.

Initial swing is characterized by a toe drag with very inadequate knee and hip flexion (Figure 15.17e). This limited function represents the delay in initiating limb advancement, the absence of pre-swing flexor assistance, a lack of quick selective control, and possible antagonistic muscle action. These are the elements of a *stiff knee gait*.

In mid swing there is good floor clearance by the foot, because all three joints are meeting the minimal demands (Figure 15.17f). Ankle dorsiflexion approaches neutral but is slightly limited by inversion, allowing the lateral side of the foot to drop. This could be a sign of strong tibialis anterior muscle action in the presence of the mild ankle plantar flexion contracture that was suspected earlier. The limitation in hip and knee flexion suggests dynamic obstruction at the knee.

Terminal swing knee extension is accompanied by a loss of ankle dorsiflexion (Figure 15.17g). This implies dependence on a primitive extensor pattern to meet the demands of stance.

Electrogoniometric recordings of the ankle and knee show very different rates of motion by the two joints. The 20° ankle plantar flexion present at initial contact progressively decreases during stance until the maximum dorsiflexion (0°) is attained in pre-swing, when the body alignment is maximally forward (Figure 15.17h). During swing, the ankle then progressively plantar flexes to 20° again.

Measurements at the knee showed abrupt changes in the direction of motion. During stance, the 15° flexion present from initial contact (IC) until the end of loading response abruptly reverses to 10° hyperextension with the onset of full weight bearing (Figure 15.18i). This persists until the limb is unlocked at the end of pre-swing. A rapid but limited arc (30°) of knee flexion develops in initial swing, and this is irregularly maintained through mid swing. In terminal swing knee flexion decreases to 15°.

The addition of dynamic electromyography to the motion data clarifies the causes of the patient's gait deviations. There are two abnormal modes of ankle control (Figure 15.17h). Premature (IC onset) and persistent soleus action, which has a clonic quality, inhibits ankle dorsiflexion from initial contact through terminal stance. A strong burst of tibialis anterior muscle action in initial swing fails to maintain the neutral dorsiflexion gained passively in pre-swing, despite relative inactivity of the soleus and gastrocnemius. This suggests the presence of an elastic contracture that yielded under body weight, but is stronger than the tibialis anterior pull. Failure of the tibialis anterior to maintain its high level of dorsiflexion activity allows the foot to drop into increasing plantar flexion. The imbalance between persistent tibialis anterior EMG and the rate of foot drop also indicates a contracture. The insignificant

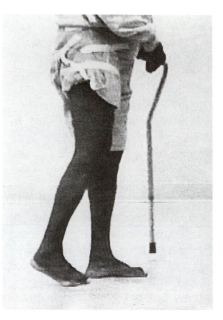

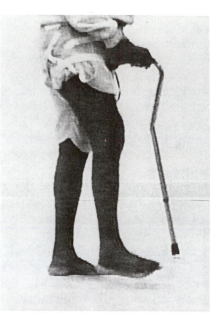

Figure 15.17e Initial swing begins with inadequate knee flexion, limited hip flexion and a toe drag. The ankle is in normal plantar flexion.

Figure 15.17f Mid swing hip and knee flexion are sufficient for the slightly equinovarus foot to clear the floor.

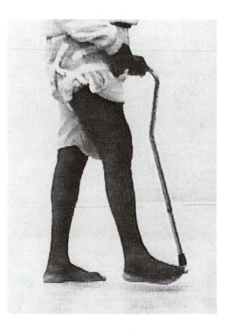

Figure 15.17g Terminal swing alignment of the foot is in greater plantar flexion while the knee is almost fully extended.

level of gastrocnemius muscle action shows that this muscle is not an automatic synergist of the soleus. One effect of this inequality is the absence of a force to counteract the inversion torque of the soleus (evidenced by the early Mt5 foot switch pattern).

Knee hyperextension has a dynamic quality and is also a reaction to inadequate ankle mobility. The intensity of the vasti EMG (VML, VI and particularly the VL) exceeds that required to support a flexed knee (Figure 15.17i). Hence, it is imposing a hyperextension force. Prolongation of the vasti muscle action through terminal stance adds a direct knee extensor force to a knee already positioned in recurvatum. Also, the intensity of the gastrocnemius activity is markedly less than that of soleus and, therefore, no synergistic posterior protection of the knee is provided.

Inadequate knee flexion in swing is consistent with the prolonged and intense action of the rectus femoris (RF) throughout swing. This is augmented by lesser levels of vastus intermedius (VI) and vastus medialis longus (VML) action.

The use of a locked ankle orthosis (AFO) demonstrates the extent to which the patient's excessive plantar flexion contributed to his poor progression. Initial contact by the heel is gained, and the patient takes a slightly longer step (Figure 15.17j). The resulting heel rocker in loading response generates excessive knee flexion because there is no ankle plantar flexion range to dissipate the effect of the heel rocker (Figure 15.17k). In terminal stance a vertical tibial alignment is attained, but not a forefoot rocker (Figure 15.17l). Knee hyperextension is not prevented, but the forward femur increases step length slightly. Initial swing knee flexion has not been improved because the pre-swing forefoot rocker action still is lacking and there is dynamic obstruction by the rectus femoris and vasti (Figure 15.17m).

Patient N. Knee hyperextension secondary to rigid plantar flexion is this patient's primary gait deviation. The muscles and their intrinsic fibrous tissues create an unyielding posterior tie between the foot and tibia.

Initial contact is by the forefoot (Mt5), as a result of excessive ankle plantar

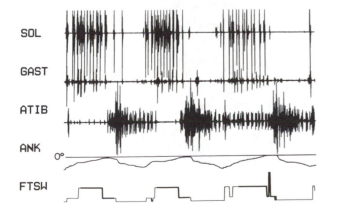

Figure 15.17h Dynamic electromyography and motion of the ankle. SOL = soleus; GAST = Gastrocnemius; ATIB = tibialis anterior; ANK = electrogoniometer at the ankle; FTSW = foot switches for reference limb.

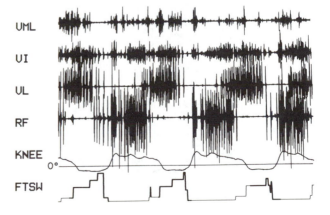

Figure 15.17i Dynamic electromyography and motion of the knee. VML = vastus medialis longus; VI = vastus intermedius; VL = vastus lateralis; RF = rectus femoris; KNEE = knee electrogoniometer.

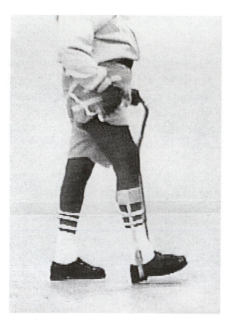

Figure 15.17j An orthosis (AFO) locking the ankle at neutral provides initial contact with the heel.

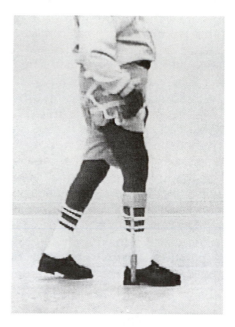

Figure 15.17k Loading response with the locked AFO causes increased knee flexion.

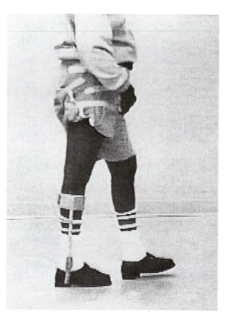

Figure 15.17l Mid stance AFO stabilization of the tibia in an erect posture does not prevent knee hyperextension.

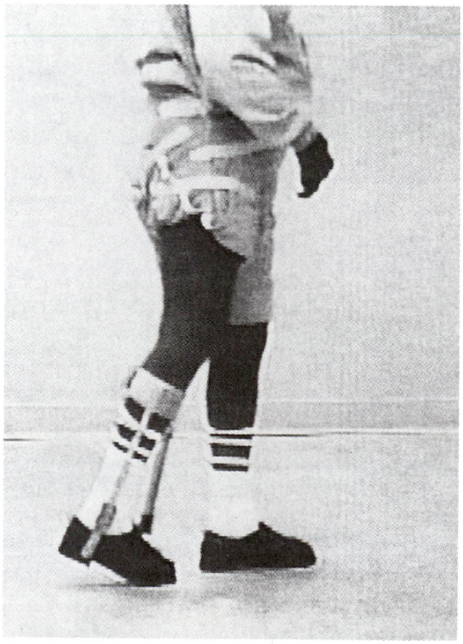

Figure 15.17m Initial swing still has a toe drag despite the AFO because knee flexion still is very inadequate.

flexion, a fully extended knee, and limited hip flexion (Figure 15.18a). The very short step accentuates the limb's vertical alignment for forefoot contact. Loading response shows a delayed heel contact that results in a foot flat posture without any reduction in the ankle plantar flexion. The knee is in significant hyperextension (Figure 15.18b). These actions imply forceful retraction of the tibia as a result of the foot and ankle loading posture. Mid stance advancement of the opposite limb fails to draw the stance limb tibia forward (Figure 15.18c). No additional advancement in limb posture is gained by pre-swing (Figure 15.18d). The persistent heel contact and double limb stance with the feet parallel confirm the lack of a progressional forefoot rocker. Relieving the limb from total body support reduces the knee hyperextension, but does not initiate knee flexion for swing.

Lacking a trailing limb posture in initial swing, there is no need for the usual large knee flexion arc. Instead, the patient merely needs sufficient hip and knee flexion to clear the floor with the plantar flexed foot. Hence, the only limb advancement actions are those characteristic of mid swing (Figure 15.18e). To accommodate the increased amount of lift imposed by the plantar flexed ankle, lateral trunk lean is used to augment the limited limb flexion observed. A comparison of the mid swing and initial contact limb positions indicate use of a past retract maneuver in terminal swing to gain full knee extension at the onset of stance.

Electrogoniometric recording of the ankle motion shows an almost unvarying posture of approximately 25° PF (Figure 15.18f). There are no notable changes between swing and stance. The knee maintains hyperextension throughout stance. This varies from 15° in loading response to 25° in terminal stance. With the onset of swing the knee flexes 15°.

The foot switch records identify that the fifth metatarsal is the primary area of foot support during stance. There is a brief interval of foot flat (H,5,1) in terminal stance. The persistent Mt5 foot switch pattern (Figure 15.18g) indicates an unstable weight-bearing posture and consequent short stance time. Inability to effectively flex the limb is consistent with the short swing interval.

Dynamic electromyography of the foot and ankle muscles shows almost a complete lack of phasing (Figure 15.18g). The soleus and gastrocnemius have only sparse, low-intensity action. While nearly continuous, sparsity of the EMG indicates only a few motor units are active. Thus, this muscle is not providing a major plantar flexor force. The brief moment of dense EMG in the soleus at the end of terminal stance is consistent with this being a period of peak dorsiflexion stretch. The dense period of the low gastrocnemius EMG during the first half of stance suggests a reaction to stretch at the knee that exceeds the soleus experience. This action, however, decreases at the time of peak knee hyperextension, suggesting posterior knee protection is not a primary stimulus for the gastrocnemius. The combination of low gastrocnemius and soleus EMG with persistent, excessive plantar flexion indicates the primary restraining force is a contracture. Two of the perimalleolar muscles (flexor hallucis longus and peroneus longus) might be adding some tibial restraint by their continuous and intense action. However, the effect is very limited, since neither muscle has the bony lever arm nor size to hold the ankle in 25-30° plantar flexion against the body weight torque that is sufficient to hyperextend the knee (Figure 15.18h).

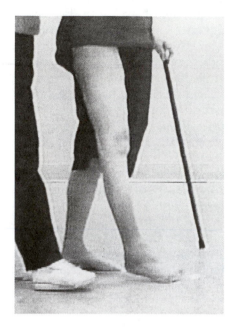

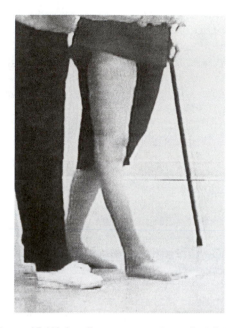

Figure 15.18 Patient N: Rigid equinus and hyperextension (Hemiplegia).

Figure 15.18a Initial contact with the forefoot. The foot is in equinovarus, knee hyperextended and hip flexion limited.

Figure 15.18b Loading response shows foot flat contact, persistent ankle plantar flexion and increased knee recurvatum. The femur as well as the tibia is retracted.

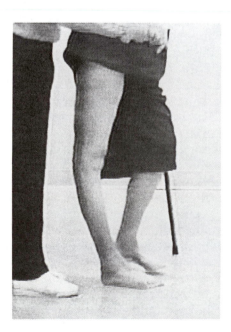

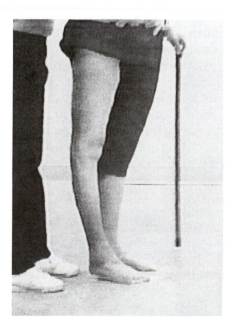

Figure 15.18c Mid stance ankle and knee position are unchanged and foot flat continues.

Figure 15.18d Pre-swing double limb support shows less knee hypertension from weight sharing. The other foot is opposite the reference foot.

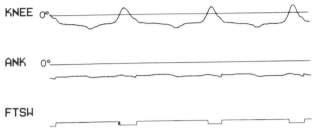

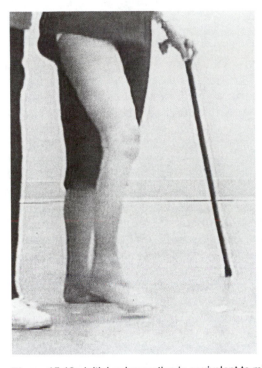

Figure 15.18e Initial swing motion is equivalent to mid swing. Knee flexion is very inadequate, but the forward position of the limb allows floor clearance by the foot.

Figure 15.18f Electrogoniometer recordings show minimal motion. The ankle remains in 25° plantar flexion throughout the stride. At the knee there is almost continuous hyperextension of 15°.

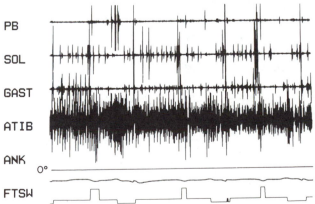

Figure 15.18g Dynamic electromyography of the ankle muscles. SOL = soleus; GAST = gastrocnemius; ATIB = tibialis anterior; PB = peroneus brevis; FTSW = foot switches of that limb.

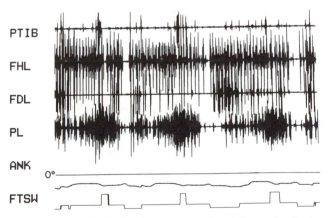

Figure 15.18h Dynamic electromyography of the perimalleolar muscles. PTIB = posterior tibialis; FHL = flexor hallucis longus; FDL = flexor digitorum longus; PL = peroneus longus.

Two factors contribute to the varus. Most prominent is the intense continuous activity of the anterior tibialis muscle. This EMG implies the muscle is exerting an active attempt to advance the tibia. The muscle, however, lacks the mechanics to move the tibia against the existing plantar flexing forces, but is a strong inverter of the foot. The soleus contracture also induces inversion, as its point of insertion on the os calcis has a medial orientation to the subtalar joint. There is no significant action by the posterior tibialis.

In summary, this patient's limited performance indicates a profound loss of selective control without the emergence of primitive locomotor patterns for muscle activation. The functional result is general limb weakness during both swing and stance. Aggravating this is the presence of a severe ankle plantar flexion contracture.

Stiff Knee Gait (Spinal Cord Injury)

The unique characteristic of spinal cord injury is that there are three types of function. Above the level of the lesion, control is normal. This offers the patient maximum substitution capability. A lower motor neuron lesion occurs at the level of the cord damage. Flaccid paralysis occurs within these segments. Distal to the site of injury, the impaired control is that of an upper motor neuron lesion. Now function represents an individual mixture of spasticity, impaired selective control and primitive locomotor patterns. While spinal cord injuries tend to be bilateral, the functional involvement on the two sides can differ markedly in severity and the neural tracts included.

Patient O. This SCI patient has regained a community level of ambulation (velocity = 37m/min, 42% normal). His gait, however, is significantly limited by inadequate knee flexion during both limb loading and swing.

Initial contact is normal (Figure 15.19a). As the heel contacts the floor, the forefoot is well elevated by the neutrally aligned ankle, extended knee and flexed hip. During loading response, the knee fails to flex (Figure 15.19b). This extended knee position continues through single stance. In terminal stance, the patient displays prolonged heel contact (Figure 15.19c). Progression is gained by increasing ankle dorsiflexion. Pre-swing knee flexion is severely limited, though unloading the limb allowed a late heel rise (Figure 15.19d). Initial swing knee flexion is very limited and there is poor advancement of the thigh (Figure 15.19e). Toe drag is avoided by a slight lateral trunk lean and ankle dorsiflexion to neutral. In mid swing, floor clearance is gained by the well-dorsiflexed ankle (Figure 15.19f). Hip flexion is notably greater than knee flexion. Hence, there is excessive knee extension. Terminal swing shows good limb control, with selective ankle dorsiflexion while the knee is extended (Figure 15.19g).

Motion analysis shows the primary functional deviations involve both the knee and ankle (Figure 15.19h). Loading response lacks the normal plantar flexion. Instead, beginning from a neutral position at initial contact, the ankle progressively dorsiflexes through the weight-bearing period until a peak angle of 15° is reached in late terminal stance. Slightly excessive dorsiflexion (10°) is maintained through initial and mid swing. The ankle then drops to neutral in terminal swing.

Knee motion is independent of the ankle. The extended position (5° flexion) at initial contact is maintained through the stance phases until pre-swing. In this double support period, knee flexion begins, reaching 20° by the onset of initial swing. Further flexion during initial swing is minimal (5°). Beginning in mid swing, the knee extends to a terminal position of 5° flexion.

The thigh follows a normal pattern throughout the stride, while there is a progressive anterior pelvic tilt in stance. Hip flexion at initial contact is limited (20°). From this point the joint progressively extends, reaching slight hyperextension (5°) shortly before an early toe-off.

The foot switches show a brief heel only support interval (H) that quickly progresses to foot flat (H,5). Heel contact is maintained until the other foot is loaded. Toe-off is premature, occurring at 54% GC (versus the normal 62% GC). This is related to a short single stance time (27% GC versus 40%). The other limb has an extended SLS (49% GC). These differences reflect limited progression in stance and difficulty advancing the limb in swing.

Dynamic EMG of the muscles about the knee shows continuous activity of all the vasti. It is most marked in the vastus medialis longus (VML) and vastus intermedius (VI) (Figure 15.19i). While the intensity is greater during stance, there also is highly significant extensor muscle activity in swing. Conversely, there is no rectus femoris action in either gait period. A brief burst of biceps femoris short head action occurs at the onset of initial contact, but the muscle is too small to counter the multiple vasti (Figure 19.19j). There also is no significant hamstring activity to decelerate knee extension in terminal stance or to assist the heel rocker flexion thrust in loading response.

Thus, during stance a fully extended limb, locked by continually active vasti, rolls forward across the ankle. Excessive dorsiflexion substitutes for a forefoot rocker. This signifies gastrosoleus muscle weakness. An erect trunk posture is maintained by an anterior pelvic tilt, compensating for restricted hip mobility (25° versus the normal 40° arc).

Spastic Cerebral Palsy

There are two characteristic gaits of children with spastic paralysis of diplegic, quadriplegic or paraplegic origin. These are a crouch and genu recurvatum.

The *crouch gait* is a bilateral impairment typified by excessive hip and knee flexion, excessive ankle plantar flexion and anterior pelvic tilt (Figure 15.20a). Even the vertical alignment of mid stance fails to correct the basic gait deviations, though their magnitude may decrease (Figure 15.20b). The two limbs may vary in the severity of their posturing. One variant is an apparent reduction in equinus, as the subtalar joint everts under the forces of body weight (Figure 15.20c). Swing shows an exaggeration of the flexion needed to clear the floor as the equinus persists (Figure 15.20d). This difficulty indicates ankle control is not a part of the patient's flexor pattern.

Primitive patterning with excessive flexor muscle action at the hip and knee is the basic control deviation. Overactivity and contracture of the hamstrings is

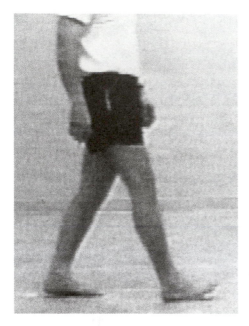

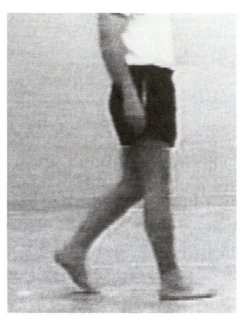

Figure 15.19 Patient O: Stiff knee gait (Spinal Cord Injury).
Figure 15.19a Initial contact by the heel with normal limb alignment.

Figure 15.19b Loading response lacks knee flexion. Limb position, otherwise, appears normal.

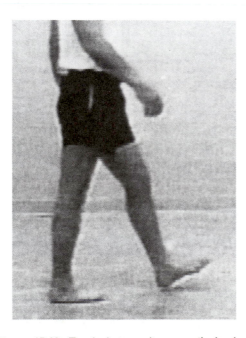

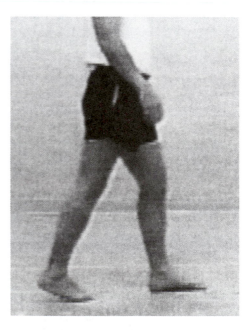

Figure 15.19c Terminal stance has a continuing heel contact. The ankle is dorsiflexed, knee extended. Step length is shortened by the body center remaining over the foot.

Figure 15.19d Pre-swing lacks knee flexion and the ankle is excessively dorsiflexed. There is a good heel rise and a trailing thigh.

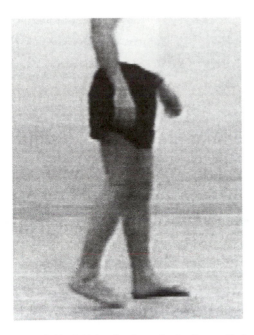

Figure 15.19e Initial swing knee flexion is very limited and the ankle is dorsiflexed to neutral (excessive). Contralateral trunk lean assists floor clearance.

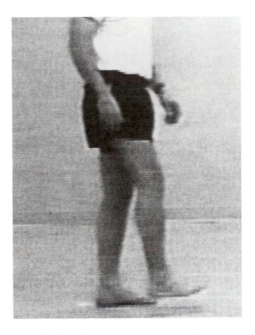

Figure 15.19f Mid swing knee flexion is inadequate (less than hip flexion).

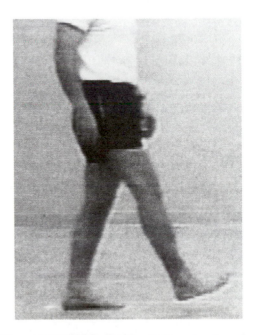

Figure 15.19g Terminal swing limb posture is normal except for slight knee flexion. The foot is higher than normal because the other limb has not rolled the body forward.

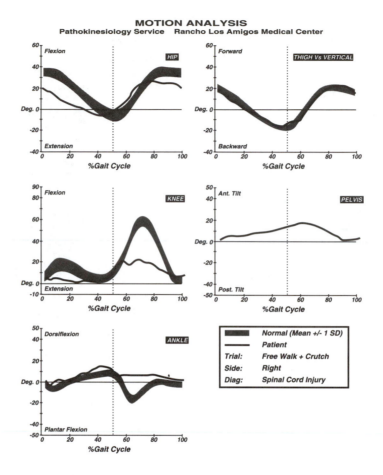

Figure 15.19h Vicon motion analysis. The vertical axis is degrees of motion (flexion is positive). The horizontal axis is the percent of the gait cycle. The vertical dotted line divides stance and swing (toe-off). Gray area indicates the 1 standard deviation band of normal function. Black line is patient data.

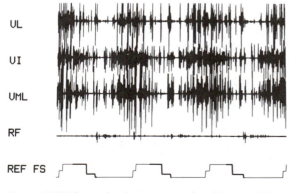

Figure 15.19i Dynamic electromyography of the quadriceps. VML = vastus medialis longus; VI = vastus intermedius; VL = vastus lateralis; RF = rectus femoris; FTSW = foot switches for the reference limb.

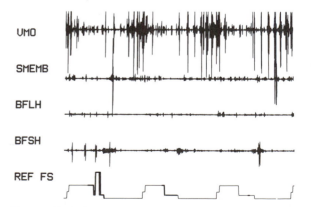

Figure 15.19j Dynamic electromyography. VMO = vastus medialis oblique; SMEMB = semimembranosis; BFLH = biceps femoris long head; BFSH = biceps femoris short head; FTSW = foot switches.

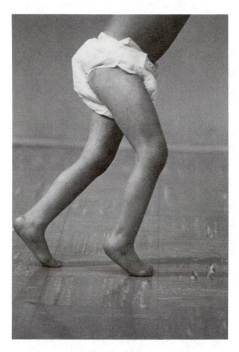

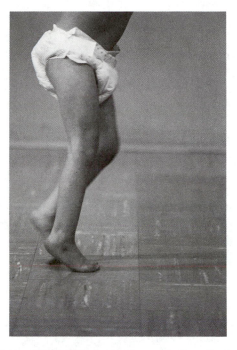

Figure 15.20 "Typical" Cerebral Palsy diplegia.
Figure 15.20a Loading response with bilateral excessive ankle plantar flexion, inadequate knee extension, excessive hip flexion and anterior pelvic tilt.

Figure 15.20b Mid stance excessive knee flexion is less severe. Excessive ankle plantar flexion and the anterior pelvic tilt persist.

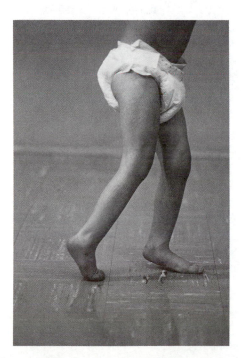

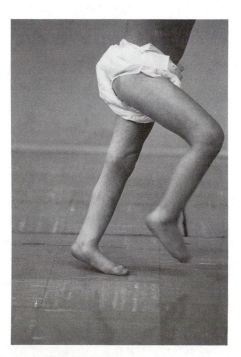

Figure 15.20c Terminal stance shows continuing severely excessive ankle plantar flexion. Apparent ankle plantar flexion is reduced by foot eversion.

Figure 15.20d Mid swing shows excessive plantar flexion as a continuous deviation. Hip and knee flexion are excessive and greater than is needed for floor clearance. The ankle did not join the flexor pattern.

a particularly common finding.[12] The position of the ankle varies with the severity of calf muscle action. Individual patients, however, show considerable variation from the *typical* crouch gait model. Consequently they have to be studied carefully, and often the functional diagnosis depends on instrumented gait analysis.[3]

Patient P. The most conspicuous aspects of this patient's crouch are the excessive heel rise and knee flexion. The thigh also lacks a trailing posture.

Initial contact is made with the forefoot (Mt5) and a notably high heel rise (Figure 15.21a). There is excessive knee flexion, with a normal hip posture, and the foot position suggests excessive ankle plantar flexion. The loading response moves the ankle into neutral dorsiflexion and reduces hip flexion slightly, while the excessive knee flexion shows no change (Figure 15.21b). The trunk is forward. Mid stance advancement of the body over the supporting foot leads to a premature heel rise. Knee flexion decreases slightly, while the ankle continues to slowly dorsiflex and the hip to extend (Figure 15.21c). In terminal stance, as the body moves ahead of the forefoot support area, limb stability is lost. This is evident by excessive heel rise, rapid ankle plantar flexion, increased knee flexion and posterio-lateral pelvic drop (Figure 15.21d). The thigh remains in flexion, as it fails to reach a trailing position. Unloading the limb in pre-swing allows the thigh to advance, and the knee moves into additional flexion (Figure 15.21e). There is a high heel rise, but the ankle is in slight dorsiflexion. During initial swing, knee flexion is inadequate and thigh advancement is delayed. Nor does the pelvis fully recover from the earlier drop. Consequently, the foot displays a brief toe drag (Figure 15.21f). By the end of mid swing, full hip flexion is attained while excessive knee flexion persists (Figure 15.21g). In preparation for initial contact, there is moderate knee extension and full dorsiflexion of the ankle, while the position of hip flexion is unchanged (Figure 15.21a).

Motion analysis identified that excessive knee flexion is the patient's major gait deviation. At initial contact the equinus posture of the foot includes an ankle that is plantar flexed less than 5° (Figure 15.21h). Hence, the primary source of the heel rise is the 40° knee flexion. The position of maximum stability is attained by mid stance (25% GC). At this time, the limb posture includes a premature heel rise with 30° knee flexion, 5° ankle dorsiflexion and 5° thigh flexion. Conversely, the unstable alignment that develops during terminal stance includes 60° knee flexion with 5° ankle plantar flexion and 10° thigh flexion. (Hence, there is no passive stability.) This early positioning of the knee in 60° flexion meets the requirement for initial swing, but the knee maintains its flexed position in mid swing. The resulting delay in tibial advancement contributes to the inadequate knee extension (40° flexion) at the end of terminal swing.

The ankle is minimally (3°) plantar flexed at initial contact. As weight is applied to the limb, the joint slowly dorsiflexes, reaching 5° DF by late mid stance. When forward alignment of the body on the forefoot rocker creates stance instability (40% GC), the ankle rapidly plantar flexes, reaching 15° by toe-off. In swing, the ankle slowly dorsiflexes, reaching neutral by the end of terminal swing.

Throughout the gait cycle, the thigh is in excessive flexion. This is significant in two intervals. During late mid stance and terminal stance, persistent flexion prevents the thigh attaining a trailing posture (10° flexion versus 15° extension). Step length is correspondingly shortened. In swing, the thigh continues its excessive flexion but at a rate slower than normal. Peak thigh flexion (40°) occurs late (90% GC). Throughout the stride, the pelvis has a continuous posterior pelvic tilt of 10° that reaches 25° in pre-swing.

Dynamic EMG shows abnormal function at both the hip and knee. Knee flexor muscle action is a synergy of semimembranosus, biceps femoris long head (BFLH) and gracilis muscle action occurring in two periods of the gait cycle (Figure 15.21i). These three muscles begin their activity with initial contact and continue through mid stance. Hamstring intensity is moderately high. Opposing these flexor muscles is the continuous action of the quadriceps (VI and RF) (Figure 15.21j).

A second synergy of the same three knee flexors (GRAC, SMEMB, BFLH), accompanied by the biceps femoris short head (BFSH), starts in late terminal stance and continues through initial swing. Now knee flexion increases to 65°. During the rest of swing, there are low levels of muscle action by the original flexor synergy (GRAC, SMEMB, BFLH).

Hip flexor muscle action is another contributor to the flexed knee. The iliacus begins it normal phasing in initial swing and continues into terminal swing. During this same period, the gracilis is contributing to flexion of the hip as well as the knee. Through mid and terminal swing, the rectus femoris increases its effort. At the end of terminal swing, the adductor longus begins intense action that continues, unabated, through the weight-bearing period into terminal stance.

Hip control is contradictory. Dynamic flexor action (iliacus and gracilis) to advance the thigh in pre-swing and initial swing is opposed by the extensor action of the hamstrings. Presumably, the latter muscles are striving to facilitate knee flexion (the actual arc of motion is only 20°, even though the desired posture is reached). Action by rectus femoris (RF) assists hip flexion while opposing knee flexion. Out-of-phase adductor longus action in terminal swing helps overcome the delayed hip flexion to attain a longer step than might otherwise occur. Hence, while ill timed it is useful. Continuation of adductor longus action in stance adds to the flexed knee posture, however, by maintaining thigh flexion.

The conclusion is that inappropriate timing (and contracture) of the hamstrings is creating excessive knee flexion. Activity of the adductor longus and rectus femoris is inappropriate. There is also undesirable swing phase action of the vastus intermedius. The iliacus and biceps femoris short head (BFSH) are functioning appropriately. This is primarily true for the gracilis. At the ankle, the 5° plantar flexion contracture is useful rather than obstructive. Early knee stance stability is probably aided by the plantar flexor control of the tibia, while the heel rise is small. Further progression over the forefoot accelerates tibial advancement, and this source of passive stability is lost. Heel rise reflects excessive knee flexion, not ankle equinus.

Patient Q. The gait of this nine-year-old diplegic cerebral palsy child is characterized by excessive knee flexion and ankle dorsiflexion during stance

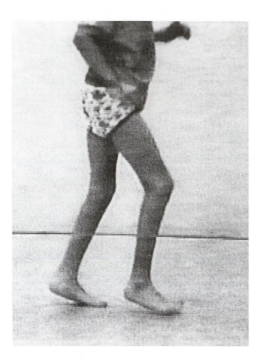

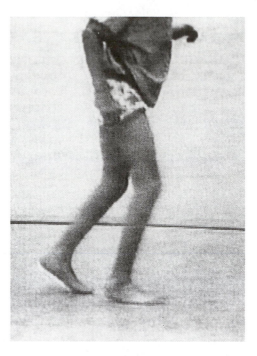

Figure 15.21 Patient P: Excessive Knee flexion (Cerebral Palsy Diplegia).
Figure 15.21a Initial contact with the forefoot, excessive knee flexion, mild ankle equinus.

Figure 15.21b Loading response shows flat foot support, excessive ankle dorsiflexion, excessive knee flexion and forward trunk lean.

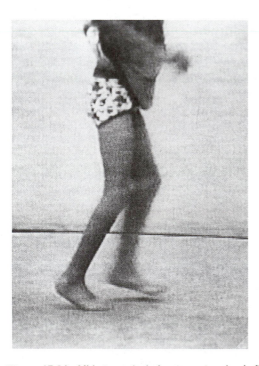

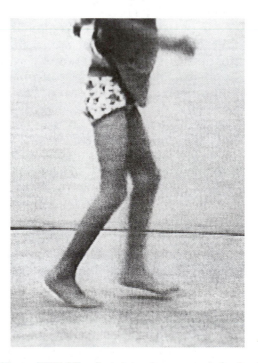

Figure 15.21c Mid stance includes premature heel off, excessive knee flexion, vertical thigh and less forward lean.

Figure 15.21d Terminal stance has an excessive heel rise, neutral ankle, significantly excessive knee flexion, thigh remains vertical.

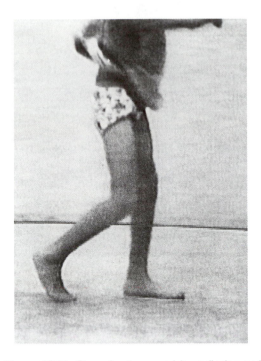

Figure 15.21e Pre-swing has good knee flexion and heel rise. The ankle is excessively dorsiflexed (at neutral) and the thigh normally positioned.

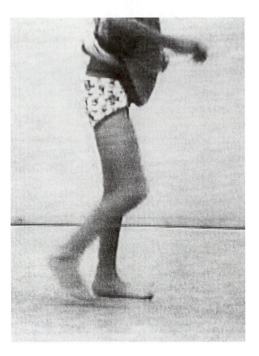

Figure 15.21f Initial swing is normal except for a lack of the usual ankle plantar flexion.

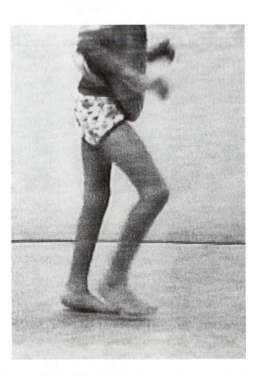

Figure 15.21g Mid swing has excessive knee flexion compared to the hip and knee positions.

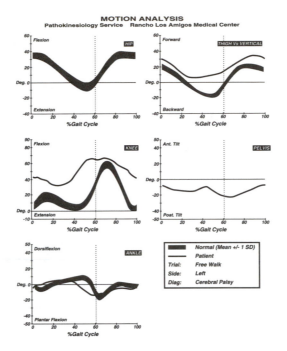

Figure 15.21h Vicon motion analysis.The vertical axis is degrees of motion (flexion is positive). The horizontal axis is the percent of the gait cycle. The vertical dotted line divides stance and swing (toe-off). Gray areas indicate the 1 standard deviation band of normal function. Black line is patient data.

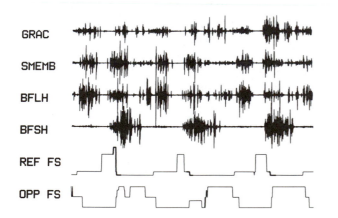

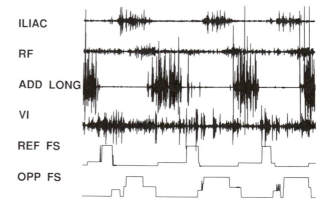

Figure 15.21i Dynamic electromyography, spastic diplegia. GRAC = gracilis; SMEMB = semimembranosis; BFLH = biceps femoris long head; BFSH = biceps femoris short head; REF FS = reference foot switch; OPP FS = opposite foot.

Figure 15.21j Dynamic electromyography, spastic diplegia. ILIAC = iliacus; ADD LONG = adductor longus; RF = rectus femoris; VI = vastus intermedius; REF FS = reference foot switch; OPP FS = opposite foot.

(Figure 15.22). Initial contact will be made with a very low heel rocker despite good ankle dorsiflexion and thigh advancement since the patient is unable to fully extend the knee in terminal swing (Figure 15.22a). Loading response increases knee flexion to a posture that is excessive for this phase, yet the available dorsiflexion range allows the tibia to be vertical (Figure 15.22b). Mid stance advancement of body weight over the foot reduces the knee flexion a little (Figure 15.22c). Ankle dorsiflexion above neutral allows the tibia to roll forward, but a trailing thigh posture is not attained. The position of the limb in pre-swing implies inadequate terminal stance mechanics (Figure 15.22d). Continuing heel contact with excessive ankle dorsiflexion and knee flexion fails to provide a functional increase in limb length. Consequently, there is an ipsilateral pelvic drop. In initial swing, there is a foot drag because of the inadequate knee flexion and incomplete correction of the pelvic drop (Figure 15.22e). The equinus position of the foot relates to the trailing position of the tibia; the ankle is not plantar flexed. Mid swing foot clearance is more than adequate as the ankle is fully dorsiflexed and the hip appropriately flexed, although extension of the knee is delayed (Figure 15.22f). This knee extensor lag is the basis of the inadequate knee extension in terminal swing (Figure 15.22a)

Motion analysis confirms the magnitude of the patient's excessive knee flexion (Figure 15.22g). From the 25° flexed posture at initial contact, the loading response increases the knee flexion to 35°. Mid stance advancement of the limb over a flat foot only reduces knee flexion to 20°. Then, in terminal stance, knee flexion progressively increases, reaching 40° at toe-off. This position is maintained rather than increased in initial swing. Hence, the toe drag noted earlier. Terminal swing knee extension only reduces the flexed knee posture to 25°.

At the ankle, there is excessive dorsiflexion present throughout the stride. Beginning with 5° at initial contact, the ankle progresses to 15° DF in mid stance and continues through terminal stance. Even in pre-swing the ankle remains dorsiflexed 5°. This increases to 10° during swing, a sign of excessive joint mobility (and lack of posterior tissue tension).

Hip motion, measured between the pelvis and femur, is slightly greater than normal (45°) from mid swing through loading response. The significant functional deficit occurs in terminal stance where excessive flexion is marked (20° flexion). The consistent 20° anterior pelvic allows the thigh to follow a normal path during the flexion phases, but it is insufficient to provide a trailing limb posture for full step length. The thigh remains flexed 5° rather than hyperextending 10°.

Dynamic electromyography (EMG) shows strong quadriceps support of the flexed knee (VI). Onset of the vastus intermedius in mid swing is premature but appropriate for this patient, because excessive knee flexion is a persistent problem (Figure 15.22h). Cessation of VI action so close to toe off limits the freedom desired for passive knee flexion in pre-swing. During initial swing, there is no significant obstruction by the VI, but the rectus femoris action is intense. The RF dynamically inhibits swing phase knee flexion, beginning in pre-swing and continuing through initial swing.

Intense, premature and prolonged hamstring activity is a dynamic source of the excessive knee flexion occurring from terminal swing through mid stance (Figure 15.22i). Action of the semimembranosus is much greater than that of the

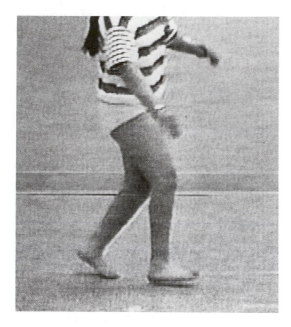

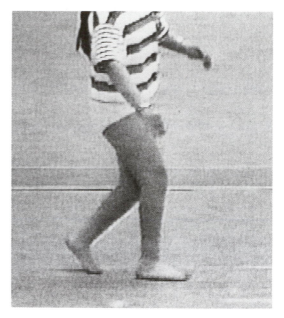

Figure 15.22 Patient Q: Excessive knee flexion & ankle dorsiflexion (Cerebral diplegia).
Figure 15.22a Initial contact will be with a flat foot. The ankle is dorsiflexed and knee extended.

Figure 15.22b Loading response has foot flat support with a vertical tibia and flexed knee.

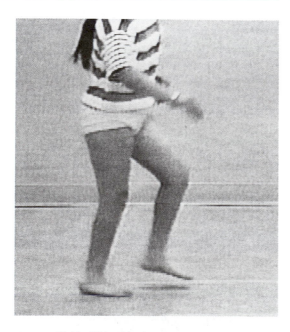

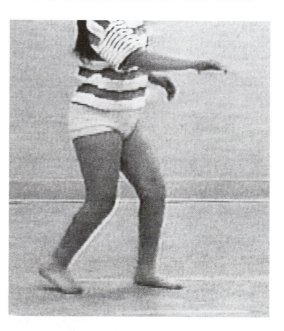

Figure 15.22c Mid stance includes excessive dorsiflexion and excessive knee flexion.

Figure 15.22d Pre-swing shows a low heel rise. The ankle is dorsiflexed and there is an ipsilateral pelvic drop, and thigh flexion is excessive. Knee flexion is good.

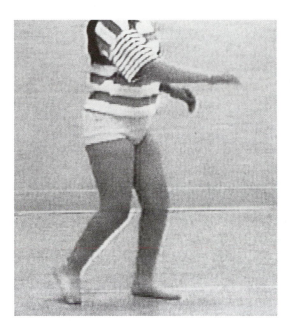

Figure 15.22e Initial swing includes a toe drag. Both knee flexion and thigh advancement are limited.

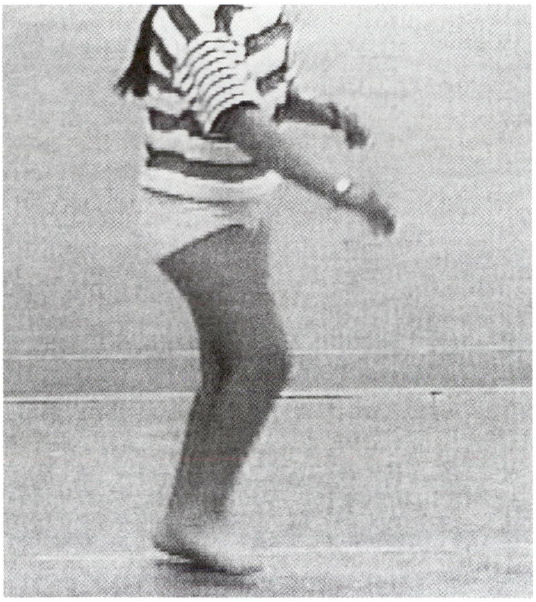

Figure 15.22f Mid swing thigh advancement exceeds knee extension. The ankle remains dorsiflexed.

biceps femoris long head. There is, however, no dynamic cause of the persistent knee flexion in the later phases of stance. The hamstrings have relaxed, and there is no significant action of the biceps femoris short head (BFSH) or gracilis muscles. Thus, inability of the strongly active quadriceps to fully extend the flexed knee, in late mid stance and terminal stance, relates to passive tibial instability. Excessive ankle dorsiflexion is the first mechanism. Flat foot contact with a flexed knee introduces a dorsiflexion torque at the ankle as the limb is loaded. The excessive ankle dorsiflexion displayed by the patient indicates an inability to restrain tibial advancement. This deprives the quadriceps of a stable base from which to extend the knee. Another possibility is the active hip flexion related to the intense adductor longus muscle action.

At the hip, two patterns of muscle control are evident. Three flexor muscles are active in swing: the gracilis, rectus femoris and adductor longus. This is good. There also are two hip extensors active: the semimembranosus and, less intensely, the biceps femoris long head. While their action as knee flexors is desirable, these muscles also are introducing hip extension. This would account for the delay in thigh advancement during initial and mid swing. During stance, the continuous activity of the adductor longus (which is aligned to flex the hip) dynamically inhibits thigh extension. The relative forward advancement of the thigh also contributes to the excessive knee flexion occurring in terminal stance. Hence, the adductor longus demonstrates inappropriate action, while the gracilis is a useful muscle. Unfortunately, the activity of the iliacus is not known, as the electrode

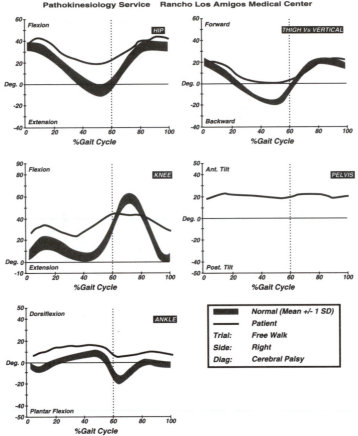

MOTION ANALYSIS
Pathokinesiology Service   Rancho Los Amigos Medical Center

Figure 15.22g Vicon motion analysis. The vertical axis is degrees of motion (flexion is positive). The horizontal axis is the percent of the gait cycle. The vertical dotted line divides stance and swing (toe-off). Gray areas indicate the 1 standard deviation band of normal function. Black line is patient data.

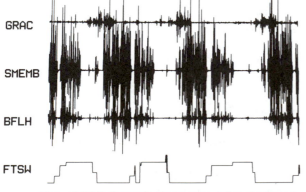

Figure 15.22h Dynamic electromyography of selected hip and knee muscles during free gait. GRAC = gracilis; SMEMB = semimembranosus; BFLH = biceps femoris long head; FTSW = foot switch of the same limb.

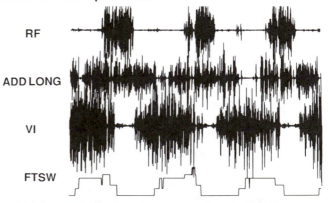

Figure 15.22i Dynamic electromyography of selected hip and knee muscles during free gait. RF = rectus femoris; ADD LONG = adductor longus; VI = vastus intermedius; FTSW = left footswitch; FTSW = right foot switch.

insertion was unsatisfactory. In terminal stance, excessive hip flexion is sustained by the premature and intense action of the rectus femoris.

The conclusions are that three situations contribute to the patient's excessive knee flexion in stance. Of primary significance is the excessive ankle dorsiflexion. The second major cause of excessive knee flexion in stance is the premature, prolonged and intense action of the hamstrings. Thirdly, there is overactivity of two hip flexor muscles, adductor longus and rectus femoris (the gracilis is appropriate and useful). Conversely, the lack of knee flexion in swing relates to the knee extensor action of the rectus femoris and the hip extensor action of the hamstrings. The neurological factors contributing to the inappropriate muscle action can be deduced from the patient's reactions to the pre-gait, upright motor control muscle tests (Figure 15.22j). Limited selective control is implied by low levels of EMG recorded during the manual muscle tests and confirmed by the high percentage of the *maximum voluntary effort* displayed by the muscles during walking (semimembranosus 85%, adductor longus 75%, rectus femoris 71%, vastus intermedius 75%). Only the VI EMG can be attributed to a high functional demand. The stretch tests identified sustained intense EMG in the RF, ADD LONG, SMEMB, and to a lesser extent the BFLH. For all four of these muscles, the high amplitude EMG persisted the entire 5 seconds of test time. In contrast, the stretch response of the gracilis, VI and BFSH, while still abnormal, was of short duration (.5sec). Hence, all the muscles exhibited spasticity, but at two very different levels, with only the highly spastic group registering obstructive action during gait. Primitive pattern control is evident in the participation of the muscles during the resisted mass flexion and extension tests

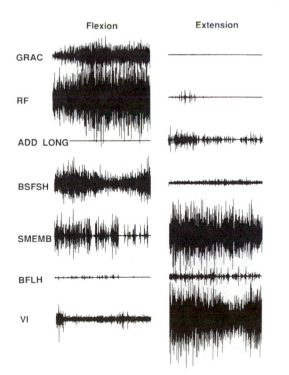

Figure 15.22j Dynamic electromyography of selected hip and knee muscles during the upright motor control tests. Flexion = resisted voluntary mass flexion of the limb; Extension = resisted voluntary mass extension of the limb; GRAC = gracilis; SMEMB = semimembranosus; BFLH = biceps femoris long head; RF = rectus femoris; ADD LONG = adductor longus; VI = vastus intermedius.

conducted with the patient standing (Figure 15.22j). Three muscles show dominant flexor action (gracilis, rectus femoris and biceps femoris short head) and their action in gait correlated. During the extensor pattern, there were two surprises, preference by the adductor longus to function with the extensor muscles, rather than the flexors and strong semimembranosus action. These findings justify the stance phase involvement of these muscle.

Patient R. Spastic genu recurvatum presents the opposite clinical picture of a crouch gait. The knee moves into hyperextension during stance, and the ankle has excessive plantar flexion. The hip still may have persistent flexion as the patient leans forward to balance over the plantar flexed foot.

For this cerebral palsy boy, incomplete knee extension in terminal swing presents a poor limb posture for stance (Figure 15.23a). Initial contact will occur at the forefoot rather than the heel, because there is inadequate knee extension and excessive ankle plantar flexion. Loading response knee motion is toward extension rather than flexion. This follows a drop of the foot into a delayed heel contact while the ankle remains plantar flexed (Figure 15.23b). In mid stance, the knee moves into hyperextension with a premature heel rise accompanied by excessive ankle plantar flexion (Figure 15.23c). Terminal stance advancement of body weight ahead of the foot continues the knee hyperextension while there is excessive heel rise and additional ankle plantar flexion (Figure 15.23d). There is a moderate trailing position at the thigh. The excessive ankle plantar flexion may be voluntary, substitutive vaulting to provide toe clearance by the other limb, which also has marked equinus and inadequate knee flexion. Pre-swing lacks knee flexion, but the hyperextension is less as advancement of body weight onto the anterior portion of the forefoot rocker rolls the foot and tibia forward (Figure 14.23e). While these postures would tend to unlock the knee, that does not occur. As a result, initial swing lacks knee flexion (Figure 14.23f). The toe drag appears to increase the ankle plantar flexion and delay advancement of the thigh. Contralateral trunk lean is needed to free the foot, due to the lack of initial swing knee flexion. In mid-swing inadequate hip and knee flexion, continue although the motions provide a vertical tibia. Failure of the limb to accommodate the excessive ankle plantar requires contralateral vaulting (Figure 15.23g).

The electrogoniometer recording of the ankle shows continuous plantar flexion of approximately 20° (Figure 15.23h). There is a minimal (5°) decrease in the ankle angle at the moment of limb loading and a second, more prolonged decrease of similar magnitude at the end of stance. Conversely, the ankle drops into its maximum plantar flexion in terminal swing. This motion recording reveals that the apparent vaulting, observed in mid stance, is not an interval of increased ankle plantar flexion.

By the electrogoniometer, the knee shows two arcs of motion (Figure 15.23i). The neutral extension present at initial contact promptly increases to hyperextension in loading response. This posture becomes maximal at the end of mid stance (20°). Then, the knee rapidly returns to neutral and moves into 5° flexion during pre-swing. No additional flexion is gained in initial swing. Once the foot becomes clear of the floor at the onset of mid swing, the

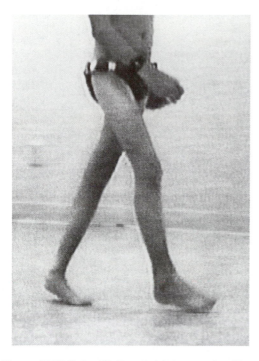

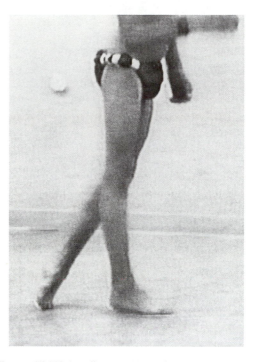

Figure 15.23 Patient R: Spastic hyperextension (Cerebral Palsy diplegia).

Figure 15.23a Initial contact by the forefoot with the ankle plantar flexed, knee flexed.

Figure 15.23b Loading response is knee extension following foot flat contact with ankle plantar flexion.

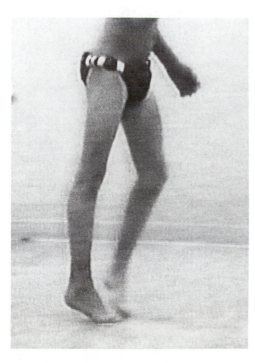

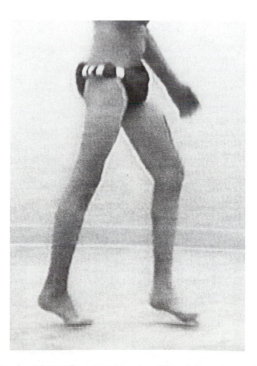

Figure 15.23c Mid stance shows knee hyperextension with excessive ankle plantar flexion and premature heel rise.

Figure 15.23d Terminal stance with a fully extended knee, excessive ankle plantar flexion and excessive heel rise. Thigh has a trailing alignment. The other limb also has excessive ankle plantar flexion.

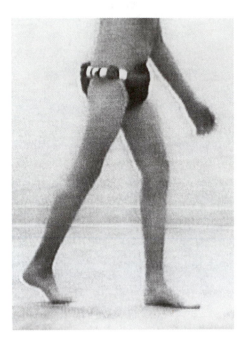

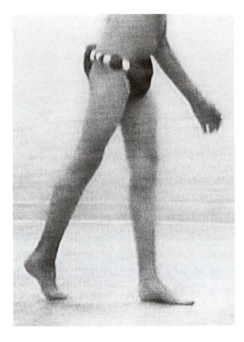

Figure 15.23e Pre-swing lacks knee flexion. Heel rise persists while ankle is only mildly plantar flexed. Weight appears to be primarily on the other foot (which now is plantigrade).

Figure 15.23f Initial swing totally lacks knee flexion and thigh advancement. The ankle is excessively plantar flexed, and there is a toe drag.

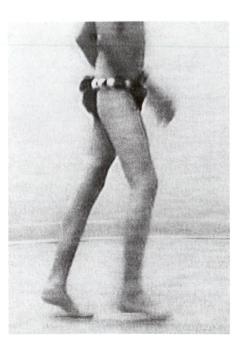

Figure 15.23g Mid swing hip and knee flexion are equal and not excessive. A toe drag from the plantar flexed ankle is avoided by contralateral vaulting.

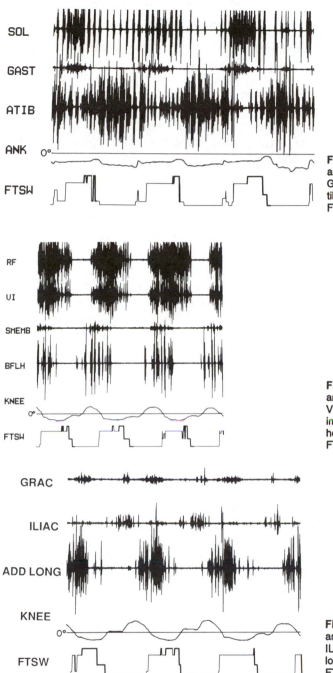

Figure 15.23h Dynamic electromyography and motion of the ankle. SOL = soleus; GAST = gastrocnemius; ATIB = anterior tibialis; ANK = ankle electrogoniometer; FTSW = foot switches for that limb.

Figure 15.23i Dynamic electromyography and motion of the knee. RF = rectus femoris; VI = vastus intermedius; SMEMB = semimembranosis; BFLH = biceps femoris long head; KNEE = knee electrogoniometer; FTSW = foot switches for that limb.

Figure 15.23j Dynamic electromyography and motion of the knee. GRAC = gracilis; ILIAC = iliacus; ADD LONG = adductor longus; KNEE = knee electrogoniometer; FTSW = foot switches for that limb.

knee flexes to a delayed peak posture of 30°. During terminal swing the knee again extends to neutral.

The EMG records demonstrate severe soleus muscle spasticity, with the clonic bursts persisting through swing as well as stance (Figure 15.23h). This spastic action is superimposed on a primitive control pattern (dense, continuous EMG), with premature onset at the beginning of stance. The significantly less gastrocnemius EMG activity (primitive phasing, but no clonus) implies limited protection of the knee from the hyperextension thrust. Accompanying the soleus is excessive action by the perimalleolar muscles during stance. The onset of the posterior tibialis, peroneus longus, peroneus brevis and flexor digitorum longus is premature and the intensity severely clonic. Hence, the foot as well as the ankle is rigid. Continual, high-intensity tibialis anterior EMG throughout the gait cycle implies strong dorsiflexion action. The muscle's small size compared to that of the soleus (20%) makes the tibialis anterior an ineffective dorsiflexor in swing, despite this being the period of major EMG. This tibialis anterior action, however, complements the soleus to cause varus, making the forefoot support less stable.[4,5] Strong PL and PB activity provide lateral stability for Mt1-5 contact.

EMG recordings of the knee muscles show intense, premature and prolonged action of the knee extensors (VI and RF) from the onset of terminal swing through terminal stance (Figure 15.23i). While having the vastus intermedius begin in terminal swing is normal, its intensity is excessive. Continuation beyond loading response is abnormal, and activity in the presence of a hyperextended posture is very inappropriate. In addition, the rectus femoris (RF) is functioning totally out of phase as well as displaying excessive intensity. The intense, spastic action of the biceps femoris long head (BFLH) and the lesser action of the semimembranosus between mid swing and mid stance are attempting to assist knee flexion in swing. At the same time the hip extensor action of these hamstring muscles is antagonistic to thigh advancement, and this is a critical element of swing phase knee flexion. In stance, contrary to expectations, the hamstrings offer no prolonged resistance to the knee hyperextension thrust imposed by the intense quadriceps action. Nor has the biceps femoris short head altered its action from swing to stance to provide protection.

Hip flexor control is provided by three muscles. It begins in initial swing with the iliacus (Figure 15.23j). Low level gracilis action is a useful synergist. Dynamic hip flexion is continued between terminal swing and mid stance by intense and excessive adductor longus action. While useful for limb advancement in terminal swing, the stance phase action of the adductor longus is the probable source of the anterior pelvic tilt.

The conclusion is that the boy's knee recurvatum results from excessive action of a highly spastic soleus and quadriceps. Hip flexor control would be adequate if the limb were unlocked. The adductor longus is serving as a useful swing phase hip flexor, but might also create undesired scissoring. The limitation of swing knee flexion relates to two EMG findings. Premature hamstring muscle action during initial swing inhibits hip flexor momentum by their hip extensor effect, and the primary hip flexor action by iliacus, gracilis and later the adductors longus provides an insufficient counterforce. Intense rectus femoris action in mid swing inhibits knee flexion by its knee extensor effect, and the less intense and smaller biceps femoris short head (BFSH) is an ineffective antagonist. The seemingly random mixture of appropriate, ill timed and out-of-phase muscle action illustrates the reasons why one cannot predict muscle activity in the spastic patient with impaired neural control.[3]

References

1. Bodian D: Motoneuron disease and recovery in experimental poliomyelitis. In Halstead LS, Weichers DO (Eds): *Late effects of poliomyelitis*. Miami, FL, Symposia Foundation, 1985, pp. 45-55.
2. Charnley J: The long-term results of low-friction arthroplasty of the hip performed as a primary intervention. *J Bone Joint Surg* 54B(1):61-76, 1972.
3. DeLuca PA: Gait analysis in the treatment of the ambulatory child with cerebral palsy. *Clin Orthop* 264:65-75, 1991.
4. Hoffer MM: Ten year follow-up of split anterior tibial tendon transfer in cerebral palsied patients with spastic equinovarus deformity. *J Pediatr Orthop* 5(4):432-434, 1985.
5. Hoffer MM, Reiswig JA, Garrett AL, Perry J: The split anterior tibial tendon transfer in the treatment of spastic varus hindfoot of childhood. *Orthop Clin North Am* 5(1):31-38, 1974.
6. McComas AJ: *Neuromuscular Function and Disorders*. Boston, Butterworths, 1977, pp. 148-150.
7. Melkoian GJ, Cristoforok RL, Perry J, Hsu JD: Dynamic gait electromyography study in Duchanne Muscular Dystrophy (DMD) patients. *Foot and Ankle* 1(1):78-83, 1980.
8. Pease WS, Johnson EW: Rehabilitation management of diseases of the motor unit. In Kottke FJ, Lehmann JF (Eds): *Krusen's Handbook of Physical Medicine and Rehabilitation*. Edition 4th, Philadelphia, W. B. Saunders, 1990, pp. 754-764.
9. Perry J, Antonelli D, Ford W: Analysis of knee-joint forces during flexed-knee stance. *J Bone Joint Surg* 57A(7):961-967, 1975.
10. Sharrad WJ: Muscle recovery in poliomyelitis. *J Bone Joint Surg* 37B:63-79, 1955.
11. Sutherland DH: *Gait Disorders in Childhood and Adolescence*. Baltimore, Williams and Wilkins, 1964.
12. Thometz J, Simon S, Rosenthal R: The effect of gait of lengthening of the medial hamstrings in cerebral palsy. *J Bone Joint Surg* 71A(3):345-353, 1989.
13. Wong MA, Simon S, Olshen RA: Statistical analysis of gait patterns of persons with cerebral palsy. *Statistics in Medicine* 2:345-354, 1983.

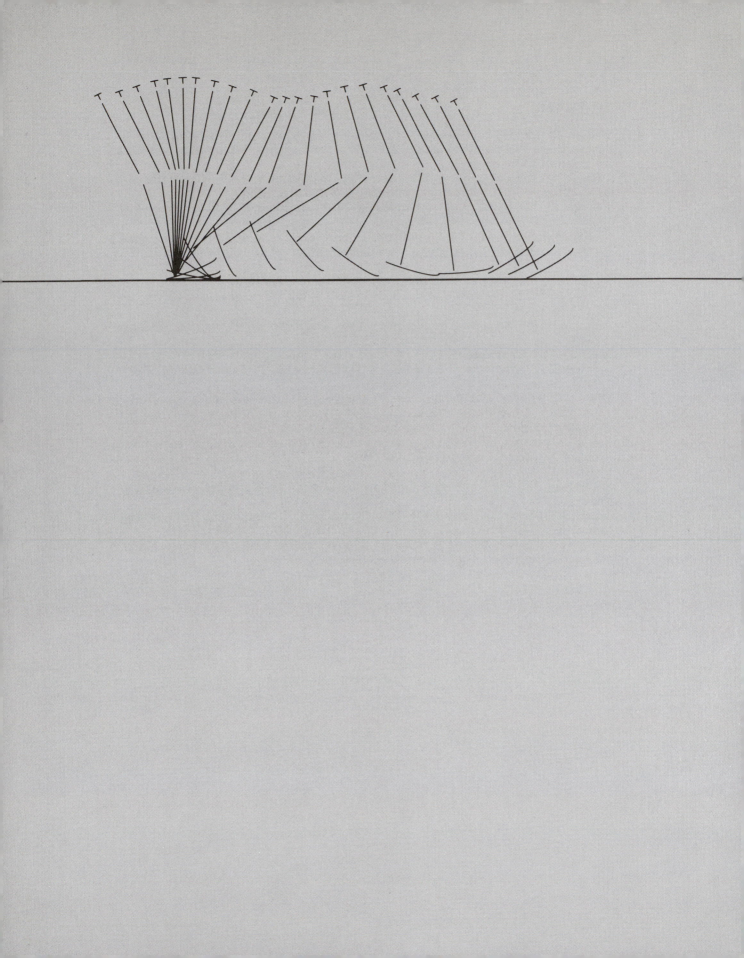

Section Four

Gait Analysis Systems

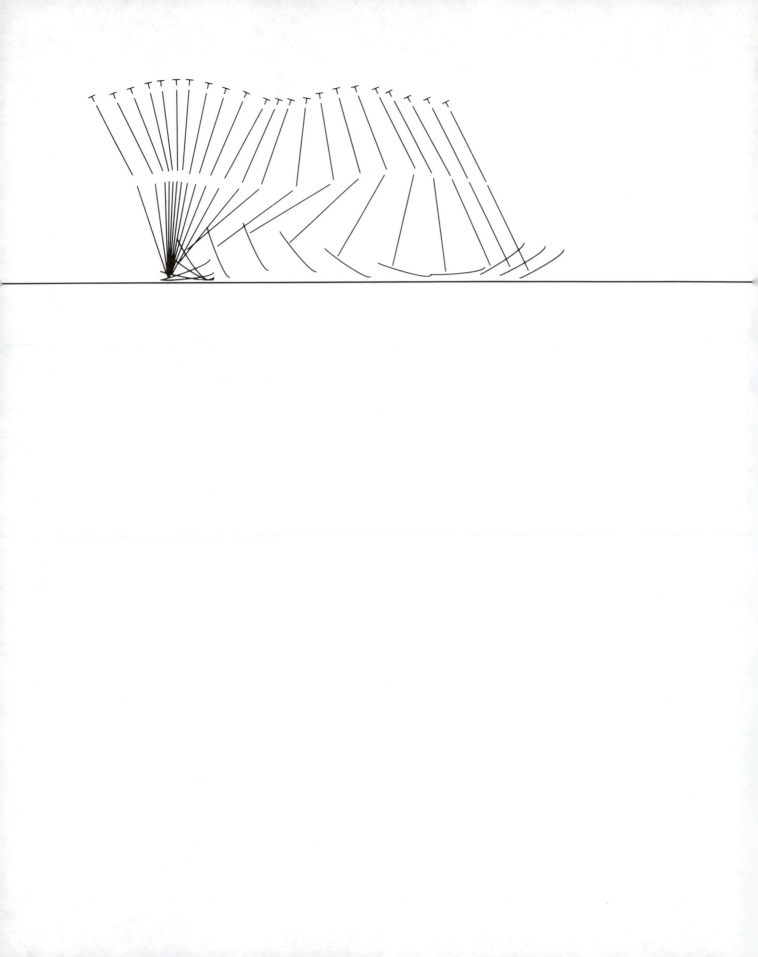

Chapter 16

Gait Analysis Systems

The complexity of walking becomes very apparent as soon as one considers either referring a patient for objective analysis or establishing your own gait laboratory. Immediately a decision must be made as to what techniques should be employed.

Basically, there are five measurement systems. Three of these focus on the specific events that constitute the act of walking. Motion analysis defines the magnitude and timing of individual joint action. Dynamic electromyography identifies the period and relative intensity of muscle function. Force plate recordings display the functional demands being experienced during the weight-bearing period. Each of these systems serves as a diagnostic technique for one facet of gait.

The two remaining gait analysis technics summarize the effects of the person's gait mechanics. To determine overall walking capability, one measures the patient's stride characteristics, while efficiency is revealed by energy cost measurements.

Within each of these five basic measurement systems

there are several choices of technique. These differ in cost, convenience, and completeness of the data provided. As there is not a single optimal system, selections are based on the needs, staffing and finances of the particular clinical or research situation. Some decisions are optional, while others are determined by the type of pathology to be analyzed. A basic aid in making these choices is skill in observational gait analysis.

Observational Gait Analysis

All professionals involved in the management of the lower extremities use some form of gait analysis. The simplest approach is a generalized screening to note the gross abnormalities of the person's walk. The observer is more likely to make the appropriate determinations, however, if the analysis proceeds in a systematic fashion. This circumvents the natural tendency to focus on the obvious events while overlooking other, more subtle deviations, which may be highly significant. In response to this need, most organizers of gait analysis courses develop a syllabus as a guide to their students.

To be complete, systematic gait analysis involves three steps. First is information organization. The second is an established sequence of observation (data acquisition). Third is a format for data interpretation.

The essential gait events and their classification for observational analysis are demonstrated by the format of the chapters in this book. Normal function is sorted by anatomical area and the phasing of the events in the gait cycle. The list of gait deviations, representing clinical experience with a wide variety of pathology follows the same anatomical and phasic organization. The observational process is facilitated by having an analysis form that guides the clinician. In addition to identifying the gait deviations, having the form designate the phases in which each gait deviation can occur focuses the observer. A further asset is the differentiation of the more significant gait deviations from the minor occurrences (Figure 16.1).[1] The usual vertical orientation of the recording form from proximal (trunk) to distal (toe) is contrary to the order of analysis, but the result is an anatomically correct summary of the patient's difficulties.

The process of observational analysis (data acquisition) is best performed in two stages. First is a gross review to sense the flow of action. Then the analysis should follow an anatomical sequence in order to sort the multiple events happening at the different joints. Clinical experience with multiple approaches has led to the practice of starting at the foot and progressing upward. Floor contact, ankle/foot, knee, hip, pelvis and trunk are assessed, in this sequence. Familiarity with normal function is developed first. At each level, the direction and magnitude of motion in each phase of gait is noted and imprinted on the observer's memory. An organized awareness of normal function is developed. From this model, pathology is identified as deviations from normal function. At each area the patient's performance is compared to normal and deviations noted. Regardless of the gross appearance of the patient's gait, the observer should follow the format of sequentially analyzing each anatomical area relative to the gait phases and determining the deviations from normal, before moving up to the next segment. Basically, the observer moves horizontally

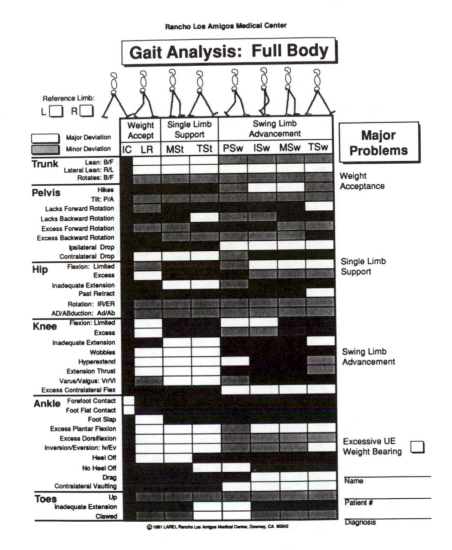

Figure 16.1 Full body observational gait analysis form (Rancho system). Rows = gait deviations; columns = gait phases. Walking dysfunction tabulated by checking the pertinent boxes. White boxes = major gait deviations; gray boxes = minor gait deviations; black boxes = not applicable.

across the gait analysis form within each anatomical area.

The findings are interpreted at two levels. Total limb function is identified by summing the gait deviations that occur in each gait phase. In this way the motions that impair progression or stability are differentiated from substitutive actions. The findings per phase then are related to the basic tasks, and the deterrents to effective weight acceptance and limb advancement are identified. The cause of these functional deterrents are deduced from the physical findings of weakness, contracture, spasticity and sensory loss. When a conclusion cannot be reached, instrumented gait analysis, such as dynamic electromyography is recommended.

Reference

1. Pathokinesiology Department, Physical Therapy Department: *Observational Gait Analysis Handbook.* Downey, CA, The Professional Staff Association of Rancho Los Amigos Medical Center, 1989.

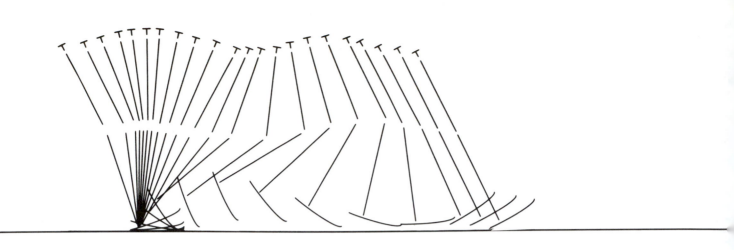

Chapter 17

Motion Analysis

Because walking is a pattern of motion, diagnosis of the patient's difficulties depends on an accurate description of the actions occurring at each joint. The customary approach has been to carefully observe the patients gait and make appropriate conclusions. While performing the observation in a systematic manner results in more agreement among observers, there still is disagreement on details. The asynchronous series of changes occurring at each joint of the two limbs presents such a maze of data that few persons can assimilate it all. The result may be premature conclusions. An alternate approach is quantitated documentation of the person's performance with reliable instrumentation that provides a permanent record of fact. The indecisions of subjective observation are avoided. Rapid and subtle events are captured. A printed record of the patient's motion pattern provides a reference base for interpreting EMG, stride, and force data.

Motion, however, is much easier to observe than measure. While the major arcs of joint motion occur in the sagittal plane, there also are subtle actions occurring in the coronal and transverse planes. These deviations from the sagittal plane of progression often are much greater in the disabled walker, and they may be of considerable clinical significance. This introduces two problems. First is the technical challenge of making the necessary measurements. The second problem is the effect of out-of-plane movement on the amount of sagittal motion that is perceived. For example,a single lateral view will underestimate the amount of flexion present if the limb is internally rotated, because the segments are foreshortened. This fact is most easily appreciated by comparing the image of a flexed knee with the limb in the sagittal plane and having it rotated 45° (Figure 17.1). The thigh, shank and bent knee define the plane in which the limb lies. When the limb is parallel with the wall, the photograph has the same angle as exists in the knee. Internally rotating the limb 45° reduces the recorded knee angle to 20°. If this were a lateral camera recording of a child walking, the reviewer would say the child lacked the normal swing phase knee flexion. There are two technical means of correcting this error: placing a goniometer on the limb and using three-dimensional camera recording. Both technics have lengthy history of instrumentation development.[20] Each technic has specific capabilities and limatations.

Electrogoniometers

The first goniometer designed to measure knee motion during walking was an electronically instrumented hinge between two bars, one strapped to the

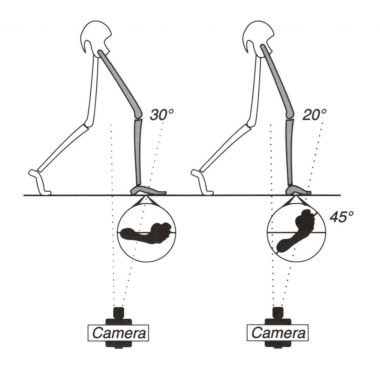

Figure 17.1 Single camera motion analysis cannot identify the effects of limb rotation. With 45° internal rotation of the limb, a knee flexed 30° is recorded as 20° flexion.

thigh and the other to the leg.[11,18] While the principle was good, alignment of the apparatus deteriorated with increasing knee flexion. The problem was the difference in the types of joint axes. The axis of the goniometer was a fixed point, while the knee has a series of instant centers that follow a curved path as the knee flexes.[12] Design of the double parallelogram system corrected this limitation.

Single Axis Parallelogram Electrogoniometers

To follow the ever-changing location of the knee joint's instant centers, the double parallelogram-type electrogoniometer designed to record finger motion[10,34] was adapted for the lower limb.[4]

Each arm of the goniometer is a slender parallelogram frame, which is free to alter its shape, so the junction between the two frames can change its location. This allows the location of the goniometer's axis of rotation to follow the path of the anatomical joint (Figure 17.2).

Changes in the angle between the two parallelograms defines the joint's position. The thin parallelogram frames are serially connected so that the distal frame is attached to a limb cuff and the proximal arm is connected to the shaft of a potentiometer mounted on the cuff of the other limb segment. Relative angular motion between the two limb segments (e.g., thigh and shank for a knee goniometer) is sensed by the potentiometer, producing a proportional electrical signal that can be recorded by any of the standard systems. Translation (nonrotational shifting) of the parallelograms caused by the changing anatomical joint center is not transmitted to the potentiometer. Moderate slack at the base of each goniometer arm accommodates the small arcs of transverse rotation and coronal angulation that also occur.

The basic single axis goniometer system has been modified three ways. It has been adapted for orthoses, adapted for other joints, and multiple units have been combined for simultaneous multiarticular recordings.

Electrogoniometers customarily are strapped to the lateral side of the limb. This same area is occupied by the uprights of orthoses. To permit the measurement of knee motion in patients dependent on orthotic assistance, a unit that crossed the joint anteriorly was designed (Figure 17.2). Roentgenographic correlation of skeletal motion and that recorded by the anterior goniometer demonstrated a mild lag in the system. With 30° of knee flexion the difference is only 1.5°. At 60° of flexion the goniometric reading is 6.8° less and 8° when the knee is flexed 90°.[31] This average 10% difference still yields motion patterns that are consistent with the output of the automated video systems,[17,33] but less than Murray's strobe light data.[27] Tilting of the thigh segment into the soft tissues is visible on roentgenograms.

Smaller units have been designed for the ankle and subtalar joint. Roentgenological analysis of ankle motion confirmed the presence of a moving axis at the ankle.[30] The interval between the leg and foot fixation points for a goniometer spans a minimum of three joints: tibiotalar, subtalar, and midtarsal. Variability in subtalar joint axis alignment implies this, too, has a shifting axis.[14] A U-shaped foot attachment excludes shoe motion in the measurements when barefoot testing is not appropriate. At the ankle, where there is less soft tissue mobility, the error documented by X-ray is only 2° (unpublished data).

The third development has been a lightweight system that provides bilateral measurements of the hip, knee and ankle.[6,7] By combining the data with foot switch information, the developers can also calculate step length.

Triaxial Parallelogram Goniometers

Extension of the goniometer concept to measure rather than just accommodate nonsagittal plane motions led to the triaxial parallelogram electrogoniometer (TPE).[9,15,16,19,21] This has parallelograms and a potentiometer for each plane of motion (sagittal, coronal and transverse) (Figure 17.3). The compound unit is strapped to the lateral side of the limb, centered over the joint of interest. Several developers have combined the TPE units into systems that simultaneously measure hip, knee and ankle. Connecting rods and body fixation straps are shared. This is the design of the commercial systems now available.

Recording accuracy of these multiaxial units has been analyzed. Simultane-

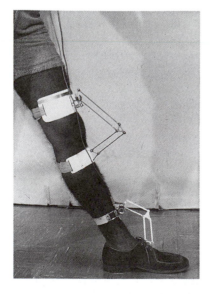

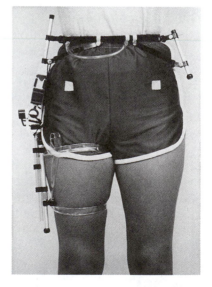

Figure 17.2 Parallelogram goniometers for the knee and ankle. The junction of the double bar shaped arms separates a change in joint angle from changes in instant center alignment. At the ankle there is a double flange that fits under the tongue of the shoe (Rancho design).

Figure 17.3 The hip electrogoniometer spans both the lumbar spine and hip joint as the proximal band is at the waist. White squares overlie the superior anterior iliac spines of the pelvis. (Courtesy Churchill Livingstone, N.Y., 1984.)

ous recordings with the anterior and lateral knee goniometers demonstrated the same discrepancy that was found by the roentgen study of the anterior unit. Hence, the data from the lateral unit matched the X-ray positions. The CARS-UBC™ triaxial goniometer that was studied used very firm strapping to the leg. Fixation on the thigh included both a groin and supracondylar strap. Recently more comfortable strapping has been substituted, but the accuracy has not been retested. Hence, there may be an exchange between comfort and recording accuracy.

Accuracy on repeated use has proved to be satisfactory. Retest of the same individual resulted in a 2° difference in hip motion.[16] Reapplication by another person increased the error to a 4° difference. The comparison of triaxial electrogoniometer data to that obtained by other measuring devices has led to mixed results, from close agreement to 10° differences in either direction. The unresolved question is which technic should be the standard?

Cross talk is another potential limitation to triaxial goniometers. The three sensors at each joint are linked in series, so motion of one could displace the connecting arm of the next. The possibility of cross talk was measured with an experimental device that controlled posturing in one plane, while allowing free motion in the other planes.[28] When the angle in the coronal or transverse plane equalled 10° or more there was a significant error in sagittal motion. Inspection of the goniometers under these complex circumstances confirmed a change in goniometer alignment. Based on the assumption that the three-dimensional dependency is consistent computer corrections of the data have been formulated.[9] Clinically the cross talk would not be significant in normal knee function, which has minimal coronal or rotatory motion, but values obtained on patients with hypermobility require the added calculations.

Measurement of hip motion should be between the pelvis and thigh, but this rarely occurs with electrogoniometers. Only with thin subjects can one truly keep a strap around the pelvis. Muscle attachments obscure all but the narrow brim of the iliac crest and a highly mobile layer of skin and fat overlie this. The pelvic band more commonly is at the waist (Figure 17.3). The resulting measurement combines lumbar spine motion with that occurring at the hip, as the points of goniometer fixation are the trunk and thigh. In the slender person with a normal gait, there is so little trunk motion that no significant error is introduced. Patients with incompetent hip musculature or joint structures, however, frequently use large arcs of trunk motion (Trendelenberg limp) to substitute for their limitations. At the same time, the pelvis often drops in the opposite direction. Hence, the pelvic electrogoniometer can track normal motion satisfactorily, but not that of the person with hip pathology. Photographic recordings during a Trendelenberg gait documented significant differences between trunk and pelvic motions, while the simultaneous electrogoniometer readings showed only minimal coronal plane motion, which approximated the average of the two opposing actions. Thus, the electrogoniometer is not a useful instrument at the hip when pathological function leads to significant displacement of the trunk.

Despite the limitations just discussed, electrogoniometers remain the most convenient and least expensive means of measuring knee and ankle motion during walking. Today, a set of goniometers (one ankle, one knee) can be obtained for approximately $6,000. The minimal supplementary equipment needed is a recorder. From this simple record, one can identify minimal and maximal arcs of motion and calculate rates of change. Another significant advantage of electrogoniometers is the immediate availability of the data, which facilitates prompt functional interpretation.

Cameras

Cameras offer a remote (noncontact) means of recording and reviewing motion of the entire body (head, trunk, arm and both lower limbs). Technology today allows recording the subject's motion for observational analysis or quantitating the data. The three basic systems available today are classified by the medium used to capture the data. These are film, visible video and automated video. The film and visible video systems can serve two purposes. Their immediate product is a visual record that is reviewed by eye. By further processing the film a digital record of the motion can be obtained. The video electronics also can be used as an automated system for direct motion quantification. A variant of this is the optoelectrical systems that use small lights (diodes) to activate the camera.

Film Photography

The most versatile means of recording joint motion, today, is film photography, but reducing the images to numerical values is a laborious task. There are two basic techniques: still photography and movies.

Still photography uses a large frame camera to record motion by multiple exposures with interrupted light, commonly called *strobe light photography*. A rotating shutter determines the rate of film exposure and, therefore, the number of images that will be recorded in that picture. Shutter speeds of 10 to 20 exposures per second are the most frequent choices (Figure 17.4a). For slow walkers such as a stroke patient, the rate may be reduced to 5 exposures per second (Figure 17.4b). The subject is clothed in black leotards and the room lights dimmed. Reflective linear markers are applied along the lateral sides of the thigh, leg and foot with additional markers on other areas as needed. The resulting photograph is a series of stick figures. A large (10 X 12) print is often made for data reduction. Then, the limb angles are either measured by hand directly or with the aid of a digitizer. The stick figures provide a good display of motion, but transposing the data to numerical values is far too inefficient for more than a limited student exercise. An alternate marker system involves the use of colored lights that display the motion as a trail of spots. Each color represents one anatomical marker.[32]

Movie cameras provide much more versatility. They have a wide range of speeds (24 through 500 frames per second is the range in common use). Their images are sharp and clear and provide accurate reproductions of rapid athletic events as well as the performance of a slow walker. Motion at all joints (head to foot) can be clearly documented. Close up filming is an easy means of getting

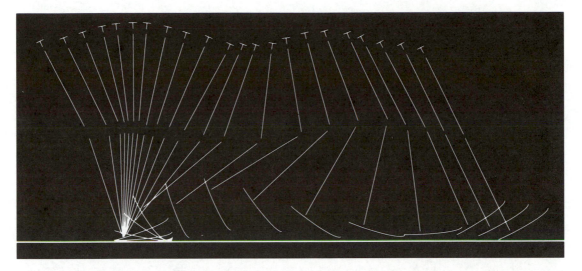

Figure 17.4a Interrupted light (strobe) photography of one stride of a normal subject. The images represent 20 samples per second. (Adapted from Eberhart HD, Inman VT, Bresler B. The principal element in human locomotion. In Klopsteg PE and Wilson PD (Eds), *Human Limbs and their Substitutes.* Hafner Pub, New York, 1968, p. 442.)

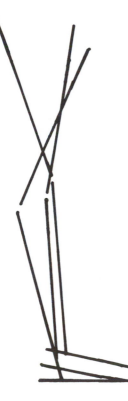

Figure 17.4b Strobe photography at a slower rate (5 frames/sec) portrays the disability of hemiplegia. Swing showing failure to extend the limb and the inhibition of progression by ankle immobility. Terminal stance flexion is rapidly reversed to knee hyperextension.

more detail. Projectors are standard equipment for display at any meeting.

Countering these many advantages is the tedious task of transferring the data from film to computer. This must be done by hand. Frame by frame, one must designate the location of each anatomical marker by placing a digitizing sensor over its center. The sonic digitizer (the most common type) then electronically assigns numerical coordinates to that spot (Figure 17.5). An established sequence is followed, so the signals are related to the correct joint marker for computer interpretation. This labor-intensive process takes about one hour to reduce just one stride of motion. One additional problem is the need to have the film developed before the data can be verified and processing begun.

The number of cameras used determines the accuracy of the motion recording. To appropriately track the body and limbs through space, one needs a minimum of two cameras. Otherwise, sagittal motions will be underestimated when joint alignment is oblique to the plane of the recording film, as described earlier.

For sagittal motion, two lateral cameras are spaced several feet apart (Figure 17.6).[2,3] By triangulation mathematics the true position of the joints is determined. This now is done with computer correlation of the data from each camera. To fully record the anterior and rotatory actions, one generally needs three cameras. The motion data are derived from tracking brilliant one-inch, black rimmed, white targets positioned over the pertinent landmarks.

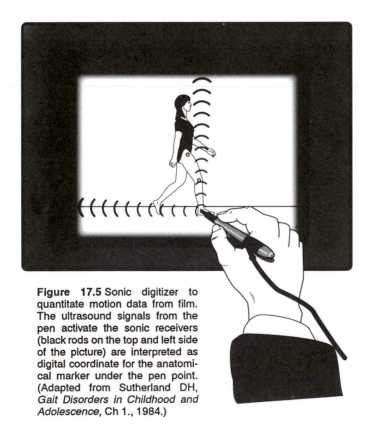

Figure 17.5 Sonic digitizer to quantitate motion data from film. The ultrasound signals from the pen activate the sonic receivers (black rods on the top and left side of the picture) are interpreted as digital coordinate for the anatomical marker under the pen point. (Adapted from Sutherland DH, *Gait Disorders in Childhood and Adolescence*, Ch 1., 1984.)

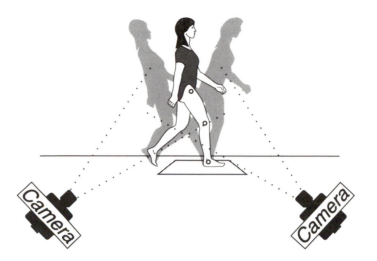

Figure 17.6 Two camera motion analysis provides a three-dimensional (3D) representation of the limb. Rotation does not alter the joint angles recorded.

While recording usually is done at 60 frames per second, to control the processing time only 20 frames within the stride are usually analyzed. This small sample size is accurate only for slowly moving patients. The speed of normal walking requires 60 samples per second to avoid missing peaks of rapid motion change. This sample rate is also sufficient for straight-line running. The sampling rate, however, must be increased to 100 or even 500 frames/second for more demanding athletic events (Centinela Hospital Biomechanics laboratory, unpublished data). Consequently, data reduction from film photography is very laborious. Correlating data from three cameras also requires considerable computer programming. A minimum of two steps are involved. First is designation of the instantaneous three-dimensional coordinates of each marker. Second is the processing of these data to formulate the graphs of joint motion. A third stage in computer programming analyzes the data for the magnitude and time of the high and low peaks of motion. Each step is a complex time-consuming process. Commercial programs have not been available. Hence, each laboratory has had to invest in the necessary engineering or computer programmer's time and skill.

Visible Video Recording

The most convenient and least costly means of documenting a patient's gait is by single camera video recording. This provides an immediate display for observational analysis. In turn, a lateral and a frontal recording can be made. The popular $1/2$ inch video systems are adequate for most clinical situations. A total system will require a video camera, recorder and monitor. For satisfactory clinical review, the recorder should have a playback system

Instead, its major mass is posterior to the femoral shaft, and normal anteversion of the femoral neck positions the head anteriorly (Figure 17.7). In an unpublished study, marker placement was compared to lateral roentgenograms of the hip, knee and ankle. The center of the hip joint (femoral head) lies 3.5cm anterior to the posterior margin of the greater trochanter. When the overlying soft tissue is included, this point corresponds to the superior, anterior margin of the greater trochanter (Figure 17.8).

Knee joint anatomy is more direct. The lateral epicondyle of the femur overlies the center of the joint. Because this bony landmark often is not very prominent even without a heavy fatty covering, the head of the fibula was investigated as an alternate guide. By the roengenographic study it was determined that the lateral femoral epicondyle lies just above a point 1.5cm anterior to the posterior margin of the fibular head.[29]

The ankle presents a minor discrepancy between the most stable location for a lateral surface marker (i.e., the lateral malleolus) and the center of the joint axis. Medially, the ankle joint axis is 5mm inferior to the medial malleolus, while the lateral landmark for the ankle axis is 3mm inferior and 8mm anterior

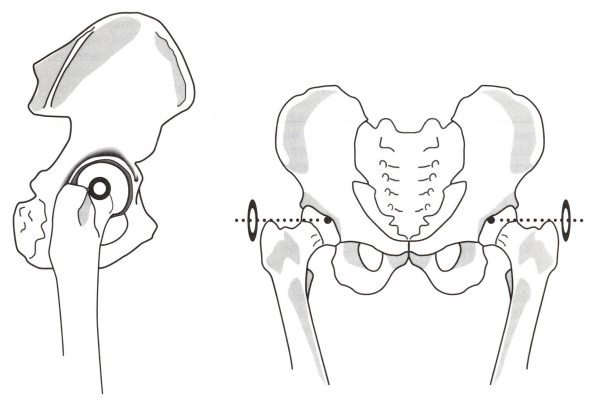

Figure 17.7 Laterally the hip marker should be at the anterior, superior margin of the greater trochanter to overlie the hip joint center.

Figure 17.8 Skin marker located at the upper margin of the greater trochanter is opposite the center of the hip joint.

to the tip of the malleolus (Figure 17.9).[14] This places the center of the line joining these two points just slightly below and anterior to the apex of the lateral malleolus. By the roentgen study, the discrepancy is about 0.5cm.[29] That is, the apex of the lateral malleolus is only 0.5cm posterior to the line between the knee center and Inman's joint axis landmark.

At the pelvis, the clinical landmarks for the sagittal (progressional) axis of the pelvis are the posterior and anterior superior iliac spines.[26] For gait analysis the posterior landmark generally is identified by a stick taped to the center of the sacrum. The anterior landmark is the calibrated center of the line between the right and left anterior superior iliac spines (ASIS). During quiet standing with normal back alignment and a vertical thigh (full-knee extension), the sagittal pelvic axis is anteriorly tilted downward approximately 10° from the horizontal (Figure 17.10).[26] This increases the measured angle between the pelvis and thigh (hip flexion) by 10°. The interpretation of thigh position during walking relative to the erect posture in stance and the contribution to step length made in swing is

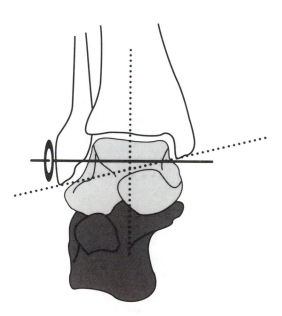

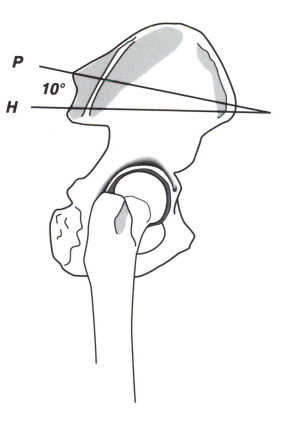

Figure 17.9 Ankle joint on the lateral protuberance of the lateral malleolus is within millimeters of the point where the ankle joint axis crosses the limb midline (center of ankle joint).

Figure 17.10 Pelvic landmarks are the posterior superior iliac spines (PSIS) and the anterior superior iliac spines (ASIS). This tilts the anterior posterior (AP) axis of the pelvis down 10° below the horizontal.

correspondingly modified. Both hip flexion and lumbar lordosis that are greater than normal can proportionally increase the tilt of the pelvic axis.

Secondary Marker Modifiers. Several additional factors reduce the accuracy of motion analysis with surface markers. Obesity hides the bony prominences at the pelvis, particularly the anterior superior iliac spines. There can be independent motion of the skin away from the joint centers. Laboratories differ in their method of establishing the zero reference position.

The Zero Position. Using the subject's quiet standing position is the easiest method of establishing the zero position, but this can introduce considerable variability. Common subtle errors can be introduced. Often it is assumed that the ankle is at 90°, yet a balanced stance requires 5° of dorsiflexion to position the body vector in the middle of the supporting foot. The knee may be either flexed or hyperextended, rather than at neutral. For example, Murray's data on men showed the knee never fully extended during walking.[27] This related to a quiet standing posture of 4° hyperextension that was called zero (M.P. Murray, personal communication).

Recording the actual standing posture as it occurs helps avoid the current inconsistency. To accomplish this the anatomical normal (neutral) alignment is the reference posture (Figure 17.11a). When the subject's limb cannot be positioned in normal alignment, the deviation is identified as a postural error and noted as an abnormal *zero* position (Figure 17.11b). The significance of motion marker location was demonstrated by a comparative study of gait motion for the same subjects obtained in three different research laboratories, which were participating in a collaborative study that included staff travel to the other centers. Results of the analysis showed that the pattern of motion recorded for each subject was the same at the different laboratories, but the numerical end points differed markedly.[8]

Independent skin motion is caused by bowstringing of the tendons and bulging of the contracting muscles pulling on the elastic skin. A radiological study of the knee and mid thigh markers showed progressive displacement as flexion was increased.[29] Posterior shift of the mid thigh marker increased from 0.9cm with 15° knee flexion to 2.8cm at the 90° position. The skin marker at the knee showed a similar pattern of displacement, being 0.6cm posterior to the lateral epicondyle at 15° and 4cm with 90° flexion. In contrast, the tight skin over the head of the fibula moved only 1.7cm with 90° flexion. There was a corresponding reduction in the knee angle recorded by the skin markers. With 90° flexion the loss was 8°, a difference that is very similar to that reported for the anterior electrogoniometer.

Coronal Plane Landmarks

Designation of abduction and adduction of the limb segments customarily relies on anterior landmarks. Pelvic alignment is designated by the two anterior superior iliac spines. The middle of the patella defined the anterior center of the knee. Similarly, the middle of the distal tibia is the marker for the ankle. These same points can be calculated from the combined medial lateral markers used in a three-dimensional system.

Foot position (subtalar motion) must be judged from behind, and close-up recording is needed. Two markers each (proximal and distal) on the heel and the tibia are used to designate the posterior longitudinal axis (Figure 17.12). The neutral position of the hind foot is difficult to define, however.

Transverse Rotation Markers

Attempts to use just the anatomical landmarks has not been successful, because the arcs of rotation, even when pathological, are too small for capture by the available camera systems. To overcome this limitation a mid segment

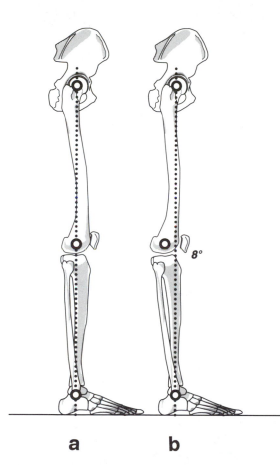

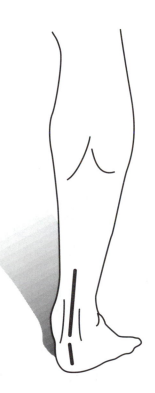

Figure 17.11 (a) The normal vertical alignment of the limb ("zero" position) is a straight line from the hip joint center, through the knee epicondyle, to the lateral malleolus. (b) Joint postures that deviate from the neutral line should be identified as abnormal. In this limb the "zero" positions are 15° knee flexion and 10° ankle plantar flexion.

Figure 17.12 Hind foot motion analysis. Angle between two lines, one each on the posterior center of the tibia and heel.

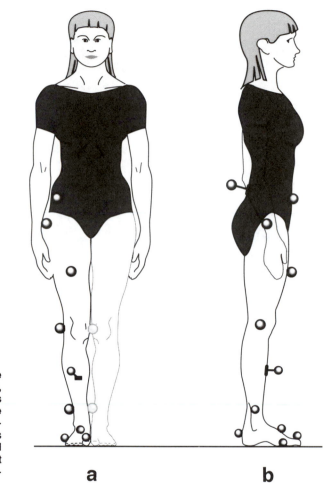

Figure 17.13 Three-dimensional surface marker system for motion analysis of hip, knee and ankle function. Dark gray balls are the gait markers. Light gray balls are the pre-gait static markers to better designate the limb segment's plane. Sticks on the sacrum, mid anterior thigh and mid anterior tibia facilitate the measurement of rotation by magnifying the arc of motion that occurs.

a   **b**

stick is used. The stick may be placed either anteriorly or on the lateral side of the limb (Figure 17.13).

Three-Dimensional Marker System

To permit simultaneous measurement of sagittal, coronal and transverse motion of the hip, knee and ankle, multiple surface markers are used. The system we are using at Rancho includes the arrangement of markers shown in Figure 17.13.

The pelvis is defined by the plane passing through the anterior and posterior superior iliac spines. Care is taken to align the marker at the tip of the stick along the ASIS-PSIS line. The plane of the thigh is designated by two systems.

For the gait recordings, markers are placed over the greater trochanter, anterior mid thigh and lateral femoral epicondyle. To relate the plane these markers define to the sagittal alignment of the limb, a temporary medial condyle marker is added for a quiet standing record. A similar system is used to identify the plane of the shank (lower leg or tibia). The gait markers are on the epicondyle, anterior mid tibia and distal shank. Supplementing these is a temporary marker on the medial shank at the same level as the lateral one. Shank markers are used instead of ones placed at the malleoli of the ankle to provide the distance needed to differentiate them from the foot markers (a minimum of 5cm). The plane of the foot is designated by gait markers on the posterior heel, laterally on the head of the fifth metatarsal and dorsum of the foot. The orienting, temporary marker is placed medially on the head of the first metatarsal. Standing records are made with the temporary markers in place, and then they are removed prior to the gait tests. Various modifications of this approach are used by other laboratories. By defining the planes of the body segments (pelvis and limb), one can identify the joint centers for force calculations and also measure joint motion.

Cluster Markers. To circumvent the difficulties of inconstant movement and location of the skin markers, the use of a mid segment cluster of markers has been introduced. The purpose is to define the plane of each segment with three

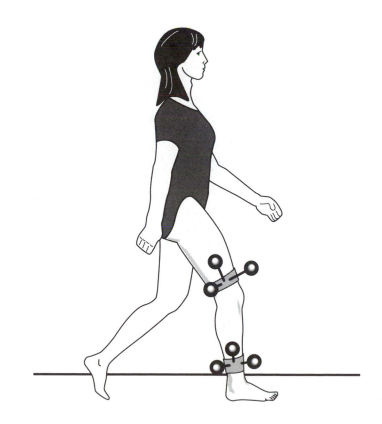

Figure 17.14 Cluster markers. Three dimensionally oriented markers are on a common base that is strapped to the center of the limb segment. It is assumed the influence of skin motion between markers is reduced.

markers and then track its movement through the basic reference planes (Figure 17.14). For the Selspot/TRACK™ motion analysis system, a shield with five markers is used.[5,24,25]

Motion Reference Scale

The final area of inconsistency that needed attention is the numerical scale used to define the arcs of motion. Designation of neutral alignment is the basic area of indecision. Is it 0° or 180°? The clinical standard of using zero was established by the American Academy of Orthopaedic Surgeons many years ago and a reference manual that now is used by many countries.[1] Periodically, neutral is called 180° to facilitate reporting the full range of hip, knee and ankle motion as a continuum of positive values. While this approach simplifies computer management of the data, it makes interpretation difficult because the reader must shift to an unfamiliar reference scale. For optimum effectiveness in information transfer, the data should be stated in the language of the clinician since the basic objective of using motion analysis is to clarify patient care.

Each lower extremity joint is capable of moving in both directions from its neutral (0°) position in each of its planes. Hence, graphically there are positive and negative values in the normal range of motion. By custom, hip flexion, abduction and internal rotation are represented as positive values (above zero), while extension, adduction and external rotation are negative values (below zero) (Figure 17.15). The knee motions are similarly represented. At the ankle, there is more confusion, because the functional neutral position is a natural right angle between the tibia and foot. Clinicians measure both dorsiflexion and plantar flexion as degrees of deviation from a zero designation of this neutral posture (even though it is a 90° angle), i.e., dorsiflexion 0° to 30° and plantar flexion 0° to 50°. Graphically, dorsiflexion beyond this anatomically neutral position is a positive value, while displacement into plantar flexion is negative.

The three-dimensional motions of the pelvis also have two directions of action. Anterior tilt, hiking and forward rotation of the reference side are presented as positive values. Conversely, posterior tilt, drop and backward rotation are treated as negative values (below the zero [0°] line). For the trunk, the positive side of the graph represents forward rotation, right lean and flexion. Extension, left lean and backward rotation are designated in the negative area. It is important, however, not to confuse a clinical discussion (text) with statements of negative or positive values, as they are generic terms. Thus, for example, negative degrees of ankle motion from a graph are still referred to as degrees of plantar flexion.

Motion Data Interpretation

The minimum information available from a motion record is the magnitude of the peak angles (high and low) experienced by the joint being studied. Because the functional demands of swing and stance are very different, the motion patterns of these two gait periods should be analyzed separately.

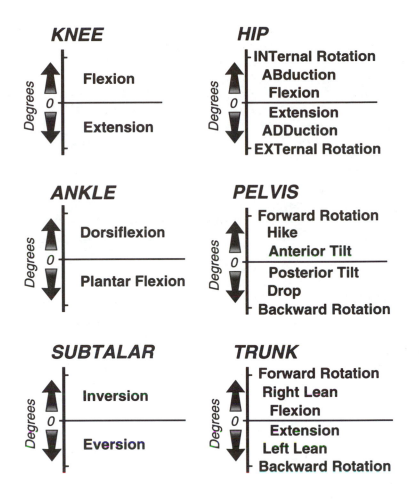

Figure 17.15 Reference scales. The direction for graphing each motion of the individual joint is identified. "0" represents the neutral position for the motion. Vertical axis indicates magnitude of motion. Arrow denotes increasing values for each direction. Horizontal axis represents the gait cycle time scale.

The magnitudes of joint motion as an independent item of information, however, may not be sufficient to identify the patient's gait abnormality, as the timing of the action may be the critical factor. Technically, identifying the time of the peak actions by the percentage points in the gait cycle is easiest, but this reference does not indicate functional significance. Expanding the analysis to define the motion occurring in each gait phase provides a much better interpretation of joint function. Now each abnormality is identified. For example, the record of a stroke patient's knee function may identify 20° stance flexion, extension to 0°, swing flexion of 50° and extension to 20° (Figure 17.16). This implies normal stance action and seemingly minor deviations in swing (flexion 50° versus 60°) and failure to complete terminal extension. In reality, the patient has a significant gait error that is identified only by noting the patient's phasic pattern. Stance phase flexion (20°) occurred at initial contact (due to inability to completely extend the knee in swing), not as a loading response event.Instead there was an extensor thrust as loading the limb caused a rapid loss of flexion. Also, this full extension persisted until toe-off. Hence, pre-swing knee flexion was lost. In swing the presumably good arc of knee flexion (50°) occurred late, that is, in mid swing rather than initial swing. This delay resulted in a toe drag, though the patient eventually advanced the limb.

The third level of analysis involves coordinating the motion patterns of the adjacent joints. Often, this alone will reveal the cause of the abnormality. In the example just cited, there was 15° equinus from terminal swing until toe-off with an associated initial contact by the forefoot (Figure 17.16). These findings indicated that the inappropriate knee motions were secondary to excessive ankle equinus, preventing the normal tibial advancement in stance, but it did not continue in swing, since the limb was advanced by a flexor pattern.

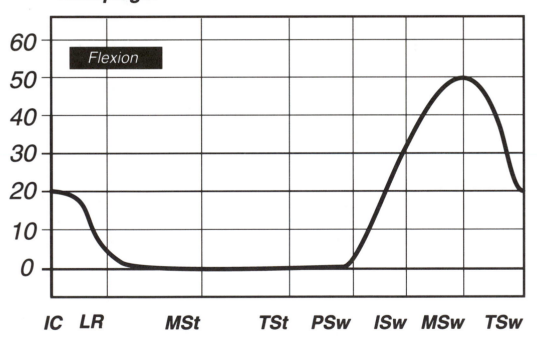

Figure 17.16 Stroke patient knee motion graph.

Summary

Motion analysis defines the person's gait. It does not identify the cause of errors, but it does delineate their magnitude, timing and phasic relationships. Through advanced reasoning, which correlates the patients performance with normal phasic function, the primary deficits can be differentiated from substitutive actions.

Film photography provides the clearest images, but one must wait for film development, and quantification involves a laborious interval of data transfer by hand. The automated video and optoelectrical systems largely circumvent the manual phase, but not entirely. More data can be processed, but there are some limitations on recording capability due to the minimum marker spacing tolerated. All the systems are costly both in equipment and data processing for gait information. As a result, a working system ranges between $150,000 and $300,000.

One unresolved problem is data storage. Experience has demonstrated that analog tapes may deteriorate after two or three years. Temperature and humidity controlled environments help but do not fully eliminate the problems. Optical disks are said to be more durable, but their history is as yet unknown because of their newness. Hence, data permanency requirements also must be considered when selecting a motion analysis system.

References

1. American Academy of Orthopaedic Surgeons: *Joint Motion—Method of Measuring and Recording.* American Academy of Orthopaedic Surgeons, 1965.
2. Andriacchi TP: An optoelectrical system for human motion analysis. *Bull Prosthetics Res* 18(1):291, 1981.
3. Andriacchi TP, Hampton SJ, Schultz AB, Galanti JD: Three-dimensinal coordinate data processing in human motion analysis. *J Biomech Eng* 101:279-283, 1979.
4. Antonelli D: Dynamic joint goniometer, in *Annual Reports of Progress.* Downey, CA, Rehabilitation Engineering Center at Rancho Los Amigos Hospital, 1975, p. 61.
5. Antonsson EK, Mann RW: Automatic 3-D gait analysis using a Selspot centered system. *Adv Bioengineering ASME*, 1979, pp. 51-52.
6. Bajd T, Kralj A: Simple kinematic gait measurements. *J Biomed Eng* 2(2):129-132, 1980.
7. Bajd T, Stanic U, Kljajic M, Trnkoczy A: On-line electrogoniometric gait analysis. *Comput Biomed Res* 9:439-444, 1976.
8. Biden E, Olshen R, Simon S, Sutherland D, Gage J, Kadaba M: Comparison of gait data from multiple labs. *Transactions of the Orthopaedic Research Society* 12:504, 1987.
9. Chao EYS: Justification of triaxial goniometer for the measurement of joint rotation. *J Biomech* 13(12):980-1006, 1980.
10. Esbkov B, Long C: A method of electromyographic kinesiology of the thumb. *Arch Phys Med Rehabil* 48(2):78-84, 1967.
11. Finley FR, Karpovich PV: Electrogoniometric analysis of normal and pathological gaits. *Res Quart (Suppl)* 5:379-384, 1964.
12. Frankel VH, Burstein AH: *Orthopaedic Biomechanics.* Philadelphia, Lea and Febiger, 1970, pp. 118- 144.
13. Gage J: Gait analysis for decision-making in cerebral palsy. *Bull Hosp Jt Dis Orthop Inst* 43(2):147-163, 1983.
14. Inman VT: *The Joint of the Ankle.* Baltimore, MD, Williams and Wilkins Company, 1976.
15. Isacson J, Gransberg L, Knutsson E: Three-dimensional electrogoniometric gait recording. *J Biomech* 19(8):627- 635, 1986.
16. Johnston RC, Smidt GL: Measurement of hip-joint motion during walking; evaluation of an electrogoniometric method. *J Bone Joint Surg* 51A(6):1083-1094, 1969.

17. Kadaba MP, Ramakaishnan HK, Wootten ME: Measurement of lower extremity kinematics during level walking. *J Orthop Res* 8(3):383-392, 1990.
18. Karpovich PV, Herden EL, Asa MM: Electrogoniometric study of joints. *U S Armed Forces Med J* 11:424-450, 1960.
19. Kettelkamp DB, Johnson RJ, Smidt GL, Chao EY, Walker M: An electrogoniometric study of knee motion in normal gait. *J Bone Joint Surg* 52A(4):775-790, 1970.
20. Krag MH: Quantitative techniques for analysis of gait. *Automed* 6:85-97, 1985.
21. Lamoreux L: Exoskeleton gonimetry. *Bull Prosthetics Res* 18(1):288-290, 1981.
22. Larsson L, Sandlund B, Oberg PA: Selspot recording of gait in normals and in patients. *Scand J Rehab Med* 23:643-649, 1983.
23. Larsson LE, Sandlund B, Oberg PA: Selspot recording of gait in normals and in patients with spasticity. *Scand J Rehab Med* 5(6):21-27, 1978.
24. Mann RW, Antonsson EK: Gait analysis—precise, rapid, automatic 3-D position and orientation kinematics and dynamics. *Bull Hosp Jt Dis Orthop Inst* 43:137-146, 1983.
25. Mann RW, Rowell D, Dalrymple G, Conati F, Tetewksy A, Ottenheimer D, Antonsson E: Precise, rapid, automatic 3-D position and orientation tracking of multiple moving bodies. In Matsui H, Kobayashi K (Eds): *Biomechanics VIII-B.* Illinois, Human Kinetics Publishers, 1983, pp. 1104-1112.
26. Mundale MO, Hislop HJ, Rabideau RJ, Kottke FS: Evaluation of extension of the hip. *Arch Phys Med Rehabil* 37(2):75-80, 1956.
27. Murray MP, Drought AB, Kory RC: Walking patterns of normal men. *J Bone Joint Surg* 46A(2):335-360, 1964.
28. Perry J, Antonelli D: Evaluation of CARS-UBC triaxial goniometer. *Bull Prosthetics Res* 18(1):225-226, 1981.
29. Perry J, Enwemeka CS, Gronley JK: The stability of surface markers during knee flexion. *Ortho Trans* 12(2):453-454, 1988.
30. Sammarco GJ, Burstein AH, Frankel VH: Biomechanics of the ankle: a kinematic study. *Orthop Clin North Am* 4(1):75-96, 1973.
31. Seibert S: The dynamic Rancho knee goniometer. *Orthopedic Seminars, RLAMC* 7:275-286, 1974.
32. Soderberg GL, Gabel RH: A light-emitting diode system for the analysis of gait. A method and selected clinical examples. *Phys Ther* 58(4):426-432, 1978.
33. Sutherland DH, Olshen R, Cooper L, Woo SLY: The development of mature gait. *J Bone Joint Surg* 62A:336-353, 1980.
34. Thomas DH, Long C: An electrogoniometer for the finger—a kinesiologic tracking device. *Am J Med Electronics* 3:96-100, 1964.

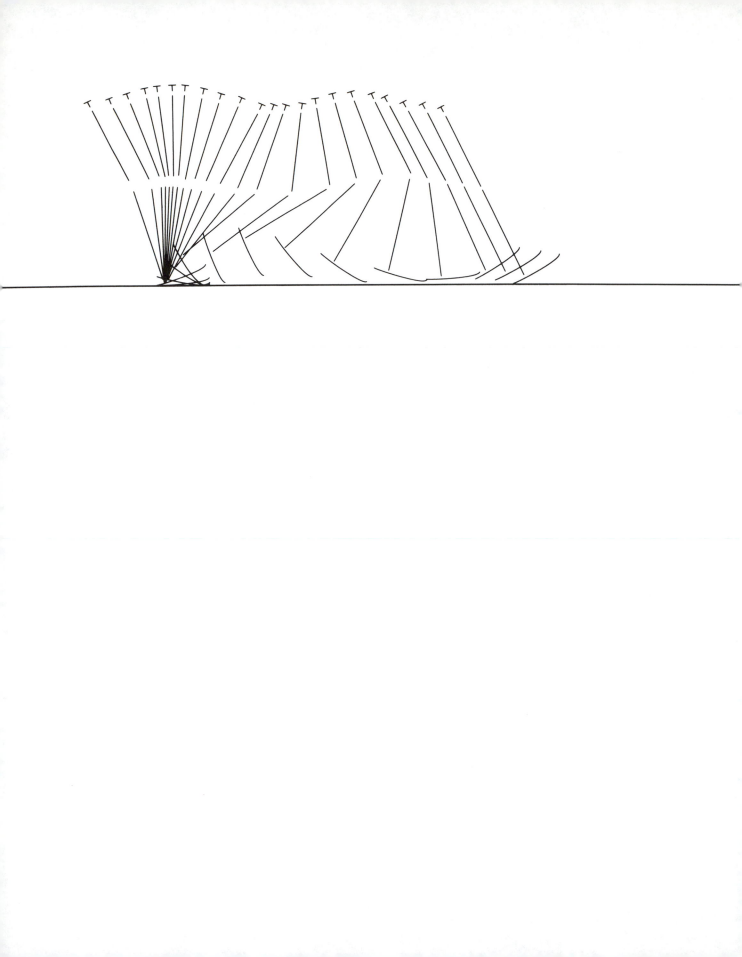

Chapter 18

Dynamic Electromyography

Muscle action, by occurring under the cover of skin and subcutaneous tissues, cannot be measured directly. The electromyogram, however, provides an indirect indicator of muscular function. The electrical signals, which accompany the chemical stimulation of the muscle fibers, travel through the muscles and adjacent soft tissues. With appropriate instrumentation, these myoelectrical signals can be recorded and analyzed to determine the timing and relative intensity of the muscular effort. Under limited circumstances one can also estimate the resulting muscle force.

EMG Origin

Muscles are composed of several thousand chains of contractile elements. Each chain (termed a muscle fiber) is under direct neural activation. The contractile elements are named *sarcomeres*. Control is simplified by having a single small motor nerve (neuron) activate a group of muscle fibers. This family of muscle fibers with their common, controlling neuron and the motor nerve cell in the spinal cord is called a *motor unit* (Figure 18.1). The EMG signal indicates motor unit activation. Effectiveness of the muscle's action is determined, primarily, by the number of motor units that are activated. Other significant factors are the size, fiber type and health of the motor units as well as intramuscular and external mechanics. Awareness of these varying qualities of the motor units provides a perspective for determining the significance of the EMG record from the different muscles.

The Motor Unit

Function as well as size of the muscles appear to influence their motor unit (MU) composition. The smallest hand muscle (lumbrical) with a responsibility for fine finger positioning has a 0.6cm^2 physiological cross-sectional area[62] that includes 95 motor units with 100 fibers each.[19] Leg muscles with a basic function of stability, rather than fine control, have a grosser motor unit anatomy. For example, the medial head of the gastrocnemius contains 579 motor units within its 28cm^2 cross section, and there are 1,784 fibers in each MU (Table 18.1). The tibialis anterior muscle that has the role of rapid foot pickup in swing is of moderate size (13.5cm^2) and contains 445 MU with 610 muscle fibers each. These three muscles with their unique functions have notably different fiber populations (10,260; 27,1450 and 1,032,936 respectively).[19]

Individual muscle fiber size is another variable. The hand intrinsic muscle fibers have a small diameter (19 to 26 microns[μ]). Fiber size in the leg ranged

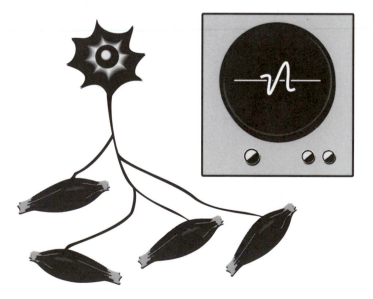

Figure 18.1 A motor unit. Left: the basic elements are the anterior horn cell, axon and branches to its muscle fibers (four displayed in this diagram). Right: a typical single motor unit EMG record display on an oscilloscope.

Table 18.1

Motor Unit Content

Muscle	Muscle Fiber size (μ)	Motor Units per Muscle	Muscle Fibers per Motor Unit	Total Fiber Count
Lumbricales	19	108	95	10,260
First Dorsal Interosseus	26	340	119	40,500
Brachialis	34	410	330	129,200
Tibialis Anterior	57	610	445	271,450
Gastrocnemius	54	1780	579	1,030,620

between 54μ and 57μ.[19] Consequently, the EMG by intramuscular wire electrode could include a considerably different number of motor units for the same sampling area.

The MU composition of the large thigh muscles has not been studied in such detail. A gross estimate can be made by relating muscle size to the motor unit pattern of the gastrocnemius, which also has a weight-bearing function. This suggests that the quadriceps, with its 177.2cm^2 cross section, could contain more than six million muscle fibers dispersed within 3,576 motor units.

Motor unit dispersion within the muscle determines the ability of intramuscular electrodes to pick up the myoelectric signals when the muscular effort is submaximal.[33] The early impression was grouping of the muscle fibers in a mosaic pattern. This was based on the patchy pattern displayed by partially denervated polio muscles.[65] Multifilament needle electrode recordings tended to support this concept as they indicated, a 9mm MU territory for the lower extremity muscles,[12,13] which included 25 MU.[12] This interpretation supports two common assumptions: (1) changes in electrode location would give totally different information, and (2) surface electrodes were necessary if one wished to sample a significant area of the muscle.

Neither situation has proved to be true. Research using glycogen depletion of muscle fibers in the motor unit demonstrated that grouping does not exist in normal muscle. To the contrary, the fibers of each motor unit are widely dispersed throughout a muscle, and their immediate neighbors are from different motor units. In the cat gastrocnemius, the motor unit territory covered as much as one third the entire volume (Figure 18.2).[14] For the tibialis anterior, the motor unit territory equaled 12% of the muscle's cross section.[11] The distances between individual fibers of the same motor unit in the biceps brachii range between 0.5mm and 6mm.[58] As a result, a single motor unit may be in contact with 50 or more other motor units. These data support the clinical experience that fine wire electrodes do not miss existing muscle action, even though their contact area is small. Generally, muscular efforts as low as 1% are recorded.

Muscle Fiber Activation

Understanding the functional significance of the electromyogram begins with an appreciation of muscle fiber action. Excitation of the muscle begins with the neurons chemically activating the motor end plates of the individual muscle fibers.[21,55] This is followed by an electrical signal spreading throughout the fiber at such speed (2-5 m/s) that all of the sarcomeres contract virtually at once.[38] The muscle fibers respond with a total contraction, which is commonly called an *all-or-none* reaction.[44] That is, if there is a signal (EMG) there is muscle fiber action generating a force to initiate or inhibit motion (Figure 18.3).

EMG Signal Management

The EMG signal of even one motor unit is a complex waveform, because the wide dispersion of its fibers throughout the muscle results in slightly different activation times. A single motor unit signal, however, is not seen during normal function, as the resulting force is too small, probably less than 0.2% of a moderately sized muscle's capability. In contrast, the clinical level of trace muscle strength is at least 1%. Voluntary isolation of a single motor unit is possible as a learned effort. It also may occur with activation of a severely

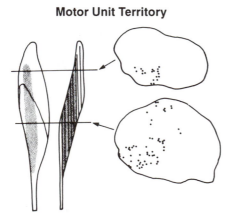

Figure 18.2 Motor unit dispersion in a muscle. Gray areas indicate the territory of the motor unit. Cross sections identify the dispersion of the motor unit's muscle fibers. (Adapted from Burke RE, Levine DN, Saloman M, and Tsairis P. Motor units in cat soleus muscle: physiological, histochemical and morphological characteristics. Vol. 238:503-514, 1974).

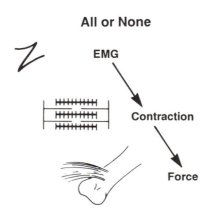

Figure 18.3 "All or None" sequence of muscle activation: Electromyographic signal, sarcomere contraction, force output.

paralyzed muscle that has no more motor units.

The typical kinesiological EMG represents the activation of multiple motor units. This record is an asynchronous series of electronic waves (action potentials) that vary in amplitude and durations due to the differences in distance of the electrode from the muscle fibers and in the length of the axon extending to the muscle fibers (Figure 18.4). The resulting electromyogram, called an interference pattern, is a composite of the two mechanisms used to increase muscle force, that is, the addition of more motor units or more rapid stimulation of the same motor units.

Each dynamic EMG contains two types of information: the timing of muscular action and its relative intensity. Timing can be determined directly from the raw EMG. This is not sufficient for the definition of relative muscular effort, since each EMG represents the relationship of the electrode to the muscles as well as the intensity of muscular action. Before meaningful comparisons can be made between muscles or subjects, the recording must be quantified and normalized. There are several technics for performing both processes.

Timing

The simplest determination from a dynamic electromyography record is the timing of muscle action. This may be identified either by visual inspection of the raw printed EMG record or computer analysis.

Defining the onset and cessation points of the muscle's activity interval remains a subjective decision, as the criteria of a minimum significant signal are still being established. Most recordings contain an occasional single spike or short bursts of extremely small signals that are functionally insignificant, as the associated muscle action would be miniscule. The experienced observer filters these out by eye. For computer analysis, 5% of the maximum effort registered on a manual muscle test was established as the minimum. This value is

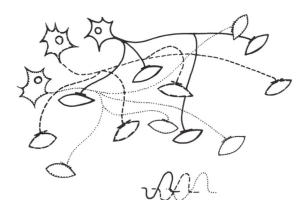

Interference Pattern

Figure 18.4 A diagrammatic representation of the normal "interference" EMG pattern. Three motor units, each with four muscle fibers, are illustrated. Below is the EMG created by their overlapping signals.

equivalent to the clinically ineffective grade 2 (poor) level of muscle action.[3] All other signals indicate pertinent muscle action.

The variability in subjective designation of the EMG endpoints was documented by a comparison of an experienced investigator to a rule-based computer analysis. While the computer showed 100% repeatability, ability of the same investigator to select the same EMG onset time after a one week interval was 51% (intrasubject repeatability).[17] Consistency in selecting the same EMG onset among three experienced, raters was 23% (intersubject variability).

Timing of muscle action also is influenced by one's definition for a significant burst of EMG. We use two criteria: the duration is at least 5% of the gait cycle and the amplitude of the sampled interval is equivalent to 5% of the maximum manual test.

EMG Quantification

The EMG signals may be transformed into numerical values either manually or by computer. These technics exchange precision for subjectivity.[22] The goal is to enable the clinician to sense the relative intensity of a muscle's action during the stride (Figure 18.5).

Manual (or descriptive) quantification usually grades the amplitude of the EMG record by an arbitrary three- or four-step scale (Figure 18.6). While greater muscular effort increases both the amplitude and density of the signal, an in-house comparison of amplitude versus density demonstrated no significant difference in the data score, as the two qualities increased almost proportionally. Hence, the inclusion of density in the subjective grading appears to be an unnecessary step in an already laborious task.

Electronic summation of the EMG signals is an old quantification technic. This has been replaced by the versatility provided by today's computers.

Computer quantification involves digital sampling (digitizing or analog to digital), rectification, and integration of the data. The digitizing rate is an important consideration, as it should be fast enough to adequately reproduce the signal, yet not so fast that the storage of large volumes of data becomes a problem. A sampling rate of 2,500 samples per second (Hz) captures all significant data. This is demonstrated by the ability to reproduce a signal pattern that is virtually indistinguishable from the original raw analog record. Hence, this is the most accurate technic, but it results in a large volume of data. To simplify data storage, many investigators use sampling rates of 1,000 or 500, even 300Hz. There is a corresponding loss of data that may be significant. One evidence of the loss is the inability to adequately reproduce the clonus seen in the raw record of a spastic patient.

Following digitization, the signal is full wave rectified to avoid the positive and negative values canceling each other out in the subsequent processing. Rectification involves transposing all the negative signals to the positive side of the zero line (Figure 18.7).

Integration consists of summing the digitized, rectified EMG signals over a time interval appropriate for the clinical function being tested. Interval duration

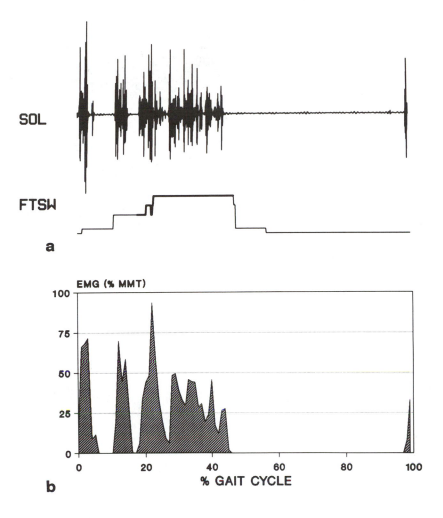

Figure 18.5 EMG representation of soleus muscle action during walking. (a) Raw EMG, (b) Quantitated EMG.

selection is based on the expected rate of change of the activity being performed. For a static situation such as an isometric test, the interval can be as long as 0.25 sec. Gait analysis requires much shorter data intervals to be compatible with the rates of joint motion and muscle function. A 0.01 second interval (approximately 1% GC for normal free gait) has been found to best correlate with the onset and cessation times displayed by the raw EMG. Reproducibility studies, however, show less variability in the EMG wave form when a 3% interval is used.[30]

Presentation of the quantified EMG may be in absolute values (millivolts) or

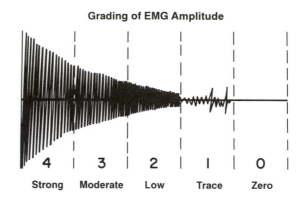

Figure 18.6 Descriptive qualitative scale. Four steps (1- 4) have been designated by amplitude ranges.

EMG Rectification

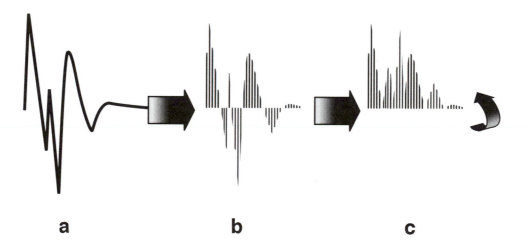

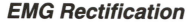

Figure 18.7 Rectification of EMG. (a) Raw EMG, (b) Negative waves delineated, (c) Negative wave assigned equivalent positive values and added to prior positive waves (full wave rectification).

as a percentage of some standard normalization. The absolute measurement (millivolts) is the most convenient, but it does not identify the clinically significant information of how hard the muscle is working (i.e., relative effort).

Normalization

The basic need for normalization is to accommodate the individual variation in the number and mixture of motor units sampled by the electrode. Despite careful electrode placement on or within a muscle, no two applications produce the same data quantitatively. Anatomical factors contributing to this situation include the small size of the muscle fibers (50μ), a varying mixture of slow and fast fiber types, wide dispersion of motor units, the fibrous tissue planes that separate the muscle fiber bundles, and variations in the contour of individual muscles. Consequently, the intensity of two muscles cannot be compared unless the EMG difference due to the motor unit sample is excluded by normalization.

The normalization technic involves treating the functional data from each electrode as a ratio (usually expressed as a percentage) of some reference value generated with the same electrode. For persons with normal neural control, the most convenient reference for the normalization process is the EMG registered during a maximum effort test. When this is generated by manual grading, the results are expressed as percents of the manual muscle test (% MMT). Maximum effort measurement with a dynamometer is more accurate but also considerably more time consuming because of the technicalities of aligning the limb and the machine. The outcome is then reported as percent maximum voluntary contraction (% MVC) (Figure 18.8) Both of these functional references differentiate the intensity of effort among muscles, as the peak value will be relative to maximum ability.

A higher strength output may be gained by training the subject to supreme exertion, but this is not practical for most testing situations. Also, this is not necessary as the repeated *spontaneous* maxima only varies about 10%.[46] Because subjects differ considerably in the way they reach their maximum effort, the common practice is to use a four or five second isometric test. Within this record the mean value for the highest one second of data is used as the reference value. This time interval is sufficiently short to avoid fatigue yet long enough to average out fluctuations in subject performance. Other investigators have found better consistency using a submaximal effort (50% max) as a defined target, rather than the spontaneous maximum (r=.83 versus .68 for 100%

SEMIMEMBRANOSUS

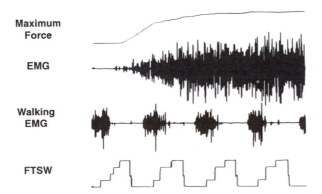

Figure 18.8 Normalization technic using maximum voluntary effort, semimembranosus data of normal subject. Maximum force = torque record; EMG = muscle action during torque test; Walking EMG = record of four strides; FTSW = foot switch records showing stance (staircase) and swing (baseline).

max).[60,66,67] This may relate to having a consistent target.

During rapid, forceful effort, the brief EMG may be greater than 100% of the reference value. An in-house analysis of the waveforms in each situation showed the amplitude of the highest potential was the same, but the number of such peak potentials was greater with the rapid, forceful effort than in the sustained maxima test. This apparently represents a trade-off between the need to preserve motor units for endurance and simultaneous motor unit activation for instantaneous force.

If an inaccurate single effort is a likely occurrence, the EMG sum for all the tests with that electrode may be used as the baseline reference value. Low-effort levels have greater signal variability, probably as a result of greater motor unit trade-off. This makes the normalizing base less consistent than using a strong or maximum effort. With either technic, the activity values are designated as a percent of the normalizing base.

A third technic often used in gait is to compare the EMG for a particular phase or event to the peak value obtained in the stride (100%). This approach has the advantage of being applicable to all test situations and being convenient.[15,41,66,67] The disadvantage is that the peak values of both weak and strong muscular activity are defined as 100% (Figure 18.9). However, this approach is particularly applicable to patients with neurological lesions that impair voluntary control such as the spastic disabilities of cerebral palsy, stroke, brain injury or spinal cord injury. They cannot reliably produce a maximum effort for the normalizing reference. In these circumstances one of the alternate approaches must be used.[31,53]

The conclusion is that normalization is an essential step in comparing activity among muscles. At present, however, there is no single best technic. Calculating the functional EMG relative to that obtained with a maximum strength test provides the most informative data when the subject can cooperate with the

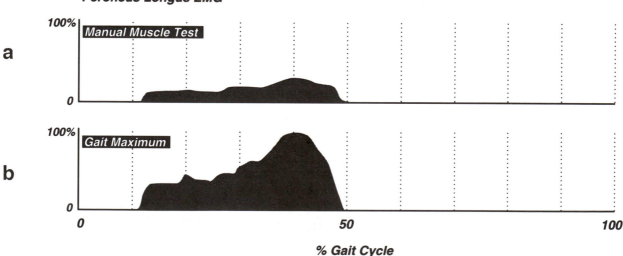

Figure 18.9 EMG normalization standard. (a) 100% = Maximum manual muscle test value (MMT); (b) 100% = Maximum EMG in the stride.

baseline test. This identifies the true intensity of the muscular effort required to walk or perform other functions.

Time Adjusted Quantification. Both timing and relative intensity are important factors in quantified gait data.[63] Individual strides show minor differences in timing of muscle action, even though their intensity profiles are similar. To combine the individual EMG data into an accurate mean-intensity profile, these timing differences must be considered (Figure 18.10). Otherwise, the mean data will have a duration longer than that of any single stride because it will start with the earliest onset and continue to the last cessation. This error is avoided by adjusting the onset and cessation times of the individual quantified records to match the mean timing. Then the mean profile is calculated. The result is a time adjusted mean profile (TAMP) (Figure 18.10).

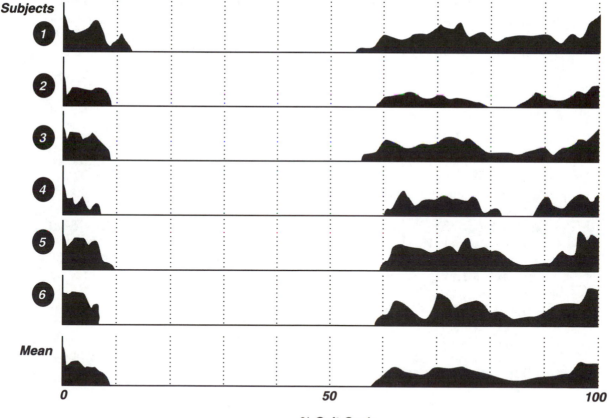

Figure 18.10 Time adjusted mean EMG profile for the group (bottom). Individual records of mean EMG of six subjects showing differences in onset/cessation times and details of amplitude pattern. Group mean amplitude profile calculated after individual records adjusted to mean timing.

EMG Interpretation

Appropriate interpretation of the timing and/or intensity of effort can identify the functional effectiveness of muscular action. From such determinations several clinical questions can be answered. When is the muscle active? How hard is the muscle working? How does the effort of one muscle compare to that of others? What is the quality of the neural control? The dynamic EMG record, however, is not a direct measure of muscle force.

Timing

Timing of muscle action in gait may be defined by three different reference scales: gait cycle interval, stance and swing periods, and the functional phases. Calculating the gait cycle interval is the simplest determination, but the designated percentage points carry no functional significance. To gain this added information, the minimum correlation would be the onset and cessation times of the EMG relative to the stance and swing periods. This has the advantage of technical simplicity by requiring only initial contact and toe-off signals. Using the eight gait phases as the reference base for the EMG interval provides the most functional significance for the data.

Relative Effort

Difference in the EMG amplitude of a single muscle represents varying levels of effort. As more muscle strength is required, additional motor units are added. Visually, the EMG record becomes denser and taller. When quantitated, the amount of signal is numerically greater (Figure 18.5).

Between muscles the differences in EMG amplitude may have a second meaning. Inequality in the number of motor units sampled by the individual electrodes is unavoidable because of the anatomical variations in muscle fiber anatomy and alignment. This means that accurate comparisons of the actions by different muscles require two processes: quantification and normalization. Quantification computes the amplitude of the analog EMG in numerical values. Normalization removes the electrode sampling differences. Following these signal management technics, the muscular effort can be designated as a percentage of the maximum registered with that electrode placement. Only then can one compare the intensity of effort during different activities and the action of different muscles.

Muscle Force

Muscles generate the force needed to provide the joint stability and motions used in walking and other physical activities. Dynamic EMG identifies the amount of muscular effort used during these activities, but does not specify the actual force, as several factors modify muscular effectiveness. The type and speed of contraction and fiber length determined by joint position directly define the force the muscle fibers can produce.

In addition, the muscle force used for a particular torque varies with the lever arm available at each joint position. The intensity of the target muscle's involvement in an activity also is modified by the contributions of synergistic muscles.

Type of Muscle Action. Muscle force varies as the stability of the myosin-actin bonding within the sarcomere and fibrous connective tissue (FCT) tension changes. Isometric contractions, by allowing no motion, have a stable sarcomere length and fixed FCT tension. This form of muscle action has long been the basic means of testing strength. An eccentric or lengthening contraction presents similar sarcomere stability and potentially greater FCT tension. Total muscle strength becomes the sum of the sarcomere force and the fibrous tissue tension. The relative strength of maximum eccentric effort has been reported both as equal to isometric[57] and exceeding it by 10-20%.[32,59] Concentric muscle action shortens the muscle. The repeated changes in actomyosin bonding result in approximately 20% less force than that generated by an equally strenuous isometric effort.[49,50,57] The strength loss varies nonlinearly with the speed of the effort.[50] Consequently the same EMG value could represent a force proportion of 1:1 (isometric or eccentric), 1.2:1 (eccentric), and 0.8:1 (concentric).

During walking all three forms of muscle action occur. Limb deceleration during stance involves eccentric contractions, while peak muscle activity generally is isometric.[69] Advancement of the limb in swing is concentric action.

The mode of increasing motor unit participation also may change during an activity. For example, the first dorsal interosseus muscle in the hand uses recruitment for the first 15% of force production and then employs increased frequency.[42-44]

Contraction Speed. The faster a muscle contracts, the less force can be attained for the same effort (Figure 18.11). Quadriceps activity, for example, shows a 38% decrease in maximum force between isometric (zero velocity) and isokinetic action at 150°/sec.[50] During maximum efforts at any speed, the EMG is relatively constant, even though the forces differ (Figure 18.12). Consequently, the force implied by the EMG differs with changes in speed.

Joint Position. As joints move, both muscle fiber length and bony leverage can change. Either factor can alter muscle torque. Shortening or lengthening the muscle from its optimum sarcomere setting leads to a corresponding reduction in force.

Strength of the quadriceps, for example, is markedly altered by changes in joint position (Figure 18.11).[34,35,38] While the intensity of the EMG remains the same, strength declines 50% between 50° and 10° flexion.[23]

Strength/Velocity

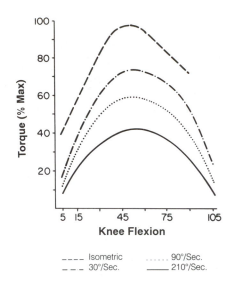

Figure 18.11 Maximum quadriceps strength (torque) during isometric and isokinetic knee extension.

Summary

In each situation the ratio between EMG and force is altered. This results in a variability in the muscle's force generation ability without a change in the number of active motor units (i.e., the EMG of maximum muscular effort in each situation remains a virtual constant, F_{EMG}). The extent to which the

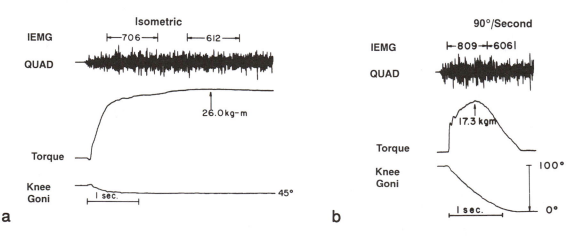

Figure 18.12 EMG (quantitated) and torque during maximum knee extension. (a) Isometric with knee at 45° flexion (Knee Goni); (b) Isokinetic (90-0° arc at 90°/sec). IEMG - integrated EMG and mean intensity over one second measured at two intervals; QUAD = raw EMG, test duration; Torque = Cybex measurement (Kilogram-meters).

optimum isometric force has been modified is reflected in the following equation:

$$F_{EMG} = F_{IM}-(K_1C+K_2L_M+K_3L_T+K_4V+K_5H),$$

where F_{EMG} = force inferred from EMG: F_{IM} = isometric force; and C, L_M, L_T, V, H represent the contraction type, muscle fiber length, tendon length, velocity of contraction, and recent muscle contraction history respectively. K_i are proportional constants.

The significance of these variables is the finding of a linear relationship during isometric efforts of increasing intensity,[27,45] yet the slope of the data line differs with the joint position tested.[5,9,40] Dynamic studies show a differing ratio of EMG to force, with variations in the speed of action.[20] When either velocity or force is kept constant, the change in the other variable is a linear relationship.[45,46] Others have reported a curvilinear relationship.[10,61,71]

An additional variable in defining the relationship between the EMG and muscle force is the electromechanical delay. That is, the electrical response precedes the mechanical reaction. Initially, Inman identified an 80ms delay. More recent studies found the interval between the EMG and resulting force to be 40ms.[37,54] The fact that the EMG signal of a single motor unit lasts only 1ms to 3ms[38] identifies muscle mechanics as the source of the delay.

Synergy is the final concern. Muscles generate force as part of a group (synergistically), rather than in isolation (Figure 18.13), to produce rotation about a joint (torques or moments). Subtle differences in alignments across the joint also give most muscles another function, so their participation in a particular activity varies with the functional demand. Thus, muscle synergy makes it impossible to accurately assign the measured torque to a particular muscle, as advocated by some investigators.[8] While designating a representative muscle simplifies the calculations, the total source of the muscle force has not been considered.

The versatility of today's computers makes it possible to include all the modifying factors in the calculations of muscle effectiveness.[47] When these

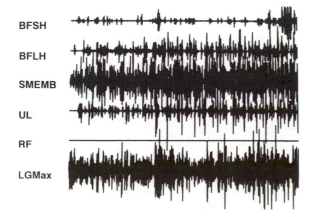

BFSH

BFLH

SMEMB

UL

RF

LGMax

Figure 18.13 Synergistic action during a standard manual muscle test of strength. Lower gluteus maximus (LGMax) was the muscle being tested. Simultaneous action occurred in the other hip extensors, biceps femoris long head (BFLH) and semimembranosus (SMEMB). Quadriceps participation (VL) implies use of mass limb extension. Biceps femoris short head suggests a low synergy with the other biceps head. Lack of rectus femoris (RF) action indicates it is a flexor and not part of the extensor synergy.

mechanical values for each of the muscles within the synergy of an activity are correlated with their quantified EMGs (defining the relative intensity of effort), the torque pattern can be reproduced (Figure 18.14). Hence, by indirect means EMG can imply force.

EMG Analysis of Pathological Gait

Errors in neurological control, muscle weakness, voluntary substitutions and obligatory posturing lead to an abnormal EMG record during walking. Both timing and intensity may be altered either for a particular phase or over the entire functional cycle.

Abnormal Timing

In the interpretation of pathological gait, relative timing of muscle action compared to normal function is highly significant.[4] Seven classifications of abnormal activity are used: premature, prolonged, continuous, delayed, curtailed, absent and out-of-phase (Table 18.2, Figure 18.15). The additional period of muscle action indicated by premature and prolonged EMG patterns has functional significance when it involves another phase of gait. This activity may represent dynamic obstruction of desired function or it may be appropriate support for an abnormal joint posture. Conversely, EMG patterns that are curtailed, delayed and absent imply the lack of desired activity. Sometimes limb posture makes the action unneeded. Continuous muscle action throughout the stride is always undesirable. Out-of-phase EMG, however, may signify a useful

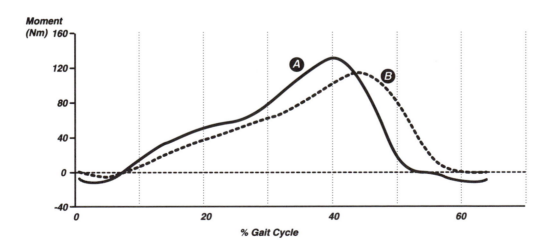

Figure 18.14 Time and intensity relationships of ankle muscle action and torque during walking. (a) Action of the ankle plantar flexors is defined by the product of their quantified EMG and their mechanical qualities (cross section area, passive elasticity, etc.). (b) Torque (moment arm times vertical ground reaction force).

Table 18.2

EMG Timing Errors

Deviation	Definition
Premature	Action begins before the normal onset
Prolonged	Action continues beyond the normal cessation time
Continuous	EMG uninterrupted for 90% or more of the gait cycle
Curtailed	Early termination of the EMG
Delayed	Onset later than normal
Absent	EMG of insufficient amplitude or duration
Out of Phase	Swing or stance time reversed

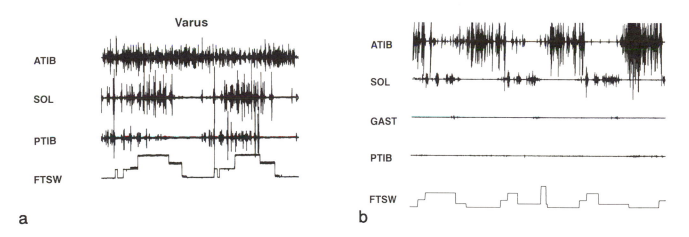

Figure 18.15 Abnormal EMG patterns occurring in clinical tests (timing). (a) Continuous (ATIB); Premature (SOL), onset in terminal swing rather than mid stance; Curtailed (PTIB), terminal stance action missing; Foot switch (FTSW) differentiates stance (steps) and swing (baseline) periods in each stride displayed. (b) Prolonged (ATIB); Premature (SOL); No significant activity (GAST and PTIB); FTSW = foot switch of reference limb.

substitution. Obstructive versus accommodating muscle action is differentiated by correlating the EMG with the accompanying motion patterns of the limb. Often, one must consider adjacent joints as well as the one being controlled by the muscles in question.

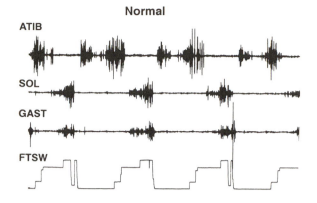

Figure 18.17 Selective control. Both the intensity and timing are proportional to the functional need. Anterior tibialis (ATIB) has two intervals of intense action: initial swing to pick up the foot and terminal swing/loading response to present and control the heel rocker. Soleus (SOL) and gastrocnemius (GAST) action controls the tibia. The low EMG in mid stance indicates the low demand of the ankle rocker. The marked amplitude increase in terminal stance correlates with the heel-off support (high demand of a forefoot rocker). Foot switch (FTSW) shows a normal sequence with a long mid stance (third step, H5-1) interval followed by heel rise (top step, 5-1). Courtesy Churchill Livingstone, NY, 1984.)

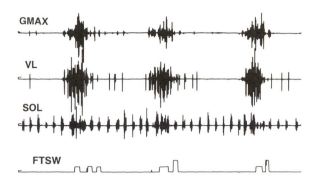

Figure 18.18 Primitive locomotor extensor synergy. Simultaneous control timing for the three muscles is indicated by the dense EMG segments: Gluteus maximus hip extension (GMax), quadriceps knee extension (VL), ankle plantar flexion (SOL). Spasticity (clonic beats) throughout swing is present in the soleus (SOL). Foot switch (FTSW) shows unstable stance on the fifth metatarsal only.

swing and vice versa (Figure 18.18). The EMG pattern varies with the rate of stretch. Slow stretch introduces a continuous pattern of EMG signals with a uniform amplitude. Quick stretch elicits a sequence of evenly spaced bursts (clonus). As the spastic response dwindles, the amplitude of the clonic bursts decrease. Both types of stretch reactions tend to be called spasticity, though the slow continuous response is technically rigidity and the fast action is true spasticity. When spasticity and voluntary muscle action signals are both stimulating muscle action, the EMG pattern can be very irregular.

EMG Instrumentation

The EMG signal displayed by the record depends not only on the intensity of the muscle action but also on the quality of the EMG instrumentation employed. While almost any system will provide an EMG record if the signal is sufficiently amplified, to assure accuracy and completeness of the information, four levels of instrumentation must be considered. These are the electrodes, signal amplification and filtering technics, signal transmission, and recording system. In addition, the ease of interpreting the record is dependent on the method of data display and processing.

Electrodes

As myoelectric signals extend through the local muscle and adjacent soft tissues, they can be recorded by three types of electrodes: needle, wire and surface. Needles are too insecure and uncomfortable for use in gait analysis. Hence, the choices lie between surface and wire electrodes. These have several different characteristics.

Surface electrodes are, basically, two small metal discs taped to the skin, each with a fine wire to attach it to an amplifier.[16] Signal reception has been improved by several developments. The type of surface electrode in greatest use today is a pair of shallow cupped, silver/silver chloride discs of varying sizes (e.g., 0.4cm to 0.94cm diameter) (Figure 18.19a).[24] The silver chloride provides a stable skin-electrode interface by diminishing the polarization,[1] while the central cup holds a saline gel for better signal transmission. For optimum signal reception, the dead epidermis is removed by alcohol and sanding and dense hair shaved to reduce impedance.[60] Electronic grounding of the system is gained by a large remote ground plate.

The distance between electrodes has been optional. Small electrodes (0.4cm) applied close together are said to best localize the signals to the target muscles. Large electrodes with greater spacing produce more signal, and this is particularly appealing to some investigators. For optimum balance between selectivity and amplitude, DeLuca recommends 1cm spacing between the electrodes.[1] Placement of the electrodes at the motor point or midway between the apex of the belly and the distal tendon also is recommended.[25,60]

Active surface electrodes have built-in amplifiers and integrated circuitry to provide optimum impedance (Figure 18.19b). They provide a cleaner (more "noise" free) signal and facilitate electrode application because all the elements are combined in a single unit, including the ground plate. Also, neither a gel nor skin preparation is needed.[1] Active electrodes are fast becoming the electrode system of choice.

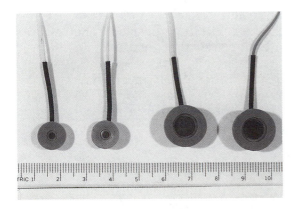
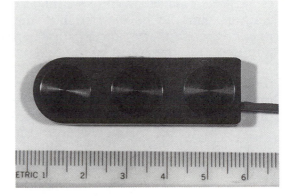

Figure 18.19 Surface electrodes. (a) Disc; (b) Active.

Wire electrodes offer a stable means of recording the myoelectric signals directly from the muscle (Figure 18.20). The most common material is nylon (or teflon) coated, nickel-chromium alloy wire (50 micron diameter). A 25μ wire also is available, but the increased flexibility makes stability a problem as the hooks yield with only small amounts of tension. Simultaneous insertion of two wire electrodes placed in a single 25 gauge hypodermic needle, is the technic of choice.[2] The end of each wire is bent into a hook and their 2mm bared tips staggered to avoid an electrical short. For sterilization, these units are packaged in small envelopes in a way that avoids tangling the wires on removal. Insertion into the designated muscle is accomplished with a quick motion, so the penetration time for skin and fascia is brief. After the needle is removed, the accuracy of electrode placement is confirmed by light electrical stimulation through the electrode wires in combination with palpation and observation of the target muscle or tendon.

Wire electrode displacement can occur with motion.[28] Radiographs demonstrated that this generally follows wire insertion. It is our practice to move the muscle through a few passive range of motion cycles as well as to have the subject exert some vigorous contractions to assure early wire fixation. In addition, to avoid pulling on the intramuscular site, a 3cm loop is formed just proximal to the fixation tape. These technics have made wire displacement an infrequent event. Whenever any muscle fails to display the expected action during the data collection procedure, an interim muscle test is performed to check electrode stability. If the signal has been lost, a second set of wires is inserted.

Occasionally the insertion site remains painful. If moving the wires does not solve the problem, a second insertion should be made, as normal function will be inhibited. On completing the test, the wires are readily removed with a quick tug that unbends the hook. Mild local bleeding at the insertion site has been identified as a cause of the discomfort.[29]

Relative Electrode Qualities

Comfort is the primary advantage of surface electrodes. Also, being merely taped to the skin they can be applied by any interested investigator. Wires, in contrast, have to be inserted into the muscle by penetrating the skin. The resulting momentary pain usually disappears with the removal of the needle. In addition, the wires must be inserted by clinical professionals.

Selectivity is the significant advantage of wire electrodes. With appropriate filtering, the EMG data can be isolated to the target muscle. Dispersion of the myoelectric signals through the tissues by volume conduction is a normal phenomenon. The signals enter adjacent muscles as well as reach the skin surface. Similarly, the signals from more than one muscle may arrive at the same surface area, though with different intensities. Hence, in its pure form, the EMG record commonly represents action of more than the designated muscle (Figure 18.21). This is muscle cross talk. Single function studies that challenge just one major muscle group are not sensitive to cross talk, since a comparison of adjacent muscle action is not involved. This has led some investigators to

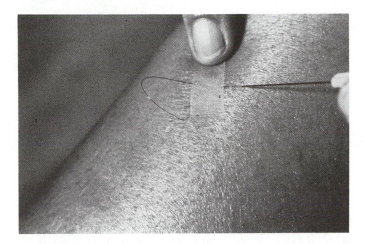

Figure 18.20 Wire electrode. Skin insertion and tension relief loop shown.

state that surface and wire electrodes give equivalent information.[7,56]

The ability to differentiate adjacent muscles depends on the frequency content of the EMG signals. Myoelectric signals are complex waveforms with a power spectrum containing a range of frequencies (Figure 18.22). Passage of the myoelectric signals through the tissues progressively lowers the frequency content of the EMG as the higher frequencies are attenuated by the tissue that acts as a low-pass filter. This makes the EMG spectra different for wire and surface electrodes. The wire data frequency range is 10 to 1,000Hz (mean = 350Hz), while the surface electrode data range is 10 to 350Hz with a mean frequency of 50Hz. For both electrode systems, the peak intensity approximates

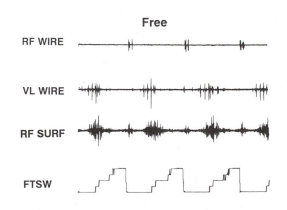

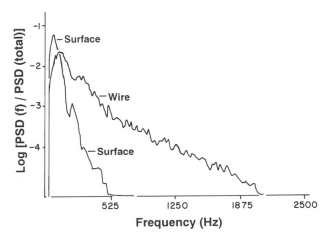

Figure 18.21 EMG cross talk during a gait record. Rectus femoris surface (RF SURF) EMG shows two intervals of action that correspond to the EMG displayed by the rectus femoris wire (RF WIRE) and vastus lateralis wire (VL WIRE). Foot switch (FTSW) shows a normal sequence of foot support.

Figure 18.22 EMG power spectrum of wire and surface EMG. Vertical axis is a logarithmic scale of EMG intensity. Horizontal scale is the signal frequency.

100Hz. The lower frequency content of signals arriving at the electrodes from more distant muscles (as the case with surface electrodes) implies that cross talk to wire electrodes from distant sources (adjacent muscles) can be filtered out using a high-pass filter.

Surface electrode cross talk from adjacent muscles has been confirmed by studies using simultaneous wire and surface recordings. Recordings of the plantar flexor muscles (gastrocnemius, soleus and tibialis posterior) showed a higher ratio of surface EMG to wire EMG during the test of the other muscles than was obtained with the target muscle's test.[52] Three muscle tests were used (Figure 18.23). Single stance heel rise with the knee flexed tested the soleus. The resulting wire EMG was maximum and the surface data one half that value. Single stance heel rise with the knee extended (the designated gastrocnemius test) produced high soleus wire and surface EMG. These findings identified two events. The soleus is strongly active in all heel rise tests, and gastrocnemius EMG was included in the soleus surface electrode data. The manual tibialis posterior test markedly reduced soleus muscle action, yet there was additional surface EMG. Again the surface electrodes picked up signals from the adjacent muscle. The conclusion was that within the EMG recorded by a soleus surface electrode only 36% of the signal represented the action of that muscle, and the rest was cross talk. A similar analysis of the gastrocnemious showed that its more superficial location increased the selectivity of the surface EMG to 60%.

A second study, using electrical stimulation of just one muscle (tibialis anterior), demonstrated EMG spread to adjacent muscles (peroneus longus and soleus).[16] The EMG cross talk was calculated to be equivalent to 16% of their peak activity. Volume conduction rather than a surface artifact was identified as the mechanism and cross correlation procedures did not exclude the cross talk.

Some of the confusion in interpreting surface data is clarified by Hof's formula ($E = [(E_A)^2 + (E_B)^2]^{0.5}$).[26] If the target muscle (E_A) is strongly active, signals from other musculature (E_B) would not introduce a significant contamination in the recorded surface EMG (E) (Figure 18.24a). In contrast, when there is little or no activity in the target muscle (E_A), cross talk from the other muscles (E_B) could provide erroneous information (Figure 18.24b). Comparisons of normal surface gait EMG data[18,64,68] to that recorded by wire EMG[39] show less discrete phasing of muscle action with the surface electrode system.

The differences in surface and wire electrode sensitivity define the appropriate uses of each system. Surface electromyography should be limited to studying group muscle action. Also, the possibility of cross talk should be recognized whenever antagonistic muscle action accompanies moderate to low-level EMG for the agonist muscle (10% to 15%). The existence of cross talk blurs the onset and cessation times of the muscles. Similarly, cross talk in surface electrode systems implies co-contraction when it is not present.

Wire electrodes are necessary whenever accurate knowledge of individual muscle action is critical to the clinical or research decisions.[16,52] Whenever it is important to differentiate the action of adjacent muscles or to make finite judgements on patients abnormal function, wire electrodes should be chosen.

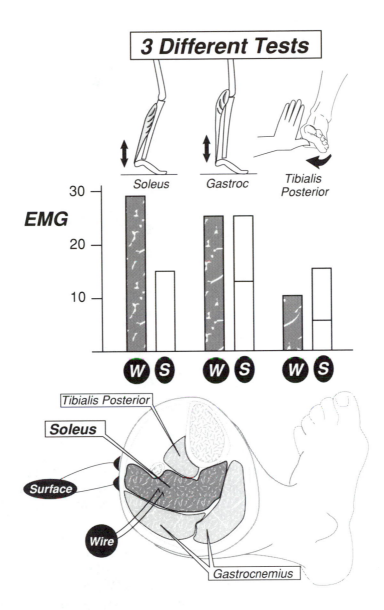

Figure 18.23 Cross talk recorded by the soleus surface electrodes (surface) during three muscle tests (top). Soleus test = flexed knee heel rise; Gastrocnemius = extended knee heel rise; Tibialis posterior = manual resistance to inversion. Quantitated EMG data (middle row)/Soleus test: wire (W, dark bar) - EMG maximum; surface EMG (S, white bar) = one half as much. Gastrocnemius test: soleus wire and surface EMG equally high. Gray bar indicates surface EMG in excess of normal surface-to-wire ratio. Tibialis posterior test: surface EMG higher than wire (gray bar = cross talk). Anatomical diagram (bottom) shows the cross section relationship of the muscles tested and the location of the electrodes (wire and surface).

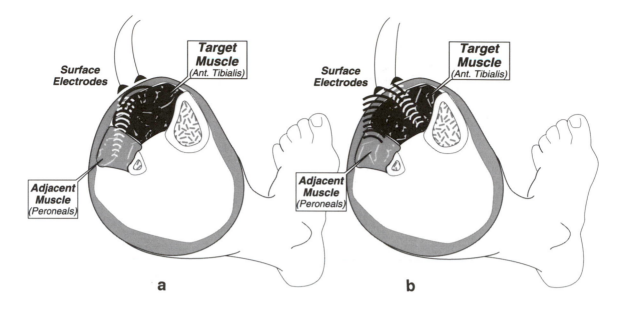

Figure 18.24 Relative significance of cross talk in surface EMG. Surface electrodes are recording tibialis anterior muscle action. (a) The primary EMG (black waves) is generated by the target muscle. Lesser signals from the adjacent muscles (gray waves from the peroneals) is a minor addition, not functionally significant. (b) Tibialis anterior has poor activity (gray waves). The major EMG (black waves) reaching the surface electrodes arise from the adjacent peroneal muscles. The result is erroneous information. The tibialis anterior is far less active than the surface EMG would indicate.

Amplifiers and Signal Filtration

EMG signals are too small (300uv to 5mv) for direct interpretation without amplification. A differential amplifier with a high common mode rejection ratio (80db or higher) should be used. This type of amplifier reduces the interference of signals from common sources such as electric power lines. The input impedance must be high (at least 1 Mohm) to adequately pick up the low-level EMG signals.

The frequency content of the signals must be considered when selecting an amplifier. The basic spectrum of myoelectric signals includes frequencies between 10 and 1,000Hz. Higher frequencies have been identified but they represent less than .01% of the spectrum.[51] To preserve the quality and quantity of the signal, the amplifier selected must have a frequency bandwidth that covers the frequency range of the myoelectric signals obtained with the selected electrode system. For wire electrodes, a high frequency response of 1,000 is more than adequate (as 90% of the energy is below 700Hz). For surface EMG, the high end of the amplifier's bandwidth should be 350Hz. The low end frequency response of the amplifier can be as low as 10Hz for both electrode systems as the actual frequency recorded is determined by the filtering technic used.

False signals (artifacts) induced by soft tissue motion and electronic noise are excluded by spectrum modifications. Signals of 10 to 15Hz and possible

25Hz are caused by muscle contraction and floor impact passively moving the electrodes and cables. These artifacts are excluded by limiting the low end of the frequency response. Some investigators use 20Hz[1] but 40Hz provides a wider margin of safety for excluding extraneous signals from the EMG. The 60Hz noise from the environment (e.g., lights, motors, etc.) not totally excluded by the differential amplifiers is filtered out by a notch filter.

To exclude the myoelectric signals representing cross talk from adjacent muscles, the Rancho system uses a 150 to 1,000Hz bandwidth for wire electrodes. This system allows one to make wire electrodes quite selective for just the target muscle. For surface electrodes the bandwidth used at Rancho is 40 to 1,000Hz. At present, there are no means of removing the cross talk from surface electrode data.

Loss of the clean baseline indicates the EMG system needs service. With visual analysis, the contaminated baseline can be partially accommodated by conscious exclusion of the faulty signals. Automatic analysis, however, will include the noise as small levels of muscle action, unless these signals are filtered prior to processing. A simultaneous blast of signal on all channels usually indicates electronic noise experienced during loss of signal transmission in telemetry systems. This needs to be excluded before the data are quantitated or interpreted.

Recorders

There are three basic ways of recording the myoelectric signals. These are strip chart recorders, multichannel analog tape, and computers. To assure storage of all the incoming signals, the recorder's frequency response must equal that of the EMG being stored, that is, 10 to 1,000Hz for wire electrode data or a capability of 10 to 350Hz for surface signals.[1]

Ink strip chart recorders are an old and relatively inexpensive approach. Their frequency capability, however, is only one-tenth that which is needed for EMG. While described as responsive to 100Hz, the pen starts lagging at 60Hz. Because the pen cannot move as rapidly as the electronic signals, much of the EMG signal amplitude is missed, with a corresponding loss of data.

The light beam galvanometer is a strip chart recorder with the necessary versatility to capture the EMG signals without alteration. A light beam imprints ultraviolet light sensitive paper. The end product is a single record that can be analyzed by eye and manual measurement. A disadvantage is that the record photographs poorly.

An analog tape recorder with multiple (4, 7, etc.) storage channels provides good versatility. The data can be transferred to any display or processing unit desired (i.e., printer or computer).

Direct, on-line recording into the computer is the preferable system today. Previously, limited memory capacity necessitated simplifying the signal (i.e., sampling at a rate of 500 rather than 2,500 per second), but modern instrumentation has reduced both the storage and financial barriers. This technical progress is fortunate, since the Nyquist frequency rule indicates full data capture requires that the recording capability be two times the peak frequency of the signal of interest to avoid some loss.

Transmission of the myoelectric signals from subject to recorder can be either by cable or telemetry. Small cables are easiest, but they introduce a drag that measurably slows the patient's walking speed.[70] Suspending the cable overhead reduces this restraint to the walking subject to an imperceptible level. Faster and more diverse activities are a problem. Telemetry is the ideal system because it offers complete subject freedom. Telemetry, however, is more costly and more demanding of service.

References

1. Basmajian JV, Deluca CJ: *Muscles Alive: Their functions revealed by electromyography.* 5th edition, Baltimore, Williams and Wilkins, 1985, pp. 19-64.
2. Basmajian JV, Stecko GA: A new bipolar indwelling electrode for electromyography. *J Appl Physiol* 17:849, 1962.
3. Beasley WC: Quantitative muscle testing: Principles and applications to research and clinical services. *Arch Phys Med Rehabil* 42:398-425, 1961.
4. Bekey GA, Chang C, Perry J, Hoffer MM: Pattern recognition of multiple EMG signals applied to the description of human gait. *Proceedings of IEEE* 65(5):674-681, 1977.
5. Bigland B, Lippold OCJ: Motor unit activity in the voluntary contraction of human muscle. *J Physiol* 125(2):322-335, 1954.
6. Bigland B, Lippold OCJ: The relation between force, velocity and integrated electrical activity in human muscles. *J Physiol* 123:214-244, 1954.
7. Bobbert MF, Huijing PA, Ingen Schenau GJ van: A model of the human triceps surae muscle-tendon complex applied to jumping. *J Biomech* 19(11):887-898, 1986.
8. Bouisset S: EMG and muscle force in normal motor activities. *New Developments in Electromyography and Clinical Neurophysiology* 1:547-583, 1973.
9. Bouisset S, Goubel F: Integrated electromyographical activity and muscle work. *J of Applied Physiology* 35(5):695-702, 1973.
10. Bouisset S, Matson MS: Quantitative relationship between surface EMG and intramuscular electromyographic activity in voluntary movement. *American Journal of Physical Medicine* 51:285-295, 1972.
11. Brandstater MF, Lambert EH: Motor unit anatomy: type and spatial arrangement of muscle fibers. In Desmedt JE (Ed): *New developments in electromyography and clinical neurophysiology.* Karger, Basel: pp. 14-22, 1973.
12. Buchthal F, Erminio F, Rosenfalck P: Motor unit territory in different human muscles. *Acta Physiol Scand* 45:72-87, 1959.
13. Buchthal F, Guld C, Rosenfalck P: Volume conduction of the spike of the motor unit potential investigated with a new type of multielectrode. *Acta Physiol Scand* 38:331-354, 1957.
14. Burke RE, Tsairis P: Anatomy and innervation ratios in motor units of cat gastrocnemius. *J Physiol* 234:749-765, 1973.
15. Cavanaugh PR, Gregory RJ: Knee joint torque during the swing phase of normal treadmill walking. *J Biomech* 8:337-344, 1975.
16. De Luca CJ, Merletti R: Surface myoelectric signal cross-talk among muscles of the leg. *Electroencephalogr Clin Neurophysiol* 69:568-575, 1988.
17. DiFabio RP: Reliability of computerized surface electromyography for determining the onset of muscle activity. *Phys Ther* 67(1):43-48, 1987.
18. Dubo HI, Peat M, Winter DA, Quanbury AO, Hobson DA, Steinke T, Reimer G:

Electromyographic temporal analysis of gait: normal human locomotion. *Arch Phys Med Rehabil* 57(9):415-420, 1976.

19. Feinstein B, Lindegard B, Nyman E, Wohlfart G: Morphologic studies of motor units in normal human muscle. *Acta Anat* 23:127-142, 1955.

20. Fenn WO, Marsh BS: Muscular force at different speeds of shortening. *J Physiol* 85:277-297, 1935.

21. Goodgold J, Eberstein A: *Electrodiagnosis of Neuromuscular Disease.* Baltimore, Williams and Wilkins Company, 1972, pp. 21-28.

22. Guth V, Abbink F, Theysohn H: Electromyographic investigations on gait. *Electromyogr Clin Neurophysiol* 19:305-323, 1979.

23. Haffajee D, Moritz U, Svantesson G: Isometric knee extension strength as a function of joint angle, muscle length and motor unit activity. *Acta Orthop Scand* 43:138-147, 1972.

24. Hary D, Bekey GA, Antonelli DJ: Circuit models and simulation analysis of electromyographic signal sources—I: The impedance of EMG electrodes. *IEEE Trans Biomed Eng BME* 34:91-97, 1987.

25. Hermens HJ, Boon KL, Zilvold G: The clinical use of surface EMG. Medica Physica 9:119-130, 1986.

26. Hof AL: EMG and muscle force: An introduction. *Human Movement Sci* 3:119-153, 1984.

27. Inman VT, Ralston HJ, Saunders JBdeCM, Feinstein B, Wright EW, Jr.: Relation of human electromyogram to muscular tension. *Electroencephalogr Clin Neurophysiol* 4(2):187- 194, 1952.

28. Jonsson B, Komi V: Reproducibility problems when using wire electrodes in electromyographic kinesiology. In Desmedt JE (Ed): *New Developments in Electromyography and Clinical Neurophysiology.* Jyvaskyla, Karger, B., 1973, pp. 540-546.

29. Jonsson B, Omfeldt M, Rundgren A: Discomfort from the use of wire electrodes for electromyography. *Electromyography* VIII:5-17, 1968.

30. Kadaba MP, Wootten ME, Gainey J, Cochran GV: Repeatability of phasic muscle activity: performance of surface and intramuscular wire electrodes in gait analysis. *J Orthop Res* 3(3):350-359, 1985.

31. Knutsson E, Richards C: Different types of disturbed motor control in gait of hemiparetic patients. *Brain* 102:405-430, 1979.

32. Komi PV: Measurement of the force-velocity relationship in human muscle under concentric and eccentric contractions, in Cerquiglini S (ed): *Biomechanics III.* Basel, Switzerland, Karger, 1973, pp. 224-229.

33. Kramer H, Kuchler G, Brauer D: Investigations of the potential distribution of activated skeletal muscles in man by means of surface electrodes. *Electromyography* 12(1):19-27, 1972.

34. Lieb FJ, Perry J: Quadriceps function, an electromyographic study under isometric conditions. *J Bone Joint Surg* 53A:749-758, 1971.

35. Lindahl O, Movin A, Ringqvist I: Knee extension. Measurement of the isometric force in different positions of the knee joint. *Acta Orthop Scand* 40:79-85, 1969.

36. Lindstrom L, Magnusson R, Petersen I: Muscle load influence on myo-electric signal characteristics. *Scan J Rehab Med* 3 suppl.:127-148, 1974.

37. Long C: *Normal and Abnormal Motor Control in the Upper Extremities.* Cleveland, Case Western Reserve University, 1970, p. 8.

38. Ludin HP: *Electromyography in Practice.* New York, Thieme-Stratton, Inc., 1980.

39. Lyons K, Perry J, Gronley JK, Barnes L, Antonelli D: Timing and relative intensity of hip extensor and abductor muscle action during level and stair ambulation: an EMG study. *Phys Ther* 63:1597-1605, 1983.

40. Metral S, Lemaire C, Monod H: Force-Length-Integrated EMG Relationships for

Sub-maximal Isometric Contractions. In Herberts P, Kadefors R, Magnusson R, et al. (Eds): *The Control of Upper-extremity Prostheses and Orthoses*. Springfield, Charles C. Thomas, Publisher, 1974, pp. 13-22.

41. Milner M, Basmajian V, Quanbury AO: Multifactorial analysis of walking by electromyography and computer. *Am J Phys Med* 50(5):235-258, 1971.

42. Milner-Brown HS, Stein RB: Changes in firing rate of human motor units during linearly changing voluntary contractions. *J Physiol* 230:371-390, 1973.

43. Milner-Brown HS, Stein RB: The relation between the surface electromyogram and muscular force. *J Physiol* 246:549-569, 1975.

44. Milner-Brown HS, Stein RB, Yemm R: The contractile properties of human motor units during voluntary isometric contractions. *J Physiol* 228:285-306, 1973.

45. Milner-Brown HS, Stein RB, Yemm R: The orderly recruitment of human motor units during voluntary isometric contractions. *J Physiol* 230:359-370, 1973.

46. Mohamed OS: *Relation Between Myoelectric Activity, Muscle Length, and Torque of the Hamstring Muscles*. Los Angeles, Doctoral Dissertation, University of Southern California, 1989.

47. Mulroy SJ, Perry J, Gronley JK: A comparison of clinical tests for ankle plantar flexion strength. *Trans Orthop Res Soc* 16:667, 1991.

48. Murray MP, Baldwin JM, Gardner GM, Sepic SB, Downs WJ: Maximum isometric knee flexor and extensor muscle contractions: Normal patterns of torque versus time. *Phys Ther* 57:891-896, 1977.

49. Osternig LR: Optimal isokinetic loads and velocities producing muscular power in human subjects. *Arch Phys Med Rehabil* 56:152-155, 1975.

50. Osternig LR, Hamill J, Corcos DM, Lander J: Electromyographic patterns accompanying isokinetic exercise under varying speed and sequencing conditions. *Am J Phys Med* 63(6):289-297, 1984.

51. Perry J, Antonelli D, Bekey GA, et al: *Development and Evaluation of a Reference EMG Signal Acquisition System. Final Project Report, N.I.H. Grant R01 GM 26395*. Downey, CA, Pathokinesiology Laboratory, Rancho Los Amigos Hospital, 1982.

52. Perry J, Easterday CS, Antonelli DJ: Surface versus intramuscular electrodes for electromyography of superficial and deep muscles. *Physical Therapy* 61(1):7-15, 1981.

53. Perry J, Hoffer MM, Giovan P, Antonelli D, Greenberg R: Gait analysis of the triceps surae in cerebral palsy. *J Bone Joint Surg* 56A:511-520, 1974.

54. Ralston HJ, Todd FN, Inman VT: Comparison of electrical activity and duration of tension in the human rectus femoris muscle. *Electromyogr Clin Neurophysiol* 16:277-286, 1976.

55. Roberts TDM: *Neurophysiology of Postural Mechanisms*. 2nd edition, London, Butterworth, 1978, pp. 37- 68.

56. Schwab GH, Moynes DR, Jobe FW, Perry J: Lower extremity electromyographic analysis of running gait. *Clin Orthop* 176:166-170, 1983.

57. Smidt GL: Biomechanical analysis of knee flexion and extension. *J Biomech* 6:79-92, 1973.

58. Stalberg E, Schwartz MS, Thiele B, Schiller HH: The normal motor unit in man. *J Neurol Sci* 27:291-301, 1976.

59. Vandervoort AA, Kramer JF, Wharram ER: Eccentric knee strength of elderly females. *J Gerontol* 45(4):B125- B128, 1990.

60. Viitasalo JT, Komi PV: Signal characteristics of EMG with special reference to reproducibility of measurements. *Acta Physiol Scand* 93:531-539, 1975.

61. Vredenbregt J, Rau G: Surface electromyography in relation to force, muscle length and endurance. In Desmedt JE (Ed): *Electromyography and Clinical Neurophysiology*. Basal, Karger, 1973, pp. 607-622.

62. Weber EF: *Ueber die Langenverhaltinisse fer Fkeuscgfaserb der Muskeln im Allgemeinen.* Math-phys Cl, Ber. Verh. K. Sachs. Ges. Wissensch., 1851.

63. Winter DA: Pathologic gait diagnosis with computer- averaged electromyographic profiles. *Arch Phys Med Rehabil* 65:393-398, 1984.

64. Winter DA, Yack HJ: EMG Profiles During Normal Human Walking: Stride-To-Stride and Inter-Subject Variability. *Electroencephalogr Clin Neurophysiol* 67:401-411, 1987.

65. Wohlfart G: Muscular atrophy in diseases of the lower motor neurons. Contribution to the anatomy of the motor unit. *Arch Neurol Psychiat* 61:599-620, 1949.

66. Yang JF, Winter DA: Electromyography reliability in maximal and submaximal isometric contractions. *Arch Phys Med Rehabil* 64:417-420, 1983.

67. Yang JF, Winter DA: Electromyographic amplitude normalization methods: improving their sensitivity as diagnostic tools in gait analysis. *Arch Phys Med Rehabil* 65:517- 521, 1984.

68. Yang JF, Winter DA: Surface EMG profiles during different walking cadences in humans. *Electroencephalogr Clin Neurophysiol* 60:485-491, 1985.

69. Yoon Y, Mansour J, Simon SR: Muscle activities during gait. *Ortho Trans* 5(2):229-231, 1981.

70. Young CC, Rose SE, Biden EN, Wyatt MP, Sutherland DH: The Effect of Surface and Internal Electrodes on the Gait of Children with Cerebral Palsy, Spastic Diplegic Type. *Journal of Orthopaedic Research* 7:732- 737, 1989.

71. Zuniga EN, Simons DG: Nonlinear relationship between averaged electromyogram potential and muscle tension in normal subjects. *Arch Phys Med Rehabil* 50(11):613-619, 1969.

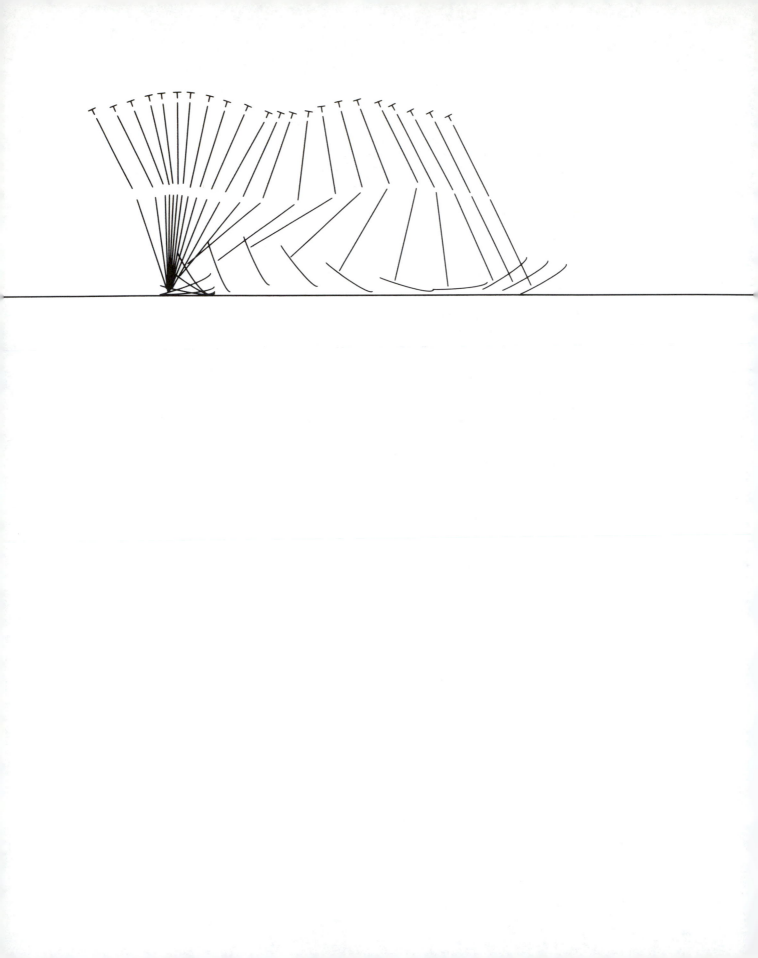

Chapter 19

Ground Reaction Force and Vector Analysis

As body weight drops onto and moves across the supporting foot, vertical, horizontal and rotatory forces are generated on the floor that can be measured with appropriate instrumentation. These ground reaction forces are equal in intensity and opposite in direction to those being experienced by the weight-bearing limb. From this information the stress imposed on the joints and the necessary muscle control can be identified.

Measurement of the ground reaction forces (GRF) is accomplished with a force plate set into the center of the walkway.[8] It consists of a rigid platform suspended on piezoelectric or strain gauge transducers fitted with strain gauges. By each supporting corner having three sensors set at right angles (orthogonal) to the others, the vertical load and horizontal shear forces in the fore-aft and mediolateral directions are measured (Figure 19.1). Through additional processing of these data, the related rotatory moments, centers of pressure, and ground reaction force vectors can

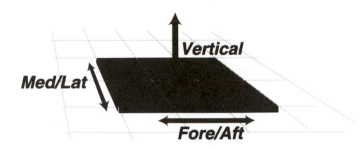

Figure 19.1 Force plate and direction of forces recorded. Vertical; Fore/Aft = forward and backward horizontal shear force (plane of progression); Med/Lat = medial and lateral horizontal shear force.

be determined. Given an accurate definition of the joint center locations, the ground reaction joint torques (moments) can be calculated.

While the force data are gathered by merely having the subject walk across the plate, several technicalities must be observed to assure an accurate outcome. It is important that the subject spontaneously load the force plate as a natural event during the course of moving along the walkway. Deliberate stepping onto the plate (called targeting) is undesirable because it causes slowing of the gait velocity and introduces artificial limb motion (A Kralj, personal communication). The result is ground reaction forces that do not represent the subject's natural walking ability. Targeting is avoided by having the plate camouflaged, mounted even with the floor surface, and covered with the same material as the rest of the floor. In addition, the subjects' awareness of the plate is minimized by focusing their attention on the far wall.

To obtain accurate data, it is essential the test foot completely contacts the plate while the other foot remains clear of the plate through the stride (Figure 19.2). This latter requirement often means repeating the test several times before the proper foot contact pattern can be attained, since the standard commercial force plate is only 45 × 60cm. A pair of long (150cm) narrow beams have been designed as a means of simplifying the force plate data collection.[5,18] This approach has not continued because fabrication is difficult and calibration more demanding.[18] A more satisfactory alternate is the use of two plates in series or even a double set (four plates) to give greater walking freedom and capture bilateral activity as well. This is a major investment, however, as the costs of the force plates plus the supporting electronics are correspondingly multiplied.

Ground Reaction Forces

Among the multitude of measurements that can be obtained with force plates, the clinical relevance differs. Those most applicable are vertical load, horizontal shear, vector patterns, joint torques and center of pressure determinations.

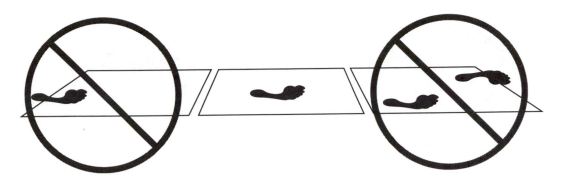

Figure 19.2 Correct and wrong foot contact patterns on a force plate. Left: Partial foot on plate (wrong); Center: Total contact by one foot on plate (correct); Right: other foot also striking plate (wrong).

Vertical Load

The normal stance phase pattern of vertical forces generated by the customary walking speed of 82m/min has two peaks separated by a valley (Figure 19.3). At this gait velocity the value of the peaks approximates 110% of body weight, while force in the valley is about 80% of body weight. Commonly, these vertical forces are designated as F_1, F_2 and F_3 (Figure 19.4). The first peak (F1) occurs at the onset of mid stance in response to the weight-accepting events during loading response. At this time the body's center of gravity is rapidly dropping, an action that adds the effect of acceleration to body weight. In late mid stance, the valley (F_2) is created by the rise of the center of gravity as the body rolls forward over the stationary foot. This valley is accentuated by the momentum of the swinging, contralateral limb, which tends to unload the force plate. The second peak (F_3), occurring in late terminal stance, again indicates downward acceleration and lowering of the center of gravity as body weight falls forward over the forefoot rocker in terminal stance. Hence, the vertical force above the weight line represents the acceleration of dropping onto the limb initially and then falling beyond the forefoot in terminal stance.

These actions can be explained mathematically by the following two equations:

$$F - w = Ma$$

$$w = Mg$$

where F is the vertical component of the ground reaction force measured by the force plate, w is the body weight, M is the person's mass, g is the gravitational constant, and a is the vertical acceleration. Combining these two equations and simplifying gives

$$F = M(g + a).$$

Since M and g are constants, the force on the force plate changes with changing

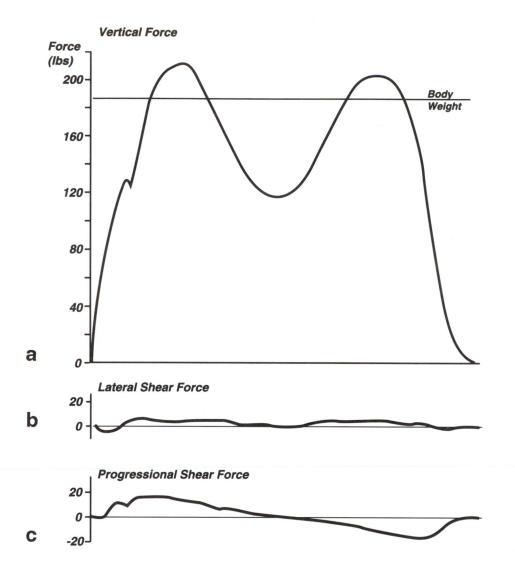

Figure 19.3 Normal ground reaction force pattern during stance. (a) Vertical force; (b) Lateral shear (horizontal); (c) Progressional shear (horizontal fore/aft).

vertical acceleration. When a = 0, the force is body weight. If a >0, the force goes up and likewise, if a < 0, the force drops below body weight. Hence, the vertical force above and below the body weight line is due to a positive and negative vertical acceleration respectively. The validity of interpreting these forces as signs of changing vertical acceleration of the center of mass is substantiated by the recording of the same vertical force pattern and comparable magnitudes of the two peaks and middle valley with an instrumented internal hip prosthesis.[18]

The magnitude of the vertical force changes with variations in gait speed.[7,14] Walking at slower speeds (<60m/min) reduces the momentum, and therefore the vertical acceleration, with a corresponding decrease in both the peaks and

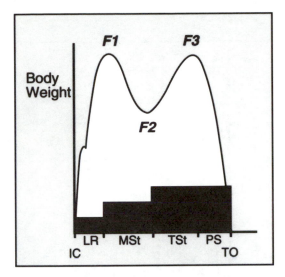

Figure 19.4 Vertical ground reaction force pattern. F1 = loading response peak; F2 = mid stance valley; F3 = terminal stance peak. Shaded base indicates foot contact pattern by step height (heel, H-5-1, 5-1). LR = loading response; MSt = mid stance; TSt = terminal stance, PS = pre-swing.

valley deviations from body weight. This results in a flat plateau at a level equal to body weight (Figure 19.5).[18] Conversely, fast walking speeds induce higher peaks and lower valleys. Running (Figure 19.5) registers peaks 2.5 times body weight.[13,14] Hence, the rate of loading the limb is the determinant of peak load, and this rate is created by gait velocity.[25]

The vertical force pattern of patients with unilateral hip pathology (degenerative disease) generally shows a reduction in the vertical loading of the disabled limb compared to that of the sound limb (Figure 19.6), but relating this to the post operative gain is difficult. The asymmetrical difference in vertical force is less than the change created by the patient's slower gait velocity, that is, within one standard deviation (unpublished data). A second common finding in the loading pattern of painful or weak limbs is an irregular series of peaks and valleys, which complicates quantification.[5] In addition, protective mechanics such as rapidly lifting ones arms may prevent the highest peak from equalling body weight. Consequently, vertical load is not a reliable clinical measure when disability is severe.[5] Better functional measures are gait velocity and single stance time.

Horizontal Shear

The forces generated parallel to the walking surface are called shear. Horizontal forces in the anterior-posterior (AP) plane occur when the ground reaction force vector deviates from the vertical. Similarly, the exchange of body weight from one limb to the other creates horizontal medial-lateral (ML) shear forces. Without adequate friction at the foot/floor interface, these shear patterns would result in sliding and potential threats to stability. However, the magnitude of the horizontal forces compared to the vertical loading is small (Figure 19.3).

However, the magnitude of the ML force is least, being less than 10% of body weight. Peak medial shear (5% BW) occurs in mid loading response. Lateral shear reaches a peak (7% BW) in terminal stance.[3]

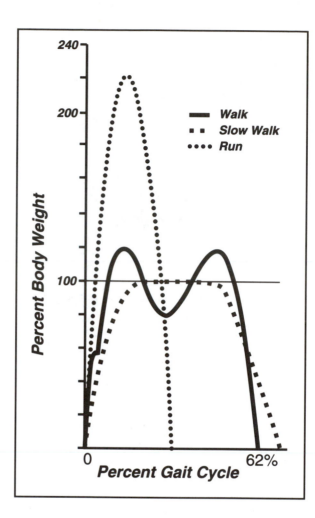

Figure 19.5 Vertical force variations with changes in walking velocity (normal). (a) Running, (b) Walking 80m/min, (c) walking 60m/min. (Courtesy of Churchill Livingstone, NY, 1984.)

The AP shear force (also called fore-aft forces) is equivalent to less than 25% of body weight. At initial contact there often is a momentary aft shear (13% BW).[3] This also was observed in half of the men studied by Skinner.[24] The action most likely reflects dynamic limb retraction to assure early weight-bearing stability. Loading the limb rapidly introduces an anteriorly directed force, which reaches a peak (13% BW) at the end of the loading response phase. This is not sustained. Mid stance is an interval with minimal sagittal shear until just before heel rise, when a posterior shear begins. There is a rapid rise in the posterior force throughout terminal stance, with a final peak equalling 23% BW.

Vectors

The ground reaction forces can be represented as a single vector that combines the simultaneous vertical, sagittal and coronal forces. This is a single

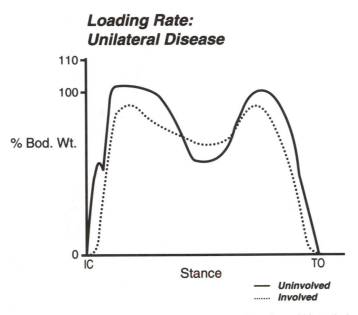

Figure 19.6 Asymmetrical vertical force pattern with unilateral hip pathology.

force line that sums the three-dimensional experience. Within this complexity, the clinically pertinent information relates to the vector patterns in the sagittal and coronal planes.

Vectors are calculated from the force plate data by combining the instantaneous vertical load and horizontal shear force into a vector sum or resultant force. The magnitude of the vector is equivalent to the hypotenuse of a right triangle with the arms being the vertical and horizontal forces (Figure 19.7). The slope of the vector is equivalent to the ratio of the vertical force to horizontal shear present. The vector intersects the force plate at the location of the instantaneous center of pressure. Fore-aft shear is used to identify the sagittal plane vectors. Frontal plane vectors relate to mediolateral shear.

Sagittal Plane Vectors. The normal sequence of vectors created during a stride subdivides into four patterns (Figure 19.8). Initial contact creates a momentary vertical force. The lack of any tilt has been considered to represent inertia of the proximal body mass.[29] A second possibility is that the high speed of the normal heel strike creates a moment without shear as body weight first drops onto the floor. This last interpretation is consistent with the isolated high-frequency vertical spike recorded by Simon et al, using a highly resonant force plate.[23]

During loading response the initial impact pattern is immediately modified by the development of an anterior shear at the foot floor interface. The effect is a posterior slope of the vectors throughout loading response similar to the beginning ribs of a fan. The base of the fan is the supporting heel.

Mid stance is an interval of nearly vertical vectors. Ankle dorsiflexion allows

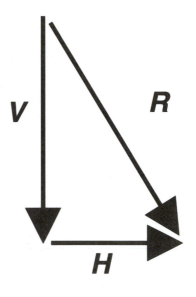

Figure 19.7 The force vector (R). A result of the simultaneous vertical (V) and horizontal (H) forces in one plane (sagittal or coronal).

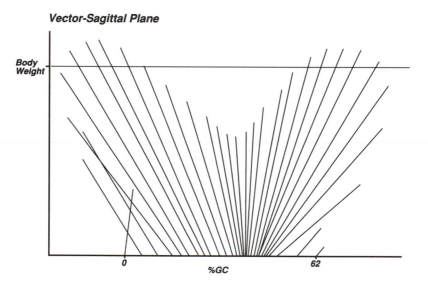

Figure 19.8 Normal pattern of sagittal vectors during a stride (5% GC intervals). The vectors form four patterns: impact, loading response, mid stance, and terminal stance.

the base of the vector (center of pressure) to advance across the foot in parallel with the progression of the body's center of mass. During this phase, the small anterior shear disappears as increasing amounts of body weight are transferred to the forefoot. When the forefoot becomes the dominant area of support, the vector reflects the beginning of a posterior shear.

During terminal stance, the increasing posterior shear causes the vectors to tilt anteriorly. Similar to the terminal edge of a fan, each vector has a greater forward slope.

Coronal Plane Vectors. Because the magnitude of the horizontal shear force is so small, the vectors in the coronal plane are dominated by the vertical force. This small shear force (typically less than 10% body weight) is in the lateral direction with two peaks having timing similar to the vertical force peaks. Consequently, the coronal vector pattern is very similar to that in the sagittal plane.

As an independent measure, ground reaction force vectors have not proved clinically useful. Use of these data, however, to determine joint torques has significantly expanded the understanding of the action of the controlling muscles.

Joint Torques

During stance the primary function of the muscles is to stabilize the joints as body weight progresses over the supporting limb. The alignment of each limb segment and *passenger unit* mass (HAT) influences joint stability. Whenever the mass center of a body segment is not vertically aligned over the joint, its weight creates a rotatory force that causes the joint to move. This is called either a moment or a torque. During stance this passive action would mean postural collapse without muscular action to restrain it. Generally, the muscular response is a yielding contraction to decelerate the motion for stability (or shock absorption), while preserving the progressional quality of walking. The intensity of this muscular action is determined by the relationship between the body weight vector and the joint center.

Two approaches have been used to designate the calculated torques. The direct technic names the torque for the type of motion it will generate if unopposed. Basically, it identifies the torque demand created by body and limb alignment (Figure 19.9a). To preserve stability, there has been an appropriate muscle response to create a counter torque (Figure 19.9b). An indirect terminology names the torque for the reaction that provided stability (the muscle action that occurred). Now the two torque stages (demand and response) are combined into one term. This complicates the clinical interpretation of pathological situations when abnormal muscle action or orthotic demands must be considered. Pathology also can introduce very abnormal postures. By designating the two stages separately, the functional situation is made clearer and therapeutic planning is simplified. For example, during loading response the body mass is behind the flexed knee. This places the vector posterior to the knee joint, creating a flexion demand torque. To stabilize the knee an extensor response is required: quadriceps action. If one needed to substitute an orthosis for inadequate quadriceps strength, knowledge of the flexor demand torque identifies the strain that will be imposed on the orthotic system. Throughout this text, the torque has been named for the functional demand created. Within joint replacement research the terms *external torque* and *internal torque* are commonly used to identify the demand and response situations respectively.

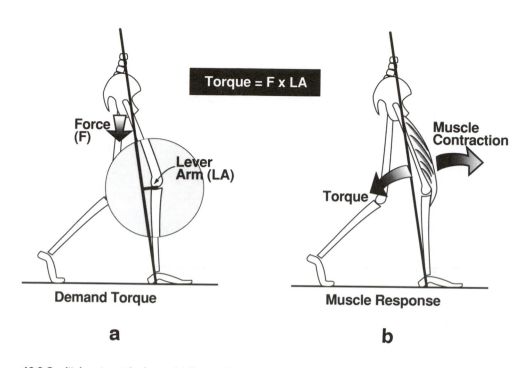

Torque = F x LA

Force (F)

Lever Arm (LA)

Muscle Contraction

Torque

Demand Torque

Muscle Response

a

b

Figure 19.9 Sagittal vector at the knee. (a) Demand torque, vector alignment behind knee creates a flexor torque. (b) Response torque, joint stability is preserved by the quadriceps creating an equal extensor torque.

Torque is defined as the product of the force and its lever arm (T = FxL).[16] The lever (or moment arm) for the joint torque presented by the body's posture is the perpendicular distance between the line of action of the vector and the center of the joint (Figure 19.9a). The vertical ground reaction is the determining force in stance. By combining motion and vector data the torques occurring throughout the stride can be calculated. Sagittal plane data define the flexion and extension torques. Coronal plane measurements identify the abduction and adduction demands.[17] Transverse moments (torques) are calculated by combining the fore-aft and mediolateral values.

Calculation of joint torques from the vector and motion data, as just described, is technically easier, but the effects of gravity and inertia are not included. Studies comparing moment calculations with and without considering the gravitational and inertial factors have shown no difference in the ankle data, but at the hip and knee there were intervals in the gait cycle where the simple vector data registered higher values.[3,15,29] The investigators have differed on the significance of these findings. Bressler and Frankel noted a brief increase in both the knee and hip values at the beginning loading response of approximately 20% and a similar difference in terminal stance for the hip.[3] Mikosz et al noted the exaggeration of the sagittal knee and hip torques (expressed in units of percent body weight × stature) was 1% each.[15] These two groups of authors concluded that for most situations, use of the unmodified vector data was adequate.[3,15] Wells, in contrast, felt the omission of the gravitational and inertial components was a grave error. His multifactorial calculations for the hip, however, differed markedly from the results of the other studies.[29]

While very significant for understanding the logic of muscular action, the resulting numbers tend to be too abstract for most clinicians. Visualization of the ground reaction force vector and walking subject by split-image photography bridges the conceptual gap. The instantaneous vector, electronically determined from the force plate, is displayed on an oscilloscope screen and recorded at the same time the walking subject is photographed (Figure 19.10).[6] Either film or video can be used. The result is a visual correlation of the instantaneous GRF vector and limb posture. From these pictures, the relative joint torques developed during the different phases of gait can be readily appreciated (Figure 19.11). This technique has been used extensively in the preceding chapters to demonstrate the force demands to which muscles must respond.

Center of Pressure

The base of the GRF vector lies within the foot, as that is the body segment in contact with the floor. This point is called the center of pressure (C/P). By tracking the path of the instantaneous centers of pressure during stance, the patient's balance and pattern of progression can be determined. While the word "pressure" is in common use, it is not correct, as the area of contact is not considered in the calculation. Center of support would be more accurate.

Each C/P point represents the mean of the vertical forces on the four

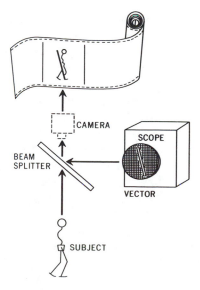

Figure 19.10 Visible vector system. Beam splitter (half-silvered mirror) allows simultaneous photography of subject and oscilloscope display of instantaneous vector. (Courtesy of Churchill Livingstone.)

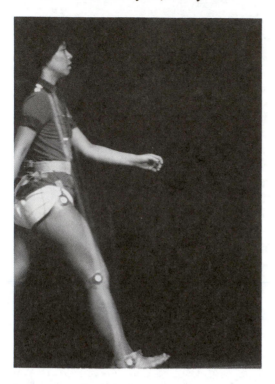 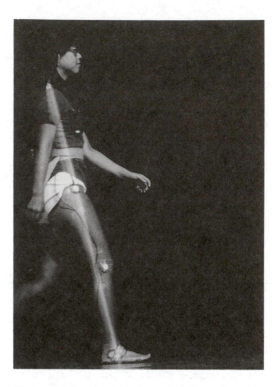

Figure 19.11 The visible vector system display of the simultaneous ground reaction force vectors and limb postures occurring in the individual phases of the gait cycle (vertical line is the vector).

Figure 19.11a Initial Contact. The vector arises from its base in the heel to pass posterior to the plantar flexed ankle and anterior to the extended knee and flexed hip. This vector alignment induces passive ankle plantar flexion, knee extension and hip flexion.

Figure 1911b Loading Response. The vector, with its base at the anterior margin of the heel, passes through the ankle joint, posterior to the flexed knee and at the margin of the hip joint. The resulting passive torques to which the muscles must respond are knee and hip flexion. At the ankle there is a transition from plantar flexion to dorsiflexion.

instrumented supporting posts of the force plate. By also defining the location of the foot on the force plate, an anatomical correlation can be made (Figure 19.12). The center of pressure is related to the plantar outline of the foot, but its location does not necessarily identify that portion of the foot receiving the greatest pressure. Only during the period of isolated heel support in loading response or the forefoot support interval in terminal stance will the C/P have any anatomical significance. Even then, the C/P point represents an average of all the forces on either the heel or forefoot, not the site of maximum pressure. During mid stance the anatomical correlation is misleading. This interval of support is shared by the heel and forefoot. The mean of the support forces provided by these two anatomical structures generally lies within the midfoot. Hence, the C/P is located in an anatomical area that makes little or no contact with the floor.

Photographing the image of the foot through a transparent force plate is a means of identifying the pressures. The camera is in a box under the force plate.[12,28]

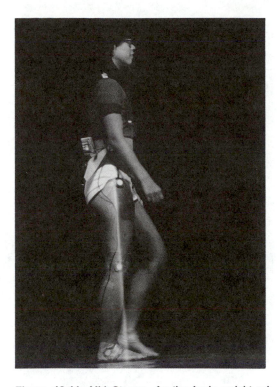

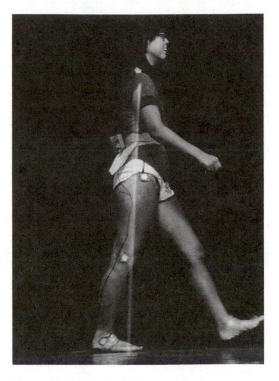

Figure 19.11c Mid Stance. As the body weight advances to the mid foot the vector lies anterior to the ankle, through the knee axis, and posterior to the hip center. The passive torques created by this vector alignment are ankle dorsiflexion torque, knee extension and hip extension.

Figure 19.11d Terminal Stance. Advancement of the vector to the forefoot increases the passive torque at each joint; that is, maximum ankle dorsiflexion, knee extension and hip extension.

Intrinsic Foot Pressure

To determine the pressures experienced by the different structures within the foot, there must be a means of limiting the recording to discrete anatomical areas.[2] Currently three approaches are in use: segmented force plates, pedographs, and an array of individual pressure sensors.

The simplest segmented force plate is a mat with a surface of multiple small projections, which, when covered with ink, imprints an overlying sheet of paper. Primarily designed for static measurement, the relative pressure is indicated by the density and size of the inked area.[10,22]

Pedobarographs use a transparent plastic platform with a stress coating that reacts to the strain by generating a color sequence that is recorded by a video camera under the plate.[1,9,21] Commercial systems are now available.

Individual pressure sensors allow anatomical designation of the testing sites.[19,20] The commercially available system uses thin (1mm) instrumented discs that are taped to the metatarsal heads and heel (Figure 19.13).[19] A significant limitation to the repeatability of the data is the anatomy of the metatarsal heads that do not provide a uniform weight-bearing surface. Instead, the posterior margin of the head is a sharp edge as it abruptly expands beyond

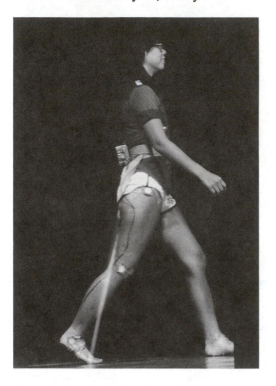

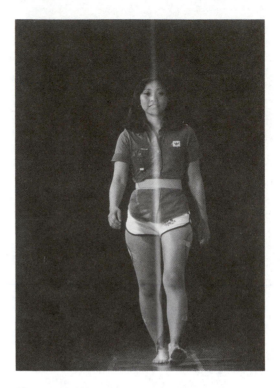

Figure 19.11e Pre-Swing. The diminished vector now is at the metatarsophalangeal joint. This aligns the vector anterior to the plantar flexed ankle and posterior to the flexed knee and extended hip. As a result the passive torques are ankle dorsiflexion, knee flexion and hip extension. The reduced height of the vector signifies unloading of the limb as body weight is transferred to the other foot.

Figure 19.11f Coronal view. The vector passes through the foot and medial to both the knee and hip and through the midline of the trunk. The effect is a passive adduction torque at the knee and hip. This late mid stance alignment is representative of other other weight-bearing phases.

the diameter of the metatarsal shaft. The rounded condyles of the metatarsal head also have a decreasing diameter anteriorly. Weight-bearing on the thin disc is very likely to cause sufficient bending to modify the pressure reading. Great care in sensor application must be taken to avoid this complication. Soames demonstrated good repeatability with his in-house strain gauge system,[26] while others have had less success.

Automated segmental force plates are the latest development. One design uses a set of twelve narrow instrumented beams laid side-by-side to divide the recording surface into 12mm strips. By repeating the test with the beams turned 90°, the sensing area is reduced to 12mm squares.[27] A segmented full-size force plate has its surface divided into .5cm areas.[4] The multisegment force plate is an advancement from earlier models, which used a series of miniature load cells.[11] Having each segment serve as an independent vertical force sensor allows discrete localization of the pressure (force/area of the sensor) within the foot. Coupled with computer technology, both numerical and color print records are produced. The advantage of the segmented force plate is its versatility, but currently it is costly ($50,000). A segmented insole also is available (Figure 19.14).

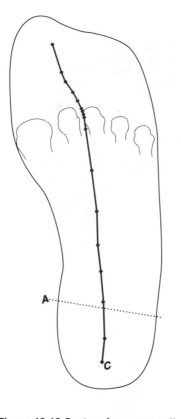

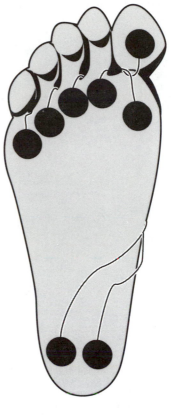

Figure 19.12 Center of pressure pattern during a normal stride. Longitudinal line (c) = path of calculated mean pressures; I = gait cycle timing of mean pressure calculations; Foot outline = tracing of subject. Horizontal line A identifies ankle joint axis. (Courtesy of SLACK Incorporated, *Orthopedics*)

Figure 19.13 Individual foot pressure sensors that allow selection of the anatomical areas to be tested. (Courtesy of of Novel Co.)

Conclusion

Loading the limb in stance initiates significant force on the floor in all three directions (vertical, progressional and lateral). As the body realigns itself over the supporting limb, the magnitude and direction of these forces change. Analysis of these forces with appropriate instrumentation can significantly contribute to the understanding of the mechanics of gait.

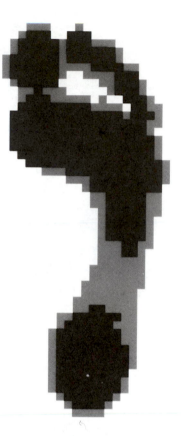

Figure 19.14 Insole containing 80 vertical force sensors for localization of the foot's weight-bearing pattern. Pressure intensity is identified by a color scale diagrammatically displayed as levels of gray; light = minimal, black = maximum. (Courtesy of Langer Co.)

References

1. Boulton AJM, Hardisty CA, Betts RP, Franks CI, Worth RC, Ward JD, Duckworth T: Dynamic foot pressure and other studies as diagnostic and management aids in diabetic neuropathy. *Diabetes Care* 6(1):26-33, 1983.
2. Brand PW, Ebner JD: Pressure sensitive devices for denervated hands and feet. *J Bone Joint Surg* 51A:109- 116, 1969.
3. Bresler B, Frankel JP: The forces and moments in the leg during level walking. *Trans of the ASME* 72:27- 36, 1950.
4. Cavanagh PR, Michiyoshi AE: A technique for the display of pressure distributions beneath the foot. *J Biomech* 13:69-75, 1980.
5. Charnley J: The recording and the analysis of gait in relation to the surgery of the hip joint. *Clin Orthop* 58:153-164, 1968.
6. Cook TM: Vector visualization in gait analysis. *Bull Prosth Res* 18(1):308-309, 1981.
7. Crowinshield RD, Brand RA, Johnston RC: The effects of walking velocity and age on hip kinematics and kinetics. *Clin Orthop* 132:140-144, 1978.
8. Elftman H: Force plate studies. In Klopsteg PE, Wilson PD (Eds): *Human Limbs and their Substitutes*. New York, Hafner, 1968, pp. 451-454.

9. Grieve DW, Rashid T: Pressure under normal feet in standing and walking as measured by foil pedobarography. *Ann Rheum Dis* 43:816-818, 1984.
10. Harris RI, Beath T: *Canadian Army Foot Survey.* Toronto, National Research Council, 1947.
11. Hutton WC, Dhanendran M: A study of the distribution of load under the normal foot during walking. *Int Orthop* 3:153-157, 1979.
12. Katoh Y, Chao EYS, Morrey BF, Laughman RK: Objective technique for evaluating painful heel syndrome and its treatment. *Foot Ankle* 3:227-237, 1983.
13. Mann R: Biomechanics. In Jahss MH (Ed): *Disorders of the Foot.* Philadelphia, W. B. Saunders Company, 1982, pp. 37-67.
14. Mann RA, Hagy J: Biomechanics of walking, running, and sprinting. *Am J Sports Med* 8(5):345-350, 1980.
15. Mikosz RP, Andriacchi TP, Hampton SJ, Galante JO: The importance of limb segment inertia on joint loads during gait. *Adv Bioengineering ASME* 1978, pp. 63-65.
16. Morrison JB: Bioengineering analysis of force actions transmitted by the knee joint. *Biomed Eng* 4:164-169, 1968.
17. Paul JP: Bioengineering Studies of the Forces Transmitted by Joints. In Kened RM (Ed): *Biomechanics and Related Bioengineering Topics.* Oxford, Pergamon Press, 1964.
18. Rydell NW: Forces acting on the femoral head- prosthesis. *Acta Orthop Scand [Suppl]* 37(suppl 88):1- 132, 1966.
19. Schwartz RP, Heath AL: The definition of human locomotion on the basis of measurement with description of oscillographic method. *J Bone Joint Surg* 29A:203-213, 1947.
20. Schwartz RP, Heath AL, Morgan DW, Towns RC: A quantitative analysis of recorded variables in the walking pattern of "normal" adults. *J Bone Joint Surg* 46A(2):324-334, 1964.
21. Scranton PE, McMaster JH: Momentary distribution of forces under the foot. *J Biomech* 9:45-48, 1976.
22. Shipley DE: Clinical evaluation and care of the insensitive foot. *Phys Ther* 59(1):13-18, 1979.
23. Simon SR, Paul IL, Mansour J, Munro M, Abernathy PJ, Radin EL: Peak dynamic force in human gait. *J Biomech* 14(12):817-822, 1981.
24. Skinner SR, Antonelli D, Perry J, Lester DK: Functional demands on the stance limb in walking. *Orthopedics* 8(3):355-361, 1985.
25. Skinner SR, Barnes LA, Perry J, Parker J: The relationship of gait velocity to the rate of lower extremity loading and unloading. *Trans Orthop Res Soc* 5:273, 1980.
26. Soames RW: Foot pressure patterns during gait. *J Biomed Eng* 7(2):120-126, 1985.
27. Stokes IAF, Hutton WC, Stot JRR: Forces acting on the metatarsals during normal walking. *J Anat* 129:579-590, 1979.
28. Sutherland DH: *Gait Disorders in Childhood and Adolescence.* Baltimore, Williams and Wilkins, 1984.
29. Wells RP: The projection of the ground reaction force as a predictor of internal joint moments. *Bull Prosth Res* 18(1):15-19, 1981.

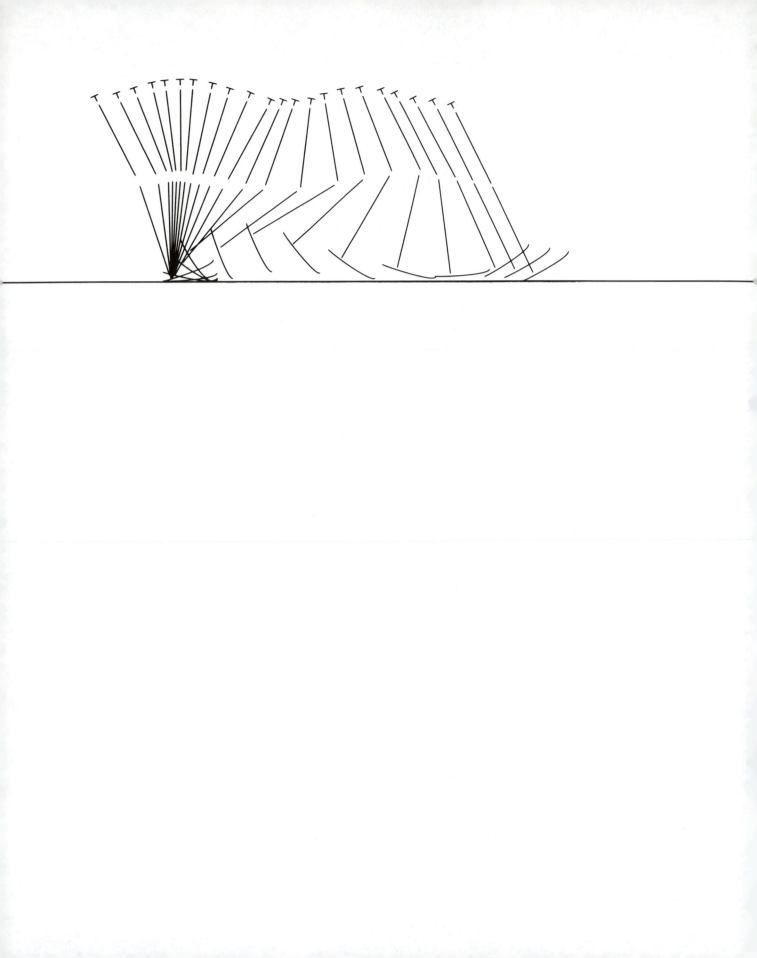

Chapter 20

Stride Analysis

The natural mix of joint mobility, muscle strength, neural control and energy leads to a customary walking speed, stride length and step rate. These time and distance factors, in combination with the swing and stance times, constitute the person's *stride characteristics*. They represent the individual's basic walking capability.

Velocity (or walking speed) is the fundamental gait measurement. Walking speed defines the person's rate of travel by identifying the time required to cover a designated distance. Technically, the term the *velocity* is the more exacting measurement as the direction of travel is a factor. The combination of direction and magnitude classifies velocity as a vector quality. This, usually, is an insignificant point, since functional testing is routinely done in the forward direction, though getting a child to walk continuously in a straight line is a challenge. The term *speed* is a numerical (scalar) value independent of direction.

By strict scientific rules, walking speed is expressed in meters per second (m/s), following the International Standards of Measurement. Many clinicians, however, prefer to express walking speed as meters per minute (m/min) in order to be compatible with the more understandable designation of cadence (steps per minute) and the custom of relating energy cost units to meters traveled. Normal persons, while able to voluntarily modify their gait velocity as needed, also have a spontaneous rate that is called either *free* or *customary walking speed* (CWS).[21] This free rate of travel designates the optimum functional balance of the person's physical qualities.

Normal free gait velocity on a smooth level surface averages 82 meters per minute (m/min) for adults. Men are 5% faster (86m/min) than the group mean (Figure 20.1a). Women's walking velocity (77m/min) is 6% slower (Figure 20.1b). These laboratory values are similar to those of Murray[13,15] and two studies involving the covert observations of pedestrians.[7,8] The range of mean values among these studies was 80 to 91m/min for the men, and among the women it was 73 to 81m/min. Stride analysis during 5 minute energy cost measurements on an outdoor, 60-meter track led to similar results (mean 80m/min, men 84m/min and women 76m/min).[21]

The primary determinants of gait velocity are the length and repetition rate of the person's stride.[1,4,11,13,19,20] This relationship tends to be linear and quite consistent for individual subjects. In practice, steps rather than strides are counted. Step rate commonly is called cadence. Hence, the determining relationship is as follows.

$$\text{Velocity} = \text{Stride Length} \times 0.5\ \text{Cadence}$$
$$(V = SL \times 0.5C)$$

Stride length for normal persons averages 1.41 meters. Men have a 14% longer stride length than women. The men average 1.46m and women 1.28m (Figure 20.2). Children have a significant increase in stride length for each year of growth until they reach 11 years of age. After this, the changes were minor.[2]

Cadence (step rate) of women (117 steps per minute) is faster than that of men

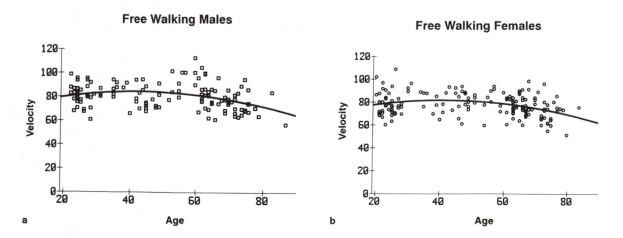

Figure 20.1 Normal velocity during free pace walking. (a) Males (N = 135); (b) Females (N = 158). Vertical scale = meters/minute; Horizontal scale = age (20 to 85 yrs).

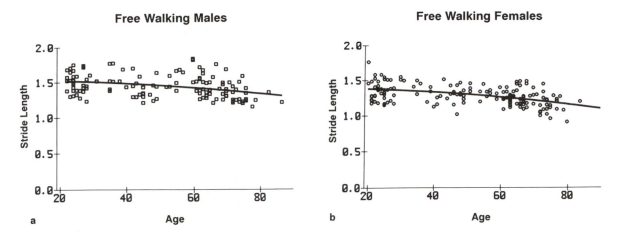

Figure 20.2 Normal stride length during free pace walking. (a) Males (N = 135); (b) Females (N = 158). Vertical scale = meters; Horizontal scale = age (20 to 85 yrs).

(111s/min) (Figure 20.3). This nearly compensates for their shorter stride length. The mean adult cadence (men and women) is 113 steps/min. Children reduce their cadence with age.[2]

Normal Variability

Normal adults show a moderate variability in their free walking velocity. One group of 60 subjects ages 20 to 65 years showed a 7% standard deviation during indoor testing following pretraining to a common cadence.[13] Another 111 persons ages 20 to 80 tested on an outdoor track displayed a 4% deviation.[21] Two identifiable sources of this variability are age and height (or limb length).

Age

Studies of aged gait in adults show a notable difference in velocity (14%) when arthritis and other disabilities are allowed as natural events.[9] With healthy subjects the influence of age is less, but increases as years beyond 65 are added. The decrease in mean velocity was just 3% for a 60- to 65-year-old group.[14] This increased to 9% when the study group included ages 60 to 80 and 11% with the upper age limit of 87 years.[4] The Rancho study of 247 persons ages 20 to 84 showed the significant decline in walking ability began after age 70 years.

Limb Length

In the growing child, the increase in leg length is obvious. Between the ages of 1 and 7 years the mean leg length increases 194% (31.6cm to 61.5cm, r =

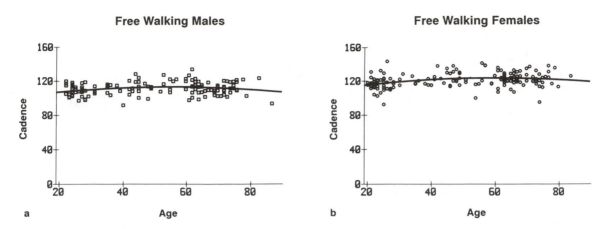

Figure 20.3 Normal cadence during free pace walking. (a) Males (N = 135); (b) Females (N = 158). Vertical scale = steps/minute; Horizontal scale = age (20 to 85 yrs).

0.95).[19] Variability also doubles (standard deviation increasing from 2% to 4% of the mean). There is a corresponding increase in stride length and walking speed. The ratio between stride length and leg length progressively increases between ages 1 and 4 (1.36 to 1.48) and then stabilizes (age 7 = 1.57). Within this age range, the correlation between leg length and stride length is strong (r = 0.95)

A similar relationship between stature and stride length has been assumed to exist in adults[6,10] but the supporting data are weaker. Grieve found a modest mean ratio between stature and stride length (r = 0.53); consequently one can attribute only 28% (r[2]) of the change in stride length to stature. Men, women, adolescents and older children showed similar correlations (r = 0.51 to 0.59). Murray found a 4% difference (r = 0.46) in the group means of tall, medium and short men (40 each). The relationship was stronger during fast walking. This is consistent with the higher correlation (r = 0.71) found during treadmill endurance running. Endurance during running was also found to decrease 7% when the stride length was altered (tests used SL = +.60 and −.80 leg length).[17] These studies, thus, have identified that leg length can influence stride length, but the relationship is weak during walking (r[2] = 0.21 to 0.28) and moderate in an endurance run (r[2] = 0.49). Hence, the recommendation that stride length should routinely be defined as a ratio of stature lacks a sound factual basis.[10,22] Das also opposes this recommendation because relative values do not present a clear picture of the distance covered.[5] Thus, the standard measurements should be the basic data, with relative anatomical values added if they contribute to the topic.

Voluntary Variability

Normal persons have a wide range of safe and relatively comfortable walking speeds. One study of men showed a 45% increase in gait velocity with equal gains in stride length and cadence (18% each).[14] Similar testing of women registered a 35% increase in walking speed, while voluntary slowing reduces the velocity by 41%. Again the changes in stride length and cadence were about equal.[15] A Rancho effort to get the slowest normal velocity resulted in a 50% reduction. Slower trials led to a disruption in the walking rhythm.

The standard deviations for normal free walking is approximately 10% of the mean value.[13,21] The preceding data indicate 4% of this deviation is related to leg length. Age has no significance until the person is past 60 years. Thus, the larger factor appears to be spontaneous variability.

Stride Measuring Systems

Several technics now are available for measuring a person's stride characteristics. They are both direct and indirect approaches. The indirect technics consist of measuring the stride characteristics from the motion recording. A particular foot or ankle marker is tracked for its pattern.

Direct technics use the foot contact pattern with the floor. Both time and distance are significant to the direct measurements. A transparent force plate will display the relative contact times of the different foot areas, as the skin changes color and shape with weight bearing. The analysis of these data is by subjective observation. Foot pressure systems automatically provide the timing data from which stride characteristics can be calculated. Foot switch systems allow measurement of the stride characteristics and floor contact pattern in either the laboratory or clinical environment with less comprehensive equipment.

Stopwatch

The simplest means of measuring a person's walking ability is with a stopwatch. Either cadence or velocity can be determined in this manner. Velocity measurements require a designated walking distance as well as timing. To minimize the effect of the examiner's reaction time, the measured walking distance should be at least 50 feet (31m). An additional 10 feet (3m) should be available before and after the measurement areas to exclude the variability of starting and stopping. Counting the number of steps taken during the timed interval provides cadence. If one has both cadence and velocity, stride length can be calculated. One can use footprints on a walkway for direct step or stride measurements.

Automated stride analysis instrumentation offers more precision in the measurements. Several types of measuring systems have been designed.

Foot Switch Systems

Commercially available foot switches are either instrumented insoles or a set of individual sensors. Many laboratories also fabricate their own foot switches. The in-house systems commonly include only one or two sensors (heel with or without the toe), with the limited purpose of differentiating stance and swing or just the gait cycle timing.

Individual Sensor Systems

The sets of small (1.5cm^2) discs designed as pressure sensors can also serve as foot switches to identify the floor contact times of the heel, individual metatarsal heads and great toe (Figure 19.13). The sensors are taped to the sole of the foot over the bony prominences of the heel and metatarsal heads. The data provided by the accompanying processor vary with the system. Basically, the duration of floor contact and the stride characteristics are identified. Portability depends on the type of recorder and analyzer used.

Insole Footswitch System

Each insole contains a large compression closing sensor in the areas of the heel (4 × 6cm), fifth and first metatarsal heads (3 × 4cm), and great toe (2 × 2cm). The sensors provide on/off signals (Figure 20.4). One may either slip the insole foot switch assembly into the shoe or tape it to the barefoot. There are six standard sizes for adults and a range of smaller insoles for children. The heel and forefoot sections are separated to allow minor size variations.

To avoid inadvertent activation by shoe pressure, foot switch sensitivity is approximately 8 psi (4 psi for children). This introduces an average 2% GC delay in the registered onset of stance and a correspondingly premature cessation compared to simultaneous force plate recordings (Figure 20.5). To determine the true stance and swing periods, the computer program includes a 2% correction factor to allow for the switch closure/opening delay. Reapplication assessment of the foot switches did not show a variation in the gait measurements beyond that found with simple repeated testing (unpublished data).

The signals from each individual sensor have a specific voltage to differentiate its floor contact time from the others. These have been processed by the computer to provide two types of clinical information: foot support sequence and gait cycle timing of the individual foot support area. Several forms of presentation have been developed. The initial approach, which remains very useful, is a diagrammatic representation of the foot/floor contact sequence through stance. A normal sequence is displayed as a four-step staircase for easy recognition. Increasing voltage levels (of equal increments) are assigned for the four support areas from isolated heel (H), through the two stages of foot flat (H-5, H-5-1), to the final area of forefoot only (5-1) or heel-off (Figure 20.6) Abnormal support patterns of just the fifth (5), the first metatarsal (1), or the heel and first metatarsal (H-1) are assigned half-step voltages. These continue to be a part of the EMG recording system (Figure 15.17h). The same information is also provided in an alphanumeric mode by the stride analyzer printer or as time bars by the EMG analyzer (Figure 11.18). Computer analysis can also specify the

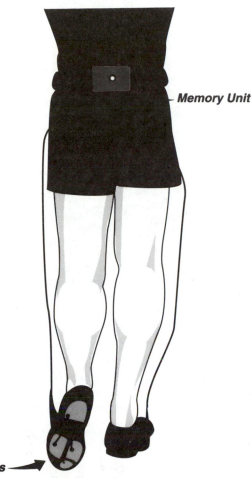

Memory Unit

Foot Switches

Figure 20.4 Insole foot switch system. Foot switches = diagram of compression switches that are contained within an insole for application within shoe or on its sole. Cable from foot switch insoles plug into memory unit. Memory unit stores foot switch signals and timer. (Adapted from Perry J. Integrated function of the lower extremity including gait analysis. Cruess RL and Rennie WRJ, *Adult Orthopaedics,* Churchill Livingstone, New York, 1984.)

duration of floor contact by the individual sensors (e.g., heel, fifth metatarsal, etc.), both in milliseconds and the gait cycle interval.

Instrumented Walkways

Walkways containing on/off sensors have been developed to avoid applying any apparatus on the subject. The basic design uses a series of electronically instrumented slats to register floor contact time (Figure 20.7). Velocity, stride

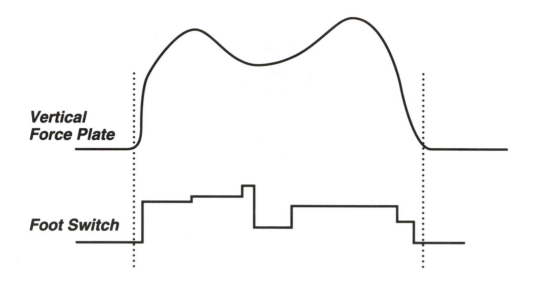

Figure 20.5 Foot switch timing compared to a simultaneous force plate record. Foot switch sensors have a 2% GC delay in onset and cessation. Horizontal scale = gait cycle. Vertical scale not significant.

length, cadence, step length, swing and stance duration, and the foot support pattern are determined by the sequence of slat contact by the two feet. This concept has been used in a few centers but the system is not commercially available. The walkways have the convenience of total subject freedom, but they also commit a significant floor space to the device.

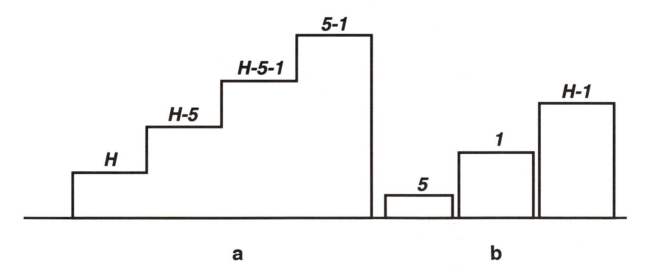

Figure 20.6 Diagrammatic scale to display individual sensor sequence and timing. Normal sequence is a stair case. Half steps designate abnormal modes of foot contact. Timing is indicated by length of step. H = heel, 5 = fifth metatarsal, 1 = first metatarasal, T = great toe.

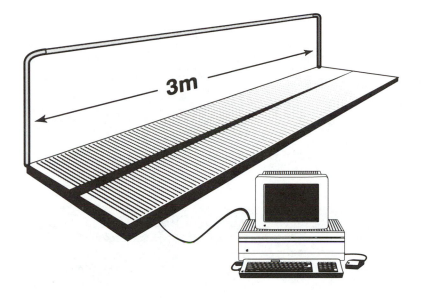

Figure 20.7 Instrumented walkway. Mat, 3 meters long, consisting of narrow instrumented slats divided into right and left halves.

Testing Procedure

The testing distance varies among the different laboratories. Space availability is a common determinate. The essential component is having sufficient distance that several strides can be recorded. The subject must feel free to walk at his/her usual pace, and there must be an interval before and after the data segment to absorb the irregularities of starting and stopping. At Rancho we found a ten-meter walkway with the middle six meters delineated for data analysis was a convenient compromise between space, patient endurance and data need (Figure 20.8). To accommodate the longer strides of normal men a 15-meter distance is used. The data interval is designated at each end by a photoelectric cell that transmits its signal to the recording instrumentation. In-house studies demonstrated that longer approach distances (6 and 12m) did not alter the data. The probability of a three-meter data collection area being too short is implied by the significantly slower normal velocity data obtained with a walkway of this distance compared to the data obtained over longer distances in other laboratories.[3,12,18]

Gait analysis is an unfamiliar experience for most subjects (normal or patients). This was confirmed by the finding of greater variability in data between the first and second walks (7% error) compared to later trials. After the first walk, retest inconsistency averaged 3%. Usually the first walk was significantly slower. Hence, an unrecorded trial is indicated before any data are stored.

The signals from the foot switches may be transmitted by telemetry or cable to a strip chart recorder for a printed record or to a computer for immediate processing. Another option is a portable system (Figure 20.9). The foot switch and time signals are collected by a microprocessor memory unit fastened to the waist

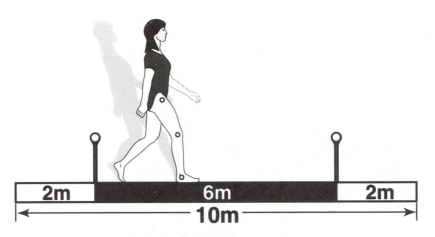

Figure 20.8 Gait recording walkway. Total length 10 meters. Middle 6 meters for data collection (black length). Photoelectric sensors (vertical objects) designate ends of data intervaal.

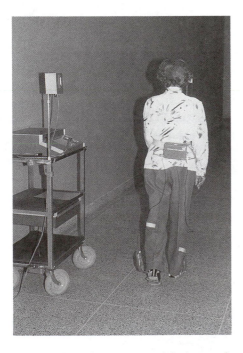

Figure 20.9 Portable foot switch system. Cart contains calculator printer. Lamp above cart is one of a pair set at the ends of data walkway (6 meters). Memory unit is on the waist belt.

band. After the test, a cable is used to transmit the data to the calculator, where the stride characteristics are determined and a printed record provided.[16] The output is based on a testing distance of six meters. This latter design allows testing in any environment having a ten-meter walking distance available.

References

1. Andriacchi TP, Ogle JA, Galante JO: Walking speed as a basis for normal and abnormal gait measurements. *J Biomech* 10(4):261-268, 1977.
2. Beck RJ, Andriacchi TP, Kuo KN, Fermier RW, Galante JO: Changes in the gait patterns of growing children. *J Bone Joint Surg* 63(A):1452-1456, 1981.
3. Berman AT, Zarro VJ, Bosacco SJ, Israelite C: Quantitative gait analysis after unilateral or bilateral total knee replacement. *J Bone Joint Surg* 69(9):1340-1345, 1987.
4. Crowinshield RD, Brand RA, Johnston RC: The effects of walking velocity and age on hip kinematics and kinetics. *Clin Orthop* 132:140-144, 1978.
5. Das Rn, Ganguli S: Preliminary observations on parameters of human location. *Ergonomics* 22(11):1231- 1242, 1979.
6. Dean CA: An analysis of the energy expenditure in level and grade walking. *Ergonomics* 8:31-48, 1965.
7. Drillis R: Objective recording and biomechanics of pathological gait. *Ann NY Acad Sci* 74:86-109, 1958.
8. Finley FR, Cody KA: Locomotive characteristics of urban pedestrians. *Arch Phys Med Rehabil* 51:423-426, 1970.
9. Finley FR, Cody KA, Finizie RV: Locomotion patterns in elderly women. *Arch Phys Med Rehabil* 50:140-146, 1969.
10. Grieve DW, Gear RJ: The relationship between length of stride, step frequency, time of swing and speed of walking for children and adults. *Ergonomics* 5(9):379-399, 1966.
11. Inman VT, Ralston HJ, Todd F: *Human Walking.* Baltimore, MD, Williams and Wilkins Company, 1981.
12. Kroll MA, Otis JC, Sculco TP, Lee AC, Paget SA, Bruckenstein R, Jensen DA: The relationship of stride characteristics to pain before and after total knee arthroplasty. *Clin Orthop* 239:191-195, 1989.
13. Murray MP, Drought AB, Kory RC: Walking patterns of normal men. *J Bone Joint Surg* 46A(2):335-360, 1964.
14. Murray MP, Kory RC, Clarkson BH: Walking patterns in healthy old men. *J Gerontol* 24:169-178, 1969.
15. Murray MP, Kory RC, Sepic SB: Walking patterns of normal women. *Arch Phys Med Rehabil* 51:637-650, 1970.
16. Perry J: Clinical gait analyzer. *Bull Prosthet Res* Fall:188-192, 1974.
17. Shields SL: The effect of varying lengths of stride on performance during submaximal treadmill stress testing. *J Sports Med Phys Fitness* 22:66-72, 1982.
18. Steiner ME, Simon SR, Pisciotta JC: Early changes in gait and maximum knee torque following knee arthroplasty. *Clin Orthop* 238:174-182, 1989.
19. Sutherland DH, Olshen R, Cooper L, Woo SLY: The development of mature gait. *J Bone Joint Surg* 62A:336-353, 1980.
20. Sutherland DH, Olshen RA, Biden EN, et al.: *The Development of Mature Walking.* London, Mac Keith Press, 1988.
21. Waters RL, Lunsford BR, Perry J, Byrd R: Energy-speed relation of walking: Standard tables. *J Orthop Res* 6(2):215-222, 1988.
22. Winter DA, Quanbury AO, Hobson DA, Sidwall HG, Reimer G, Trenholm BG, Steinkle T, Shlosser H: Kinematics of normal locomotion—a statistical study based on T.V. data. *J Biomech* 7(6):479- 486, 1974.

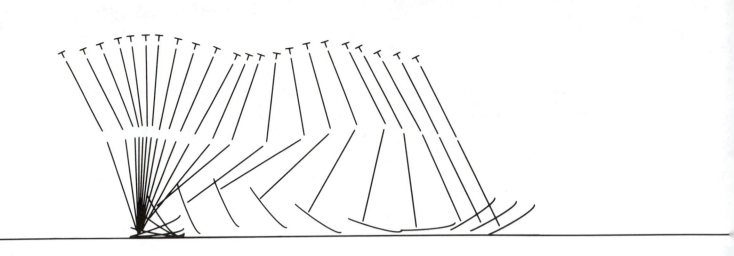

Chapter 21

Energy Expenditure

Robert L. Waters, MD

Introduction

Walking is the most common form of exercise and provides the only means of physical exertion for many sedentary individuals. Limb movement requires energy for muscular contraction. Measurement of the metabolic energy expenditure provides global information on overall gait performance and a means of quantifying the overall physiologic penalty resulting from pathological gait.[39]

A number of investigators have performed physiological energy measurements on normal subjects and patients with gait disabilities while walking using a variety of methodologies and testing equipment. Consequently, it is often difficult to compare the results. For these reasons, the majority of the data presented in this chapter were obtained by the author in the RLAMC Pathokinesiology laboratory using the same test procedures.

Work, Energy, and Power

In physics *work* is the product of force times the distance through which the force acts. This definition can cause confusion in biological situations. For example, if a muscle exerts a force under isometric conditions, there is no mechanical work since the length of the muscle remains constant; however, metabolic energy is expended, and the subject experiences physiological *effort*.

Energy is the capacity to perform work. Energy involved in the production of work is called *kinetic energy*. Energy that is stored is *potential energy*. There are six different forms of energy: chemical, mechanical, heat, light, electrical and nuclear. Transference of one form of energy to another is according to the *law of conservation of energy*. The law states that in the process of conversion, energy can neither be gained nor lost. The energy in food is biochemical energy and is converted by contracting muscles during movement to mechanical work and heat.[2]

Power is the term used to express the rate at which work is performed. Power is, therefore, a unit of time. If one man can lift a load over a given distance twice as fast as another, he is twice as powerful.

Efficiency in physiological exercise is defined as the percentage of energy input that is transformed into useful work. Studies performed in optimal situations where work is performed, such as walking on an inclined treadmill or cycling, generally demonstrate that humans can achieve an efficiency of 20 to 30%.[23] Since the law of conservation of energy states that energy cannot be lost, the metabolic energy that is not converted to mechanical work appears as heat energy, causing a rise in the body temperature.

The heat production of a maximally exercising subject may be 50 times the resting rate. Therefore, the physiological temperature controlling mechanisms that transport heat from the muscles to the skin are extremely important to prevent hyperthermia.[2]

Calorimetry

The basic unit of heat energy is the *gram-calorie* (cal) or the *kilogram-calorie* (kcal). A gram-calorie is the amount of heat necessary to raise the temperature of one gram of water one degree centigrade.

Because of the law of energy conservation, the amount of energy that is released by the complete metabolic degradation of food is the same as by its ignition and combustion with O_2 in a bomb calorimeter. Approximately 4.82 kcal of heat is liberated when a typical diet of carbohydrate, fat, and protein is burned in one liter of oxygen.[23]

Physiological energy expenditure at rest or during exercise can be measured by determining the body's heat and work production. This method is called *direct calorimetry*. However, measurement of body heat by direct calorimetry is complex and impractical for most exercise laboratory situations.

Indirect calorimetry is a simpler method of determining energy expenditure and is the equivalent of direct calorimetry. Indirect calorimetry depends on the premise that the aerobic metabolic pathways are the principle method for generating adenosine triphosphate (ATP) during prolonged exercise. By measuring O_2 consumption, the energy expenditure is indirectly determined, since the anaerobic contribution to energy production is small under this condition.

Energy Units

In most recent literature, O_2 gas volume in milliliters (ml) is reported without converting the data to calories. Since body size affects the amount of oxygen consumed, the volume of oxygen is divided by body weight to enable intersubject comparisons.

The volume of oxygen consumed in exercise studies is generally reported under standard conditions of temperature (0° centigrade), pressure (760mm Hg), and dry (no water vapor).

The O_2 *rate* is the amount of O_2 consumed per minute (ml/kg·minute). As will be discussed, the O_2 rate determines the intensity of sustained exercise and is related to the length of time exercise can be performed.

The O_2 *cost* (ml/kg·meter) describes the amount of energy used to perform the task of walking. It indicates the amount of energy needed to walk a standard unit of distance (one meter). The O_2 cost equals the O_2 rate divided by the speed of walking.

It is often useful to compare the O_2 cost of two individuals to determine their relative biological efficiency. One individual is more efficient than another if he has a lower O_2 cost. For this review, the definition of *gait efficiency* of pathological gait is as follows.

$$\text{gait efficiency} = \frac{100 \times O_2 \text{ cost (normal)}}{O_2 \text{ cost (patient)}}$$

Since the O_2 cost for a patient is nearly always greater than normal, the gait efficiency is less than 100%, depending on the degree of disability.

It is extremely important to clearly distinguish the difference between O_2 rate (ml/kg·minute) and O_2 cost (ml/kg·meter). The O_2 rate (ml/kg·minute) indicates the intensity of physical effort during exercise and is a time-dependent parameter. The O_2 cost (ml/kg·meter) is not time dependent. An individual may have a high O_2 cost, due to a gait disability, but a low O_2 rate. In this case walking can be sustained for a prolonged time, since the low O_2 rate indicates the intensity of exercise is low. On the other hand, an individual with a gait disorder resulting in a high O_2 rate may only be capable of walking a short time before the onset of fatigue, regardless of the value of the O_2 cost.

Energy Metabolism

Transfer of energy from the metabolism of foods is by way of biochemical reactions along the chains of the different metabolic pathways through chemical bonds. The final biochemical energy unit is adenosine triphosphate (ATP). When ATP is converted to adenosine diphosphate (ADP), free energy is liberated, which can be transferred to other molecules.[23]

$$ATP \rightarrow ADP + P + Energy$$

This energy shortens the contractile elements in muscle.

The amount of ATP stored in the cells is small and can only sustain muscle contraction for several seconds. In muscle, a limited amount of energy for ATP synthesis can be supplied anaerobically by creatine phosphate (CP).

$$ADP + CP \rightarrow ATP + C$$

Although the quantity of CP in muscle is three to five times more than the amount of ATP, the majority of energy to reform ATP during sustained muscle activity is actively generated from other sources.

Aerobic Oxidation

During prolonged exercise, aerobic oxidation of carbohydrate and fat are the principle food sources for generating ATP. These substrates are oxidized through a series of enzymatic reactions leading to the production of ATP. The net equation for the aerobic metabolism of glucose is

$$C_6H_{12}O_6 + 36ADP + 36P + 6O_2 \rightarrow 6CO_2\uparrow + 36ATP + 42H_2O$$

Similar equations summarize the aerobic oxidation of fats.[23]

Anaerobic Oxidation

A second type of oxidative reaction called the glycolytic cycle is available that does not require oxygen. In this pathway, carbohydrates or fats are converted to pyruvate and lactate. The net equation for the glycolytic metabolism of glucose is

$$Glucose + 2P + 2ADP \rightarrow 2\ Lactate + 2ATP$$

Bicarbonate buffers lactate in the blood leading to the formation of CO_2, which is exhaled in the expired air and summarized by the following reactions.

$$Lactate + NaHCO_3 \rightarrow Na\ Lactate + H_2O + CO_2\uparrow$$

The utilization of either carbohydrate or fat in both the aerobic and anaerobic pathways is dependent upon the type of muscular work (i.e., continuous, intermittent, brief or prolonged, intensity of work in relation to muscle groups involved), the individual's training level, diet, and state of general health.

Aerobic versus Anaerobic Metabolism

During continuous exercise there is an interplay between the aerobic and anaerobic metabolic pathways that depends on the work load. During mild or moderate exercise the oxygen supply to the cell and the capacity of aerobic energy producing mechanisms are usually sufficient to satisfy ATP requirements. During strenuous exercise, both anaerobic and aerobic oxidation processes occur and the serum lactate level rises, reflecting the additional anaerobic activity.

The amount of energy that can be produced anaerobically is limited. As reflected in the above equations, approximately 19 times more energy is produced by the aerobic oxidation of carbohydrates than by anaerobic oxidation. Anaerobic oxidation is also limited by the individual's tolerance to acidosis resulting from the accumulation of lactate. From a practical standpoint, the anaerobic pathway provides muscle with a method for supplying energy for sudden and short-term strenuous activity.

If exercise is performed at a constant rate at which the aerobic processes can supply the necessary ATP production, an individual can sustain exercise for a prolonged time without an easily definable point of exhaustion.[2] The serum lactate does not rise since the amount of anaerobic metabolism is minimal.

When exercise is performed at more strenuous work rates, the serum lactate rises, reflecting the contribution of anaerobic energy production required to meet the additional ATP demands. The point of onset of anaerobic metabolism is heralded by a rise in the serum lactate, a drop in the blood pH, and a rise in the ratio of expired carbon dioxide (CO_2) to inspired oxygen (O_2).[23] Since the metabolic contribution of anaerobic pathways, as well as the individual's tolerance for acidosis is limited, the endurance time progressively shortens and fatigue ensues earlier as the intensity of the work load rises.

Respiratory Quotient and Respiratory Exchange Ratio

In the analysis of energy expenditure, the respiratory quotient (RQ), which is the ratio of carbon dioxide production to oxygen consumption at rest, relates to the type of food that is metabolized. Interpretation of the RQ rests on the assumption that analysis of air exchange in the lungs is the same as gas exchange at the cellular level and reflects the oxidation of specific food sources. The RQ for a pure carbohydrate diet is 1.00. The RQ for a pure fat diet is 0.70. A typical mixed diet consisting of 60% metabolized fats and 40% metabolized carbohydrates results in a RQ of 0.82 at rest and the caloric equivalent is 4.8 cal per ml O_2.[23]

The respiratory exchange ratio (RER) is calculated the same as the RQ, and this term is used under exercise conditions. Sustained strenuous exercise resulting in a RER greater than 0.90 indicates anaerobic activity.[2] A ratio greater than 1.00 indicates severe exercise. From a practical standpoint, the RER provides a convenient, noninvasive method of determining whether significant anaerobic metabolism is occurring.

Maximal Aerobic Capacity

The maximal aerobic capacity (VO_2 max) is the highest oxygen uptake an individual can attain during exercise. It is a time-dependent parameter and is expressed in the same units as the O_2 rate, (ml/kg·minute). It represents an individual's maximal aerobic energy production capability and is the single best indicator of work capacity and physical fitness.[39] Generally, an individual is able to reach his VO_2 max within two to three minutes of exhausting exercise.

Age influences the VO_2 max. Up to approximately 20 years of age, the maximum oxygen uptake increases. Thereafter, the maximum oxygen uptake declines primarily due to a decrease in both maximum heart rate and stroke volume and a more sedentary life-style.[1]

Differences in body composition and hemoglobin content are factors that account for a difference in the VO_2 max between the sexes. The ratio of VO_2 max to the fat-free body mass is not significantly different between men and women. However, due to generally larger body composition and greater hemoglobin concentration in men, and greater adipose tissue in women, the VO_2 max is 15 to 20% higher in males than females.[2]

Arm versus Leg Exercise

The maximal aerobic capacity also depends on the type of exercise performed. The oxygen demand directly relates to the muscle mass involved. The VO_2 max during upper limb exercise is lower than with the lower limbs. For any given work load, however, heart rate and intra-arterial blood pressure are higher in upper limb exercise than lower limb exercise.[3] In the trained athlete, the VO_2 max is the same whether maximally running or bicycling.[3]

Deconditioning

A sedentary life-style decreases the VO_2 max.[31] Not only does atrophy of peripheral musculoskeletal structures occur but there is a central decline in stroke volume and cardiac output, and an increase in resting and exercising heart rate as a result of inactivity. Any disease process of the respiratory, cardiovascular, muscular, or metabolic systems that restrict the supply of oxygen to the cell will also decrease the VO_2 max. Bed rest for three weeks can result in a 27% decrease in the VO_2 max in normal subjects by decreasing cardiac output, stroke volume, and other factors.[31]

Training

A physical conditioning program can increase the aerobic capacity by several processes: improving cardiac output, increasing the capacity of the cells to extract oxygen from the blood, increasing the level of hemoglobin, and increasing the muscular mass (hypertrophy). All the above lead to increased fat utilization as the primary source of energy.[23] As a result, less lactate is formed during exercise and endurance is increased. Other effects of aerobic training include a decrease in resting and submaximal heart rate, blood pressure, and an increase in stroke volume and, therefore, cardiac output.

Endurance

If exercise is performed at a rate at which the aerobic processes can supply the necessary ATP production, an individual can sustain exercise for a prolonged time without an easily definable point of exhaustion.[2] When exercise is performed at more strenuous rates, anaerobic metabolism assists aerobic metabolism in meeting the demands of sustained strenuous exercise. The contribution of anaerobic metabolic pathways normally begins when the exercise work rate reaches between 55 and 65% of the VO_2 max of healthy untrained subjects, but can occur at over 80% of the VO_2 max in highly trained endurance athletes.[9,23] Anaerobic metabolism is heralded by a rise in the serum lactate and a rise in the RER.

It appears both the VO_2 max and the point at which anaerobic processes begin are determined by different factors. Training, muscle fiber type, capillary density, and alterations in the muscle's oxidative capabilities determine the percentage of the VO_2 max that can be sustained in endurance exercise without triggering anaerobic metabolism.[17,23] An experienced endurance athlete tends to compete at an exercise level just above the point of onset of blood lactate accumulation. Since the metabolic contribution of anaerobic pathways is limited, as well as the individual's tolerance for acidosis systemically and in the muscle, endurance progressively shortens and fatigue ensues earlier as the intensity of the work load rises.

Oxygen Pulse

Measurement of the VO_2 max requires the willingness of the subject to work to exhaustion and may be unsafe or undesirable for some subjects, particularly older individuals. When it is not possible or appropriate to directly measure the VO_2 max, considerable information on the level of physical conditioning is obtained by calculating the O_2 pulse.

The oxygen pulse is the ratio of the O_2 rate to the heart rate. In the absence of cardiac disease, there is a linear relation between the O_2 rate and heart rate, although there is considerable variation in the slope between individuals related to differences in physical conditioning, the muscles utilized and whether exercise is performed with the arms or legs. It is desirable to compare the O_2 pulse when subjects are exercising at approximately the same heart rates. As with the VO_2 max, the oxygen pulse is higher during arm exercise than leg exercise.[3] Because training can increase the cardiac stroke volume and increase the efficiency of the extraction of O_2 from the blood by muscle, the oxygen pulse increases with training. Conversely, the oxygen pulse decreases with deconditioning.

Metabolic Energy Measurement

Steady State

After approximately two or three minutes of exercise at a constant submaximal work load, the rate of oxygen consumption reaches a level sufficient to meet the energy demands of the tissues. The cardiac output, heart rate, respiratory rate, and other parameters of physiologic work load reach a plateau and a *steady state* condition is achieved. Measurement of the rate of oxygen consumption at this time reflects the energy expended during the activity.

Spirometry

O_2 uptake can be measured by either closed or open spirometry techniques. In closed systems, air is rebreathed after absorption of CO_2 in exhaled air in a lime canister. This method requires the subject to be adjacent to a large spirometer. Most closed systems have considerable airway resistance when conducting high volumes of air and therefore are not used in exercise studies, although they are commonly used for pulmonary function studies in hospitals.

Open spirometry is the preferred method for most exercise studies. In open spirometry, the subject does not rebreathe air, as in closed spirometry. Ambient air (oxygen 20.93 percent, CO_2 0.03 percent, nitrogen 79.04 percent) is constantly inhaled. Measurement of the volume and the percentage of O_2 in the expired air is used to calculate the amount of O_2 consumption.

Test Procedures/Treadmill or Track

Measurement of O_2 consumption in normal subject's can be performed on a treadmill with adjacent O_2 measurement apparatus. This method requires the least amount of laboratory space and also enables continuous, breath-by-breath, gas analysis.

Normal subjects easily adapt to walking on a treadmill or on a track. When asked to walk around a circular track at their comfortable speed, normal subjects and minimally disabled patients choose a self-selected velocity that remains relatively constant for a given individual over a sustained walking trial.[36,37,46] Because air resistance is minimal at functional walking velocities, there is no difference in the rate of O_2 consumption measured on a treadmill or on a track at the same speeds.[28]

Unlike normal subjects, patients with moderate or severe gait impairments may have difficulty or be unable to adapt to treadmill walking or adjust to speeds other than their customary walking speed (CWS). Those requiring walking aids, such as crutches or a walker, may be unable to walk on a treadmill. Thus, treadmill data may not reflect the true energy expenditure under the patient's customary walking conditions. For these reasons and safety, we prefer testing on a stationary track.

Measurement of O_2 consumption can be performed with a portable spirometer carried by the subject. The volume of expired air is measured and a sample of gas collected for later O_2 and CO_2 analysis. Portable spirometers are most useful for situations requiring considerable freedom of body movement such as in skiing, cross-country running or mountain climbing.

The *Douglas Bag* technique is the classic method of O_2 analysis. This method enables highly accurate gas analysis. Expired air is collected in a large portable bag over a fixed time interval. At the completion of testing, the volume of air is measured and tested for O_2 and CO_2 content on highly accurate bench apparatus.

To enable continuous gas analysis while subjects walked around a track, Corcoran developed a velocity-controlled motor driven mobile cart carrying the gas measurement apparatus.[8] Since the gas analysis apparatus is not carried by the subject, weight was not a factor and accurate instrumentation was used that enabled continuous data analysis.

Pathokinesiology Laboratory Methods

The method of gas analysis used in the RLAMC Pathokinesiology laboratory is a modification of the Douglas Bag technique. This selection is based on the simplicity, high reliability and accuracy of this method. The system is harnessed to the subject's shoulders (Figures 21.1a and 21.1b). A multiported valve enables multiple collected gas samples in nonporous polypropylene bags while the patient walks around a circular, 60.5 meter, outdoor track (Figure 21.2).

The subject breathes through a well-fitted mouthpiece and wears a nose clip to prevent air leakage. The directional flow of inspired and expired air are controlled by two large diameter, one-way "J" valves mounted over each shoulder. The large diameter design of the J valve results in a highly competent valve (insignificant retrograde airflow) without adding significant airway resistance even at the high rates of airflow obtained during intense exercise. The two valves are mounted over each shoulder and connected by large diameter flexible tubing to a "T" piece attached to the mouthpiece.

It is desirable to minimize the "dead space" in the air collection system to prevent rebreathing since the inhalation of expired CO_2 in sufficient quantity causes hyperventilation. For this reason, a third valve is mounted inside the T piece. This valve does not add significant airflow resistance and is sufficiently competent to prevent CO_2 rebreathing.

A thermistor placed in the T piece just beyond the mouthpiece detects the difference in temperature of inspired and expired air, enabling monitoring of respiratory rate. Electrocardiographic leads are taped to the subject's chest to record the heart rate. A foot switch worn inside the shoe detects step frequency. Heart rate, respiratory rate, and step frequency data are telemetered via a radio transmitter. The total weight of the entire system is less than 1.5kg.

Resting and Standing Metabolism

The basal metabolic rate (BMR) is the minimum level of energy required to sustain the body's vital functions in the waking, resting state.[23] The BMR

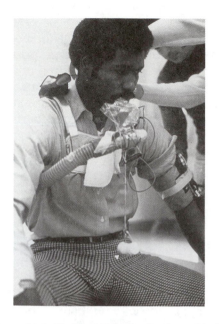

Figure 21.1a Modified "Douglas Bag" used in Pathokinesiology Laboratory. Multiported valves connected to multiple nonporous polyethylene bags.

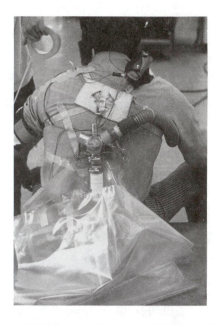

Figure 21.1b A nose clip and carefully fitted rubber mouthpiece prevent air leakage. A low-competence valve just distal to the mouthpiece minimizes rebreathing expired air. One-way J valves mounted over each shoulder control the flow of inspired and expired air. Heart rate, respiratory rate, and step frequency data telemetered from radio transmitter attached to subject's chest.

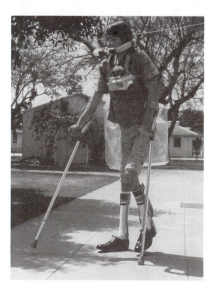

Figure 21.2 Subject walking around 60.5 meter, circular outdoor track and self-selected velocity.

generally varies according to the diet, body surface area, as well as the percentage of body fat, and this in part accounts for a 5 to 10% difference between females and males. As a function of age, the BMR decreases approximately 2% every decade through adulthood.[23]

In the recumbent position, the basal metabolic rate and resting values of O_2 consumption are approximately the same.[11] Oxygen uptake in the sitting position is slightly increased.[25] Quiet standing further elevates the rate of oxygen consumption by approximately 22%, equalling 3.5 ml/kg·minute for males and 3.3 ml/kg·minute for females (Figure 21.3).[20]

Electromyographic studies demonstrate minimal muscular activity is required for normal standing.[21] This is consistent with the fact that in the standing posture, the force of gravity acting on the centers of gravity of the different body segments passes close to the axes of rotation of the spine, hip, knee, and ankle. This is an example of the principle of energy conservation applied to the design of the musculoskeletal frame and the standing posture.

Normal Gait

Range of Customary Speeds

In a study of adult pedestrians 20 to 60 years of age who were unaware they were observed, the mean walking speed for males, 82 meters/minute was significantly higher than for the females, 74 meters/minute.[13] Approximately the same mean values, 82 meters/minute and 78 meters/minute, were obtained during energy expenditure studies performed in the Pathokinesiology labora-

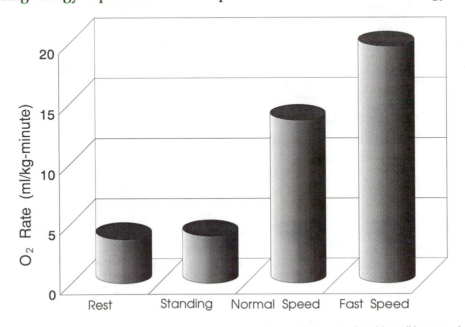

Figure 21.3 Rate of O_2 consumption at rest, standing, walking at comfortable walking speed (CWS) and fast walking speed (FWS).

tory around an outdoor, circular track when subjects were instructed to walk at their comfortable walking speed (CWS) (Table 21.1).[40] These findings support the conclusion that the gait of normal subjects tested in this manner was not altered by the experimental procedure.

The average slow and fast walking speeds in adults 20 to 59 years of age was 37 meters/minute and 99 meters/minute (Table 21.2).[40] It can be concluded that the functional range of walking speeds in adults ranges from approximately 40 meters/minute to 100 meters/minute.

At speeds above 100 meters/minute, there is a choice between walking or running. Thorstensson studied adult males and found the transition speed between walking and running averaged 113 meters/minute with a tendency for longer-legged men to have a higher transition speed.[33] Running becomes more efficient than walking at speeds above approximately 133 meters/minute.[12]

Energy Expenditure at the Customary Walking Speed

At the comfortable walking speed (CWS), the O_2 rate for young adults aged 20 to 59 years and senior subjects between 60 and 80 years of age do not significantly differ, averaging 12.1 and 12.0ml/kg·minute.[40] The O_2 rate is higher in teens and children, averaging 12.9 and 15.3ml/kg·minute respectively (Table 21.3). Expressed as a percentage of the VO_2 max, the O_2 rate at the CWS requires approximately 32% of the VO_2 max of an untrained normal subject 20 to 30 years of age and nearly 48% of the VO_2 max of a senior subject 75 years of age.[1] The RER was below 0.85 for normal subjects of all ages at their CWS, indicating anaerobic metabolism is not required.

The results account for the perception in healthy subjects that walking

Table 21.1

Gait Characteristics of Unobserved Adult Pedestrians and Adult Subjects 20 to 60 Years of Age Undergoing Energy Expenditure Testing at CWS

	Finley[13]			Waters[40]		
	M	F	T	M	F	T
Velocity (meters/minute)	82	74	78	82	78	80
Cadence (steps/minute)	110	116	114	108	118	113
Strike (meters)	1.48	1.31	1.38	1.51	1.32	1.42

Table 21.2

Gait Characteristics at Customary Slow, Normal, and Fast Speeds[40]

		Velocity (meters/minute)			Cadence (steps/minute)			Stride (meters)		
		SWS	CWS	FWS	SWS	CWS	FWS	SWS	CWS	FWS
Adults (20-59)	F	37	78	99*	68	118	137	.89	1.32	1.24
	M	48	82	110*	76	108	125	1.03	1.51	1.67
	T	43	80	106	72	113	131	.97	1.42	1.47

*Indicates significant (P < .05) difference between male and female subjects at slow walking speed (SWS), customary walking speed (CWS), and fast walking speed (FWS).

Table 21.3

Energy Expenditure at Comfortable and Fast Walking Speeds, the Influence of Age[40]

	Speed Meters/ Minute		O₂ Rate ml/kg·minute		O₂ Cost mg/kg·meter		Pulse Beats/ Minute		RER	
	CWS	FWS	CWS	FWS	CWS	FWS	CWS	FWS	CWS	FWS
Children (6-12)	70	88	15.3	19.6	.22	.22	114	127	.84	.87
Teens (13-19)	73†	99	12.9†	19.2	.18	.20	97	117	.76	.82
Adults (20-59)	80†	106†	12.1†	18.4†	.15†	.17	99	124†	.81	.92
Seniors (60-80)	74†	90†	12.0	15.4†	.16†	.17	103	119†	.85	.92

†Indicates significant (P < .05) difference between preceding value in younger age group.

requires little effort. It is significant that with advancing years older individuals have progressively smaller aerobic reserves due to a decline in the VO_2 max to accommodate to any added physiologic penalties imposed by gait disorders.

Energy Expenditure at the Fast Walking Speed

When asked to walk at a fast walking speed (FWS), the average O_2 rate for children, teens and young adults is approximately the same, averaging 19.6, 19.2, and 18.4ml/kg·minute respectively.[40] The value for senior subjects at their FWS, 15.0ml/kg·minute, is significantly lower and corresponds to a decline in the average FWS (90 meters/minute versus 106 meters/minute). The decline in the average FWS of senior subjects parallels the decrease in the average VO_2 max that occurs with aging. The RER for children, teens, young adults, and seniors at their fast speed average .87, .82, .92 and .92 respectively.[40] These findings indicate that normal adults customarily set their fast walking speed at a level approximating the threshold of anaerobic metabolism.

Males versus Females

Investigators have reported higher rates of oxygen consumption in males while walking. Others have reported higher values in female subjects or no significant difference.[5] In a review of 225 normal subjects, we found no significant differences due to sex were observed at the customary slow, normal, or fast speeds.[40] The heart rate was higher in females than males in all age groups, consistent with other types of exercise in which higher heart rates are observed in females.[40]

Energy-Speed Relationship

Different investigators have derived second order equations to describe the energy-speed relationship, which are typified by the following:

O_2 Rate = 0.00110 V^2 + 5.9   (Ralston)[29]   Eq (1)
O_2 Rate = 0.00100 V^2 + 6.2   (Corcoran)[8]   Eq (2)

where the O_2 rate is the ml/kg·minute of O_2 and V equals the velocity.

Inspection of these equations indicates they are approximately linear within the customary range of walking speeds from 40 to 100 meters/minute (Figure 21.4). We found second or higher order regressions did not significantly improve the data fit in comparison to linear regression at velocities below 100 meters/minute. Since the functional range of walking speeds is below 100 meters/minute, we prefer the following linear regression to describe the energy-speed relationship.[40]

O_2 Rate = 0.129 V + 2.60   Eq (3)

Comparison of Equation (1) through Equation (3) indicates all generate similar values in the customary range of walking speeds from 40 to 100 meters/minute (Figure 21.3). Ralston, Eq (1), performed testing on a treadmill at controlled velocities. Corcoran, Eq (2), performed testing on a track while subjects walked along a velocity-controlled mobile cart carrying the gas analysis instrumentation. Our results, Eq (3), were obtained on an outdoor track

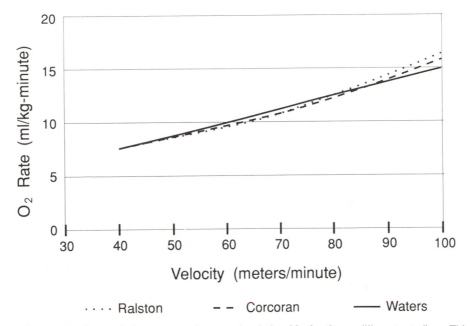

Figure 21.4 Rate of O_2 consumption-speed relationship in three different studies. This relationship is approximately linear in the range of functional walking speeds between 40 and 100 meters/minute.

at the subjects' self-selected, comfortable, slow, and fast walking speeds. The equivalency of the equations for the energy-speed relation by three different methods indicates the adaptability of normal gait to different laboratory conditions without the introduction of experimental artifact.

The above equations were not determined at extremely slow velocities. Measurement of the O_2 rate at extremely slow speeds in adults resulted in an average of 5.7ml/kg·minute.[20] This value represents the effort required to maintain the body in motion at a barely perceptible speed.

The regression equations for the energy-speed relationship in adults 20 to 59 years of age and seniors 60 to 79 years of age are the same. However, the regression equations for children and teens significantly differ from adult values as follows:

Children: O_2 Rate = .188 V + 2.61	Eq (4)
Teens: O_2 Rate = .147 V + 2.68	Eq (5)
Adults: O_2 Rate = .129 V + 2.60	Eq (6)

Interestingly, the Y-intercept (Figure 21.5) of the regression equations are essentially the same in all three groups and approximate the value for quiet standing (zero velocity).

Inherent differences in body composition and size account for the higher rate of O_2 consumption in children. The lean muscle mass in children comprises substantially greater percentage of total body weight than in adults. With increasing age, a larger percentage of total body weight becomes fat and skeleton, which are relatively metabolically inert.

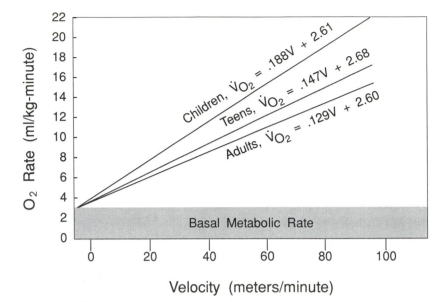

Figure 21.5 Rate of O_2 consumption-speed relationship in children, teens, and adults.

O_2 Cost-Speed Relation

The oxygen cost per meter walked is obtained by dividing the rate of oxygen uptake by the velocity. The equation for O_2 cost at different speeds can be derived by dividing Eq (4-6) by the velocity yielding the following equations.

$$\text{Children: } O_2 \text{ Cost} = .188 + 2.61 \, V^{-1} \qquad \text{Eq (7)}$$
$$\text{Teens: } O_2 \text{ Cost} = .147 + 1.68 \, V^{-1} \qquad \text{Eq (8)}$$
$$\text{Adults: } O_2 \text{ Cost} = .129 + 2.60 \, V^{-1} \qquad \text{Eq (9)}$$

It is evident that children are the least efficient walkers.

Walking Surface and Footwear

The type of walking surface has little effect on energy expenditure unless the surface is extremely rough. A 10% decrease in energy cost was found between treadmill and asphalt or cinder path walking for a young normal adult population when wearing leather combat boots.[25]

Loading

Loading the body with weights increases the rate of energy expenditure depending on the location of the loads. Loads placed peripherally on the foot have a much greater effect than loads placed over the trunk.[20] Placement of a 20kg load on the trunk of a male subject did not result in a measurable increase in the rate of energy expenditure. On the other hand, a 2kg load placed on each foot increased the rate of oxygen uptake 30%. This finding is predictable since forward foot acceleration is much greater than trunk acceleration and, therefore, greater effort is required. These findings are of clinical significance for patients requiring lower extremity orthoses or prostheses and indicate the importance of minimizing weight.[42]

Grade Walking

A number of investigators have studied walking up an incline. Bobbert combined his own data with those obtained from the literature and determined the logarithm of the O_2 rate increased linearly with the slope of the grade.[4]

Range and Duration of Customary Walking

Functional ambulation requires the individual to traverse a certain distance to perform a specific activity. The average distances for various daily living activities were measured in a cross section of different urban areas in Los Angeles, California. Most activities such as going to the post office, doctor's office, supermarket or department store necessitate less than a 300-meter walking distance from available parking (Figure 21.6).[22] Assuming automotive transport is available and the average walking speed is 80 meters/minute, it follows that most daily living activities require less than four minutes of walking for a normal individual.

Pathological Gait

It is evident that energy conservation was a major factor in the evolutionary design of the lower limbs and bipedal gait mechanism. Interruption of the normal gait cycle due to a gait disability results in increased energy expenditure. Nevertheless, a patient will adapt, if there is sufficient neurological control, by performing compensatory gait substitutions to minimize the additional energy expenditure.[20]

Joint Immobilization

Measurement of the energy expenditure after joint immobilization by surgical joint fusion or plaster casts enables determination of the energetic importance of specific lower limb joint movements to the gait cycle (Figures 21.7, 21.8, 21.9).

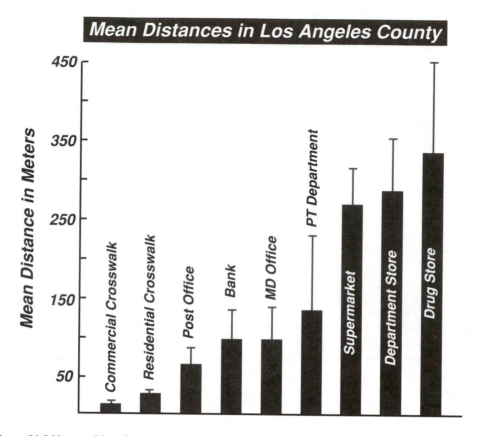

Figure 21.6 Mean walking distance in Los Angeles from available parking to different common destinations.

Ankle Fusion

Following ankle fusion, the average O_2 rate, 12.0ml/kg·minute, is approximately the same as for normal subjects, 12.1ml/kg·minute, but the CWS, 67 meters/minute, is 16% slower or 84% of normal (80 meters/minute) (Table 21.4).[36] Using Eq (3) to control for velocity, the average ankle fusion patient requires an O_2 rate 3% greater than a normal subject walking at the same speed.

Due to the slow speed, the average O_2 cost for ankle fusion patients is 0.166ml/kg·meter in comparison to 0.151ml/kg·meter for normal adults.[36] Therefore, gait efficiency is 92% of normal. The fact that there is only a 8% decrease in gait efficiency following ankle fusion is consistent with the observation that ankle fusion does not require major compensatory changes in the overall gait pattern.

Hip Fusion

Following unilateral hip fusion, the average CWS is below normal, 67 meters/minute. This is the same as the mean following ankle fusion (Table

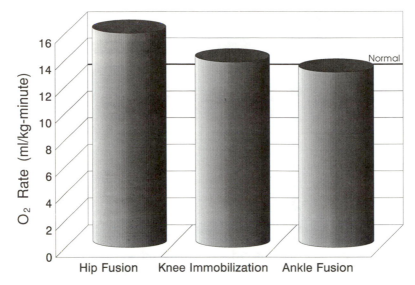

Figure 21.7 O_2 rate following knee immobilization, hip and ankle fusion.

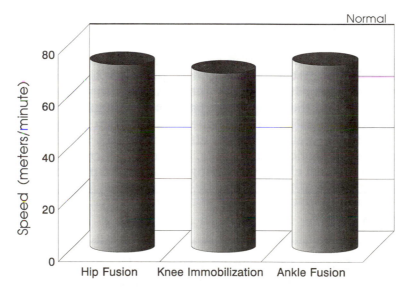

Figure 21.8 Speed following knee immobilization, hip and ankle fusion.

21.4).[36] Although there is no significant difference in the CWS, the average O_2 rate for hip fusion patients, 14.7ml/kg·minute, is significantly higher than normal or following ankle fusion. Using Eq (3) to control for velocity, this increase represents a 32% higher rate than for normal subjects.

Because of both the reduced CWS and higher O_2 rate, the average O_2 cost for hip fusion patients, 0.223ml/kg·meter, is significantly greater than following ankle fusion, 0.170ml/kg·meter. In comparison to normal walking, hip fusion patients achieve 68% gait efficiency. The elevated O_2 rate and O_2 cost indicates the importance of hip motion in the gait cycle.

stabilize the knees. Not only must the arms lift and swing the body forward in the swing phase, but they must also provide antigravity support during the stance phase if the hip and trunk extensors are paralyzed. Paraplegics may also lack motor control of lower trunk and hip flexors, further concentrating the demand on the shoulder and arm musculature to swing the body forward.

For the above reasons, it is not surprising that paraplegics with intact trunk musculature who require a swing-through gait are extremely slow ambulators. As a group, their CWS, 29 meters/minute, is approximately half the value of the fracture patients, 50 meters/minute. Despite the slow CWS, paraplegics have a high O_2 rate, 16.3ml/kg·minute and O_2 cost, 0.88ml/kg·meter. The high O_2 rate is relatively greater in consideration of the fact that the VO_2 max for paraplgics is lower than normal.[16] These findings account for the fact that few paraplegics dependent on a swing-through gait pattern continue to walk after gait training in a rehabilitation center.

Spinal Cord Injury, Reciprocal Gait

Hussey and Stauffer concluded that there is a direct relationship between motor power, the reciprocal gait and walking ability.[19] Those patients who were able to walk in the community had a reciprocal gait pattern and at least fair (Grade 3) hip flexor strength and fair extensor strength in one knee so that no more than one knee-ankle-foot-orthosis (KAFO) was required. With respect to motor strength, the principle indication for the use of a KAFO is knee instability due to quadriceps paresis. The most common indication for the use of an ankle-foot-orthosis (AFO) is ankle instability due to weakness in the plantar flexors or dorsiflexors.[45]

Ambulatory Motor Index

To further define the relationship between motor paralysis and walking ability the Ambulatory Motor Index (AMI) was developed. The AMI quantitates the extent of paralysis and relates to the physiological indices of energy expenditure and gait performance.[44] It is based on a four-grade scale derived from the standard six-grade manual motor scale. The strength of key lower extremity muscles is first determined using the standard six-grade scale (absent = 0; trace, visible or palpable contraction = 1; poor, active movement through range of motion with gravity eliminated = 2; fair, active movement through range of motion against gravity = 3; good, active movement through range of motion against gravity and resistance = 4; and normal = 5). In terms of the amount of strength needed to walk, there is no significant difference between a grade of *trace* or *poor,* since there is little difference in the amount of force generated between these muscle grades. Similarly, from a functional standpoint, a grade of *good* is sufficient to meet the demands of level walking. Therefore, the grades *trace* and *poor* are combined into a single group as were the grades *good* and *normal* yielding a four-point scale (0 = absent; 1 = trace or poor; 2 = fair; 3 = good or normal).

The AMI is calculated by adding the bilateral motor scores for hip flexion, hip abduction, hip extension, knee extension and knee flexion using the abridged scale discussed above, and the sum of these scores was expressed as a percentage of the maximum possible score (30 points). The AMI is intended for use in patients with intact trunk and pelvic strength sufficient to stabilize the trunk.

Ambulatory Motor Index and Gait Performance

In patients meeting Hussey and Stauffer's criteria for community ambulation, the AMI is greater or equal to 60% of normal strength.[46] The mean walking CWS is 56 meters/minute, mean heart rate 106 bpm, average O_2 rate 14.4ml/kg·minute and average O_2 cost 0.26ml/kg·meter (Table 21.6). In contrast, the majority of patients with an Ambulatory Motor Index less than 40% required two KAFOs to ambulate. Their mean CWS is only 27 meters per minute, mean heart rate 132 bpm, O_2 rate was 17.4ml/kg·minute, and average O_2 cost 0.98ml/kg·meter. Since ambulation for routine community activities such as shopping may require an individual to walk distances more than 250 meters,[22] the average patient in this group would need to walk at least ten minutes. At this intense exercise rate, he would arrive at his destination in a state of tachycardia (rapid heart rate), hyperhydrosis (sweating), and tachypnea (rapid respiratory rate). On the other hand, wheelchair propulsion on a level surface requires a much lower rate of energy expenditure, which is comparable to normal walking.

In a previous study performed, the average velocity of wheeling for SCI patients was 72 meters/minute, the heart rate 123 beats/minute and the O_2 rate

---

Table 21.6

Ambulatory Motor Index[46]

	AMI ≤40	AMI >40, >60	AMI ≥60
O_2 Rate (ml/kg·minute)	17.4	14.2	14.4
RER	0.80	0.89	0.85
Heart Rate (bpm)	132	123	106
O_2 Rate Increase (% norm)	216	112	49
O_2 Cost (ml/kg·m)	0.98	0.50	0.26
Velocity (m/min)	26.8	34.0	56.3
Peak Axial Load (%BW)	43.1	28.3	6.3

14.5ml/kg·meter.[41] Clearly, the high rate of physiological energy expenditure of walking compared to wheeling is the reason why many patients with severe paralysis discontinue walking as a primary means of mobility. The difference between long-term wheelchair and ambulatory patients is due to the differences in physiological demands of walking, and this physiological difference is due to degree of lower extremity paralysis.

Ambulatory Motor Index and Energy Expenditure

A comparison of the AMI to the gait velocity reveals a close linear relationship described by the equation

$$\text{Velocity} = 8.6 + (0.62 \times \text{AMI}),$$

where velocity is in meters/minute (Figure 21.10).

There are large differences in walking speed among patients, which occur because of differences in the amount of paralysis. To control for velocity, the O_2 rate for normal walking can be calculated using Eq (3) and subtracted from the patient's value. There is a close relationship between the AMI and the O_2 rate increase characterized by the equation

$$O_2 \text{ rate increase} = 257.5 - (2.82 \times \text{AMI}),$$

where the O_2 rate increase is the percent increase in the rate of O_2 consumption per minute in the SCI patient, in comparison to the value for a normal subject walking at the same speed (Figure 21.11).

The O_2 cost per meter is also strongly related to the Ambulatory Motor Index (Figure 21.12). This relationship is defined by a second order regression equation.

$$O_2 \text{ cost} = 1.39 - (0.027 \times \text{AMI}) + (0.00015 \times \text{AMI}^2)$$

Ambulatory Motor Index and Peak Axial Load

In SCI patients who can reciprocally ambulate, the relationships between O_2 rate, O_2 cost and speed are complex since the amount of force applied by the upper extremities to crutches can widely vary depending on the amount of paralysis and need for upper extremity gait assistance. To determine these relationships, the peak axial load (PAL) applied to the patient's upper extremity assistive devices was measured.[46]

As might be anticipated, there is a strong relationship between the PAL exerted by the arms on crutches, canes, and/or a walker and the Ambulatory Motor Index, which is defined as follows:

$$\text{Peak axial load} = 82.75 - (1.72 \times \text{AMI}) + (0.009 \times \text{AMI}^2),$$

where the PAL is expressed as a percent of total body weight (Figure 21.13).

In addition, the PAL is very strongly related to the O_2 rate increase.

$$O_2 \text{ rate increase} = 27.1 + (3.63 \times \text{PAL})$$

It is evident that with diminished lower limb strength, increased upper arm

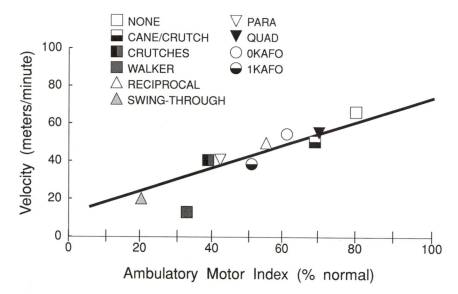

Figure 21.10 Velocity was strongly linearly related to the Ambulatory Motor Index. Velocity = 8.6 + (0.62 × AMI), [R = 0.73, p < .0001].

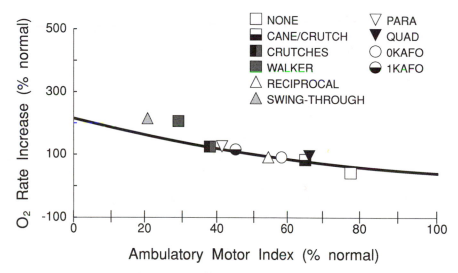

Figure 21.11 The O_2 rate increase was linearly related to the Ambulatory Motor Index. O_2 rate increase = 257.5 - (2.82 × AMI), [R = .68, p < .0001].

exertion is required and is responsible for the added rate of physiologic energy expenditure (Figures 21.13 and 21.14).

Orthotic Requirement

The division of patients into three groups, no KAFO, one KAFO or two KAFO, enables assessment of the influence of the orthotic prescription.

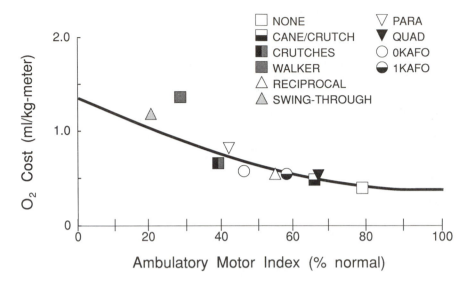

Figure 21.12 The O₂ cost was linearly related to the Ambulatory Motor Index. O₂ cost = 1.39 - (0.027 × AMI) + (0.00015 × AMI2), [R = .77, p < .0001].

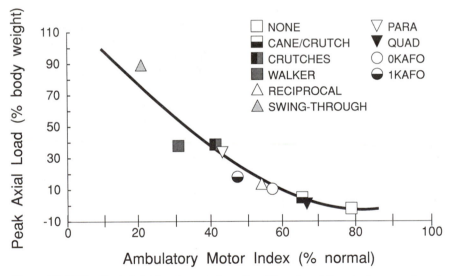

Figure 21.13 The Peak Axial Load exerted on the different assistive devices was linearly related to the Ambulatory Motor Index. PAL = 82.75 - (1.72 × AMI) + (0.009 × AMI²), [R = .73, p < .0001].

There are significant differences between these groups with regard to the dependent measures, O_2 rate increase, O_2 cost, velocity, peak axial load, and Ambulatory Motor Index. In the three groups the O_2 rate increase averaged 81%, 107% and 226%; the O_2 cost averaged 0.37ml/kg·meter, 0.46ml/kg·meter and 1.15ml/kg·meter; the velocity 48 meters/minute, 37 meters/minute and 19 meters/minute; the PAL 13.9%, 20.4% and 79.0%; and the AMI 58%, 47% and 31%. This is consistent with the fact that the orthotic

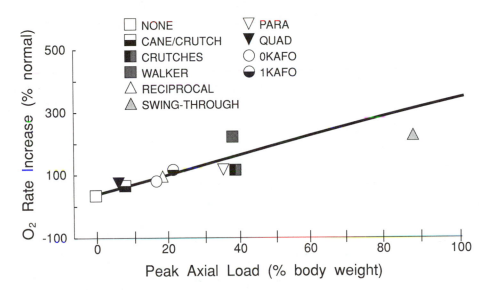

Figure 21.14 The Peak Axial Load was directly related to the O_2 rate increase. O_2 rate increase = 27.1 + (3.63 × PAL), [R = 0.91) (p < .0001].

requirement is determined by the extent of paralysis, and the AMI is related to these measures (Table 21.7).

Assistive Devices

Subdivision of SCI patients according to the need for upper extremity assistive devices also relates to the parameters of gait performance and energy expenditure. Between the four groups (none, cane or one crutch, two crutches, and

Table 21.7

SCI Orthotic Requirement

	0 KAFO	1 KAFO	2 KAFO
O_2 Rate (ml/kg·min)	15.1	14.7	14.9
RER	0.86	0.88	0.82
Heart Rate (bpm)	115	125	122
O_2 Rate Increase (% norm)	81	107	226
O_2 Cost (ml/kg·m)	0.37	0.46	1.15
Velocity (m/min)	48.1	37.1	18.9
Peak Axial Load (% BW)	13.9	20.4	79.0
AMI (% norm)	58	47	31

walker) there are significant differences in the O_2 rate increase, O_2 cost, walking speed, PAL and AMI (Table 21.8). In general these measures the parallel the need for upper extremity assistance. In the four groups, the O_2 rate increase averaged 29%, 64%, 130% and 210%; the O_2 cost averaged 0.22ml/kg·meter, 0.29ml/kg·meter, 0.56ml/kg·meter and 1.20ml/kg·meter; the velocity 66 meters/minute, 48 meters/minute, 38 meters/minute and 12 meters/minute; the PAL 0%, 7.0%, 30.8% and 39.2%; and the AMI 79%, 68%, 44% and 34%.

Table 21.8

Upper Extremity Assistive Devices

	None	Cane/Crutch	Crutches	Walker
O_2 Rate (ml/kg·minute)	14.2	14.2	15.7	12.7
RER	0.82	0.87	0.87	0.76
Heart Rate (bpm)	106	103	126	120
O_2 Rate Increase (% norm)	29	64	130	210
O_2 Cost (ml/kg·m)	0.22	0.29	0.56	1.20
Velocity (m/min)	66.5	47.9	37.8	11.8
Peak Axial Load (% BW)	—	7.0	30.8	39.2
AMI (% norm)	79	68	44	34

Level of SCI

Quadriplegic patients able to walk have incomplete neurological lesions. Their average Ambulatory Motor Index is higher than for paraplegic patients (69% versus 44%). This is because quadriplegics have varying degrees of upper extremity paralysis and are less capable of utilizing upper extremity assistive devices than paraplegics having normal upper extremities. As a consequence, the quadriplegic patients as a group require relatively greater preservation of lower extremity musculature to walk than the typical paraplegic. Thus, they demonstrate a significantly lower mean peak axial load (5% versus 29% of body weight) (Table 21.9).

Long-Term Outcome

The energy expenditure was compared at discharge from rehabilitation and at one year follow-up, using the AMI to assess motor strength.[48] At follow-up, patients walked faster, at a lower O_2 cost, had slower heart rates, and required decreased axial load on upper extremity assistive devices. Improvement was attributable to increased neurological recovery and/or physical conditioning. Patients with relative weaker lower extremities at initial and follow-up testing demonstrated a larger conditioning effect and increased O_2 pulse, when compared to patients with stronger lower extremities. Although motivation and environment have varying effects on the amount and consistency of ambulation, those patients with relatively weaker lower extremities will have larger conditioning effects if ambulation is continued, due to increased stress on the cardiovascular system by the demands of gait assistive devices.

Table 21.9

	Level of SCI	
	Paraplegia	Quadriplegia
O_2 Rate (ml/kg·min)	15.3	14.4
RER	0.87	0.83
Heart Rate (bpm)	123	109
O_2 Rate Increase (% normal)	133	66
O_2 Cost (ml/kg·meter)	0.61	0.32
Velocity (m/min)	35.6	52.0
Peak Axial Load (% BW)	28.6	4.8
AMI (% normal)	44	69

Myelodysplasia

The child with myelodysplasia has a pattern of motor paralysis that parallels traumatic SCI. There is a correlation between the orthotic requirement and the measures of energy expenditure if there is no associated neurologic impairment above the level of the spinal lesion due to hydrocephalus or Arnold-Chiari malformation or instability of the spine or hip. In general, the orthotic requirement depends on the need for knee and ankle stability and the strength of the quadriceps and ankle dorsiflexors and plantar flexors enabling division of subjects into four groups: two KAFOs, one KAFO, AFO(s), and no orthosis.

Swing-Through

Swing-through ambulation was associated with elevated heart rates greater than 140 bpm in all patient groups requiring orthotic support. Speed was slowest in patients requiring two KAFOs, 22 meters/minute. The O_2 cost progressively rose in groups requiring no orthoses (0.29ml/kg·meter), AFOs (0.41ml/kg·meter), one KAFO (0.41ml/kg·meter) and two KAFO's (0.77ml/kg·meter) (Table 21.10).

Reciprocal Walking

As expected, patients in the bilateral KAFO group had the greatest O_2 rate (18.1ml/kg·minute) (Figure 21.15), highest O_2 cost (1.35ml/kg·meter) (Figure 21.16), and slowest CWS (22 meters/minute) (Figure 21.17). Gait velocity progressively improved and the O_2 cost and O_2 rate progressively diminished in the patient groups with lesser paralysis and needing less orthotic support.

Table 21.10

Myelodysplasia Swing-Through Gait[47]

	Speed Meters/ Minute	O₂ Rate ml/kg·minute	O₂ Cost ml/kg·meter	Pulse Beats/ Minute
0-Orthosis	47	13.8	0.29	120
AFO (S)	41	15.6	0.41	147
1-KAFO	46	18.7	0.41	143
2-KAFO	22	14.9	0.77	149

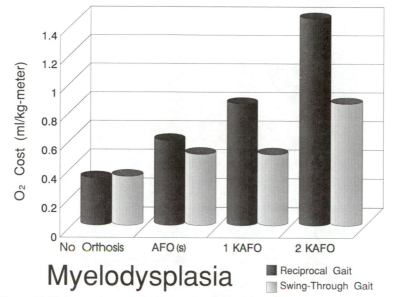

Figure 21.15 O$_2$ rate in myelodysplastic children walking with swing-through and reciprocal gait patterns requiring different types of lower extremity orthotic support.

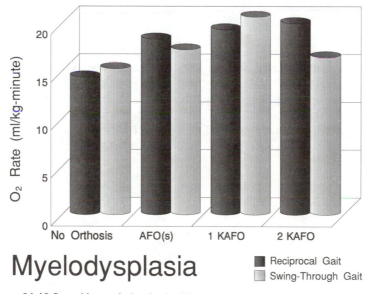

Figure 21.16 Speed in myelodysplastic children walking with swing-through and reciprocal gait patterns requiring different types of lower extremity orthotic support.

Swing-Through Gait versus Reciprocal Gait

A direct comparison of energy expenditure during both swing-through and reciprocal walking was obtained in ten children.[47] The indices reflecting physiological effort (rate of oxygen uptake and heart rate) were slightly higher during swing-through crutch assisted gait, but gait velocity was faster (Table 21.11). As a consequence, swing-through walking proved the more efficient gait (0.68ml/kg·meter versus 0.40ml/kg·meter). Not surpris-

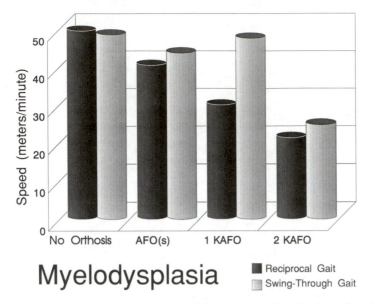

Figure 21.17 O_2 cost in myelodysplastic children walking with swing-through and reciprocal gait patterns requiring different types of lower extremity orthotic support.

ingly, seven of ten children preferred the swing-through mode of crutch use for most activities. It may be concluded that attempts to train children who prefer a swing-through gait to a reciprocal gait are probably unwarranted.

In contrast to the experience in adults with SCI, it is a common clinical experience that a swing-through gait pattern in children is functional for community ambulation outside the home. The difference in the response is due to the higher ratio of arm strength to body weight in children and their

Table 21.11

Myelodysplasia Reciprocal and Swing-Through Gait versus Wheelchair[47]

	Speed Meters/ Minute	O_2 Rate ml/kg·minute	O_2 Cost ml/kg·meter	Pulse Beats/ Minute
Reciprocal	30	15.8	0.68	138
Swing-Through	42	16.3	0.40	146
Wheelchair	65	11.6	0.17	124

higher exercise capacity and VO_2 max. Also, myelodysplastic children have proportionately lighter legs due to the effects of paralysis during the growing years.

Nevertheless, as myelodysplastic children approach maturity and gain weight, sustaining walking activity with a swing-through gait becomes more difficult and increasing reliance is placed on the wheelchair. These factors coupled with the normal decline in the maximal exercise capacity with aging account for the reason many patients choose wheeling rather than walking in later years.

Amputation

Following lower extremity amputation, the patient has a choice of walking without a prosthesis using crutches or wearing a prosthesis. A special problem confronting many older patients with dysvascular limbs is a limited exercise ability due to associated medical disease.

Prosthesis versus Crutches

The direct comparison of walking in unilateral traumatic and dysvascular amputees at the Syme's, below knee (BK) and above knee (AK) levels with a prosthesis utilizing a swing-through crutch assisted gait without a prosthesis reveals that all, with the single exception of vascular AK amputees, have a lower rate of energy expenditure, heart rate, and O_2 cost when using a prosthesis.[43] This difference is insignificant in dysvascular AK patients and is related to the fact that even with a prosthesis, most of these patients require crutches for some support, thereby increasing the O_2 rate and heart rate.[34,43]

It can be concluded a well-fitted prosthesis that results in a satisfactory gait not requiring crutches significantly reduces the physiologic energy demand. Since crutch walking requires more exertion than walking with a prosthesis, crutch walking without a prosthesis should not be considered an absolute requirement for prosthetic prescription and training.

Amputation Level

Two studies in which patients were healthy, young adults and tested under similar laboratory conditions illustrate the importance of the amputation level (Table 21.12). The first group consists of unilateral amputees at the BK, through knee (TK), and AK levels secondary to trauma.[43] The second group consists of hip disarticulation (HD) and hemipelvectomy (HP) patients following surgical amputation.[24]

The combined results of these two studies indicate that the average O_2 rate at all amputation levels when walking with a prosthesis without crutches approximates the value for normal subjects (Figure 21.18). However, as the amputation level ascends, the average CWS progressively

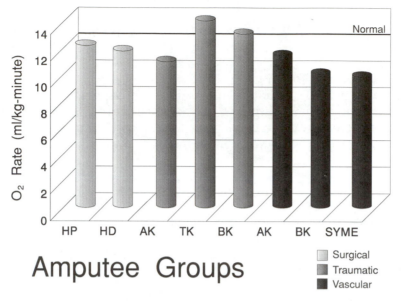

Figure 21.18 O_2 cost in normal subjects walking with progressive knee deformity.

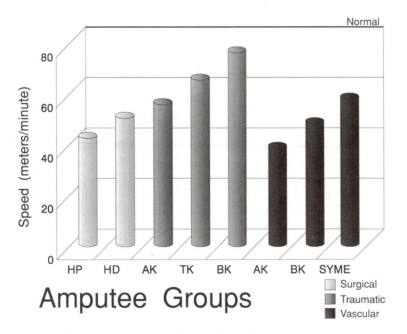

Figure 21.19 O_2 rate in normal subjects walking with progressive knee deformity.

decreases resulting in an increasing O_2 cost (Figures 21.19 and 21.20).

In summary, BK, TK, AK, HD and HP amputees progressively adapt to the increasingly inefficient gait pattern (higher O_2 cost) resulting from higher level amputations by reducing their gait velocity so that the O_2 rate does not exceed normal limits.

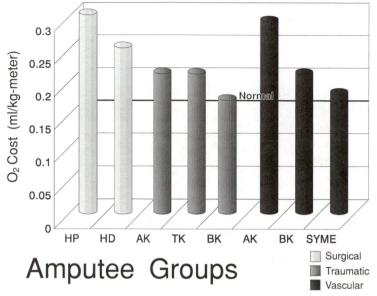

Figure 21.20 Speed in normal subjects walking with progressive knee deformity.

Dysvascular Amputees

It is important to distinguish older dysvascular amputees from their younger, usually traumatic counterparts. A comparison of the two etiologies of amputation at the BK and AK levels reveals the CWS is slower and the O_2 higher for the dysvascular BK amputee than for the traumatic BK amputees. At the BK level the CWS and O_2 cost for traumatic amputees (45 meters/ minute and 0.20ml/kg·meter) are significantly different than for traumatic amputees (71 meters/minute and 0.16ml/kg·meter). The same differences were observed at the AK level between dysvascular and traumatic amputees (36 meters/minute and 0.28ml/kg·meter versus 52 meters/minute and 0.20 ml/kg·meter). Among dysvascular amputees, Syme patients had a faster CWS and lower O_2 cost (54 meters/minute and 0.17ml/kg·meter) than BK patients (45 meters/minute and 0.20ml/kg·meter), demonstrating the same importance of the level of amputation observed in younger traumatic and surgical amputees (Table 21.12).[43]

Most older patients who have AK or higher amputations for vascular disease are not successful prosthetic ambulators. Very few are able to walk with a prosthesis without crutch assistance.[32,43] If able to walk, they generally have a very slow CWS and an elevated heart rate if crutch assistance is required.[43] It can be concluded that every effort must be made to protect dysvascular limbs early so that AK amputation does not become necessary. If amputation is mandatory, every effort should be made to amputate below the knee.

Table 21.12

Energy Expenditure—Unilateral Amputees

	Speed Meters/ Minute	O_2 Rate ml/kg·minute	O_2 Cost ml/kg·meter	Pulse Beats/ Minute
Vascular[43]				
AK	36	10.8	0.28	126
BK	45	9.4	0.20	105
SYME	54	9.2	0.17	108
Surgical[24]				
HP	40	11.5	0.29	97
HD	47	11.1	0.24	99
Traumatic[43]				
AK	52	10.3	0.20	111
TK	61	13.4	0.20	109
BK	71	12.4	0.16	106

Stump Length

Two studies examined the relationship of stump length to gait performance in BK patients.[14,18] In the first, stumps ranged from 14 to 19cm in length and in the second, stumps ranged from 9 to 24cm. Nearly all sockets were patellar tendon bearing (PTB). No significant correlations were noted between CWS and energy expenditure in either study. Of particular clinical importance, a stump as short as 9cm results in BK performance (lower O_2 cost and higher CWS) that is superior than at the TK and AK levels.

Bilateral Amputees

Not surprising, bilateral amputees expend greater effort than unilateral amputees (Table 21.13).[10,43] Dysvascular patients with the Syme/Syme combination walk faster and have a lower O_2 cost than dysvascular patients with the BK/BK combination. Traumatic BK/BK amputees walk faster and at a lower energy cost than their dysvascular BK/BK counterparts.

Considering that approximately one-third of diabetic amputees lose the remaining leg within three years, it is important to preserve the knee joint even

Table 21.13

Energy Expenditure—Bilateral Amputees

	Speed Meters/ Minute	O₂ Rate ml/kg·minute	O₂ Cost ml/kg·meter	Pulse Beats/ minute
Traumatic				
BK/BK[43]	67	13.6	0.20	112
AK/AK[43]	54	17.6	0.33	104
Vascular				
Syme/Syme[43]	62	12.8	0.21	99
BK/BK[43]	40	11.6	0.31	113
BK/BK[10]	40	7.8	0.23	116
Stubbies[35]	46	9.9	0.22	86

if the stump is short since, should a unilateral BK amputee undergo another BK amputation, energy expenditure would be less than a patient with a unilateral AK amputation.[14] Bilateral vascular amputees rarely achieve a functional ambulation status if one amputation is at the AK level.

Finally, a 21-year-old bilateral TK/TK patient with stubby prostheses was evaluated.[35] The patient attained a CWS of 46 meters/minute at an O₂ rate of 9.9 ml/kg·minute achieving an O₂ cost of 0.22ml/kg·meter. While walking on stubbies is cosmetically unacceptable for most patients (except for gait training or limited walking in the home), the data from this single patient illustrates it can be functionally useful.

Arthritis

Hip

Arthritic hip pain causes an antalgic gait pattern. Testing performed on patients with unilateral osteoarthritis of the hip prior to total hip arthroplasty (THA) reveals the average CWS, 41 meters/minute, is approximately half the normal speed and the O₂ rate, 10.3ml/kg·minute, is also below normal.[6] THA results in an improved walking speed at a reduced O₂ cost. One year following surgery, the CWS increased from 41 meters/minute to 55 meters/minute without any further increase in the O₂ rate (Table 21.14). Since the CWS improves without a corresponding increase in the O₂ rate, there is a lower O₂ cost from 0.28ml/kg·meter to 0.20ml/kg·meter indicating improved gait efficiency.

Table 21.14

Energy Expenditure—Arthritis of the Hip

	Speed Meters/ Minute	O₂ Rate ml/kg·minute	O₂ Cost ml/kg·meter	Pulse Beats/ Minute
Pre-op THR[6]	41	10.3	0.28	106
Post-op THR[6]	55	11.1	0.20	108
Girdlestone[44]	46	12.2	0.39	118
Hip Fusion[36]	67	14.7	0.22	112

It is of clinical importance to compare the results of the THA to the previously discussed results following hip fusion since both procedures can be performed for unilateral hip arthritis. Hip fusion results in a faster gait, but requires a 32 percent greater O_2 rate than THA (Table 21.4 and Table 21.14). A decreased O_2 rate is an advantage of THA over hip fusion in a patient with unilateral disease.

Girdlestone hip resection arthroplasty, resection of the hip joint, is commonly performed along with removal of the hip prothesis because of infection after THA. This is one of the most severe types of complication after joint replacement surgery. The CWS following Girdlestone arthroplasty averages 46 meters/minute, O_2 rate 12.2ml/kg·minute and heart rate 118bpm.[44] The elevated heart rate reflects the reliance of the majority of these patients on crutches for partial weight support.

Knee

Evaluation of patients with severe osteoarthritis of the knee tested prior to total knee arthroplasty reveals that the average reduction in the CWS and increase in the O_2 cost is approximately the same as in patients with osteoarthritis of the hip.[44] The similarity of these results in the two different joints is not surprising. In an effort to relieve pain, patients with arthritis at either the hip or the knee adopt many of the same strategies: decreasing the duration of the single stance phase on the involved leg to minimize the duration of loading and using upper extremity gait assist devices, which reduces the magnitude of the load.

Rheumatoid Arthritis

Evaluation of patients with rheumatoid arthritis indicates the functional benefit of total knee joint replacement surgery even in the presence of systemic illness.[44] Evaluation of rheumatoid patients with severe degeneration of the knee joint as the primary problem indicates that after surgery a significant improvement in gait velocity occurs (58 meters/minute versus 33 meters/minute) with only a slight increase in the O_2 rate (11.4ml/kg·minute versus 10.3ml/kg·minute), resulting in a marked improvement in the O_2 cost (0.41ml/kg·meter versus 0.71ml/kg·meter).

Influence of Upper Extremity Assistive Devices

The use of crutches, canes, or walkers in arthritis usually depends on the severity of pain. Forces across an inflamed joint are progressively unloaded by provision of a cane, one crutch, two crutches or a walker.

In a group of rheumatoid arthritis patients having severe knee arthritis tested prior to surgery, the O_2 rate was not elevated above the value for normal subjects at their CWS (Figure 21.21). Patients using a walker had the slowest CWS (Figure 21.22) and highest O_2 cost (Figure 21.23).[44] Speed progressively increased in the groups of patients requiring two crutches, one crutch, cane(s), or no assistive devices (Table 21.15). Conversely, O_2 cost was highest in patients requiring a walker and least in those patients requiring no upper extremity assistive devices.

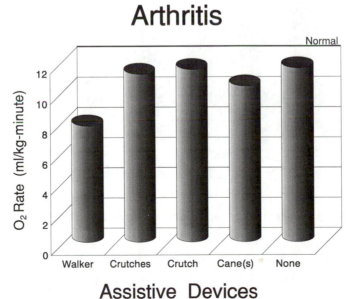

Figure 21.21 Rate of O_2 consumption in arthritis patients requiring different types of upper extremity assistive devices.

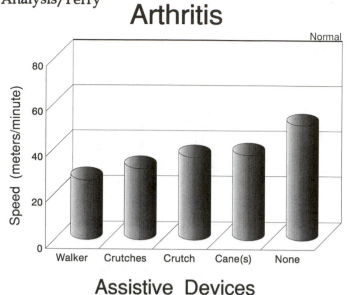

Figure 21.22 Speed in arthritis patients requiring different types of upper extremity assistive devices.

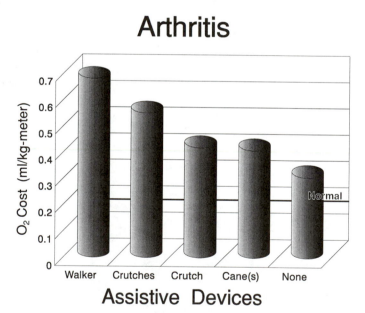

Figure 21.23 O_2 cost in arthritis patients requiring different types of upper extremity assistive devices.

Deconditioning

The oxygen pulse is lower than normal in both osteoarthritis and rheumatoid arthritis patients tested prior to surgery, even when upper extremity assistive devices are not employed.[44] These findings signify that pain leading to a more sedentary life-style and/or the systemic effects of rheumatoid disease result in deconditioning.

Table 21.15

Rheumatoid Arthritis of the Knee
Pre-Operative Evaluation
Influence Upper Extremity Assistive Devices[44]

	Speed Meters/ Minute	O$_2$ Rate ml/kg·minute	O$_2$ Cost ml/kg·meter	Pulse Beats/ Minute
Walker	21	7.2	0.63	124
Crutches	26	10.6	0.50	124
Crutch	31	10.9	0.37	102
Cane(s)	32	9.8	0.36	97
No assistive device	45	11.0	0.26	115

Hemiplegia (Stroke)

Spasticity and primitive patterns of motion characterize hemiplegic gait, and the degree of impairment depends on the magnitude of the neurological deficit.[15]

Because of a marked reduction in the speed in the typical patient, the O$_2$ rate is less than normal despite the inefficiency of the hemiplegic gait pattern and high O$_2$ cost.[15] Among ambulatory hemiplegic patients, the mean O$_2$ rate was 11.5 ml/kg·minute, slightly below the mean for normal walking. The average speed was very slow, 30 meters/minute, accounting for a high O$_2$ cost, 0.54ml/kg·meter (Table 21.16). It can be concluded that hemiplegic gait is not physiologically stressful for the typical patient unless there is severe cardiovascular disease.

Energy Expenditure of Flexed-Knee Gait

Neurological disorders such as spastic diplegia due to cerebral palsy cause the patient to walk with a flexed lower limb posture. The biomechanical requirements of flexed-knee stance are greater than normal and are associated with increased quadriceps, tibio-femoral, and patello-femoral forces.[27] The most significant increases occur at angles of knee flexion beyond 15°.

The importance of full knee extension during the stance phase of gait and the significance of knee flexion deformity is illustrated in normal subjects wearing a specially designed hinged knee orthosis that restricted knee extension but allowed full flexion.[30,42] As the amount of simulated knee

Table 21.16

Hemiplegia[15]

	Speed Meters/ Minute	O_2 Rate ml/kg·minute	O_2 Cost ml/kg·meter	Pulse Beats/ Minute
Wheelchair	37	10.0	0.27	107
Walking	30	11.5	0.54	109

flexion contracture is increased, the O_2 rate and O_2 cost progressively rise and the CWS decreases (Table 21.17). Restricting knee flexion to 30° leads to a 15% rise in O_2 rate and a 19% increase in O_2 cost (Figure 21.24). Restricting knee extension to 15° causes a 7% rise in the rate of O_2 consumption and a 13% increase in O_2 cost in comparison to normal walking (Figure 21.25). Limiting knee extension to 45° resulted in a 21% increase in O_2 rate and a 38% increase in O_2 cost (Figure 21.26).

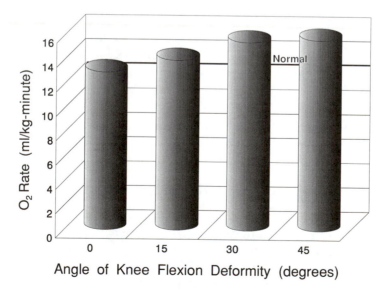

Figure 21.24 O_2 rate in normal subjects walking with progressive knee deformity.

Table 21.17

Energy Expenditure of Flexed Knee-Gait[30]

	Speed Meters/ Minute	O_2 Rate ml/kg·minute	O_2 Cost ml/kg·meter
0 degrees	80	11.8	0.16
15 degrees	77	12.8	0.17
30 degrees	75	14.3	0.19
45 degrees	67	14.5	0.22

Spastic Diplegia (Cerebral Palsy)

The child with spastic diplegia involving both lower limbs typically has spasticity and a pervasive loss of motor control, which depends on the degree of involvement. When moderate or severe disability is present, the child typically fails to fully extend the hips and knees and has a flexed hip and knee posture. In a group of spastic diplegic children between the ages of 5 and 17

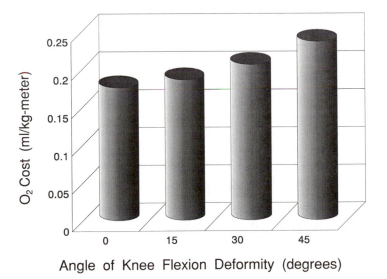

Figure 21.25 O_2 cost in normal subjects walking with progressive knee deformity.

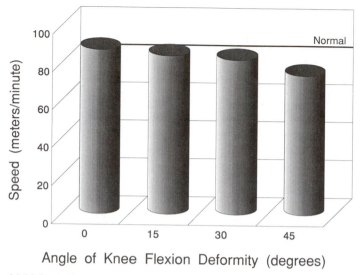

Figure 21.26 Speed in normal subjects walking with progressive knee deformity.

years, walking speed averaged 40 meters/minute.[7] The mean heart and O_2 rates were significantly higher than normal, averaging 145 bpm and 18.6ml/kg·minute. As a group, these children had a very inefficient gait, averaging 0.72ml/kg·meter (Table 21.18).

Most individuals with gait disabilities that do not require the use of upper extremity assistive devices purposefully slow their speed and are able to keep the rate of O_2 consumption from rising above normal limits. Nevertheless, elevated rates of O_2 consumption and high heart rates were consistently recorded in spastic diplegic children even when upper extremity assistive devices were not required.

Table 21.18

Cerebral Palsy[7]

	Speed Meters/ Minute	O_2 Rate ml/kg·minute	O_2 Cost ml/kg·meter	Pulse Beats/ Minute
Spastic Diplegia	40	18.6	0.72	145

The flexed hip and knee posture of the child with spastic diplegia requires considerable muscular effort by the antigravity muscles to prevent collapse even at a slow speeds. Another reason for the elevated O_2 rate is the limited motor control to perform the necessary compensatory gait substitutions since both legs are involved. In contrast, the hemiplegic can perform substitutions with the normal limb and spends approximately 80% of the gait cycle on the uninvolved leg and, during the period of single limb support on the affected side, is able to maintain the hip and knee in a relatively extended position.[26]

In normal individuals the O_2 rate decreases as the child grows older. The opposite trend was observed in children with spasticity. Their O_2 rate increased with age. This observation has clinical significance for the spastic child who complains of fatigue or the need for rest. Clinically, this is consistent with the increased body weight and size in older children and the greater difficulty of the child with impaired motor control and spasticity carrying the added weight. As a result, the older child may prefer to walk less and increasingly rely on a wheelchair.

References

1. Astrand A, Astrand I, Hallback I, Kilbom A: Reduction in maximal oxygen uptake with age. *J Appl Physiol* 35:649-654, 1973.
2. Astrand PO, Rodahl K: *Textbook of Work Physiology*, 2nd ed, New York, McGraw-Hill, Inc., 1977.
3. Astrand PO, Saltin B: Maximal oxygen uptake and heart rate in various types of muscular activity. *J Appl Physiol* 16:977-981, 1961.
4. Bobbert AC: Energy expenditure in level and grade walking. *J Appl Physiol* 15:1015-1021, 1961.
5. Booyens J, Keatinge WR: The expenditure of energy by men and women walking. *J Physiol* 138:165-171, 1957.
6. Brown M, Hislop HJ, Waters RL, Porell D: Walking efficiency before and after total hip replacement. *Phys Ther* 60:1259-1263, 1980.
7. Campbell J, Ball J: Energetics of walking in cerebral palsy. In "Energetics: Application to the study and management of locomotor disabilities." *Orthop Clin Nor Amer* 9:351-377, 1978.
8. Corcoran PJ, Gelmann B: Oxygen reuptake in normal and handicapped subjects in relation to the speed of walking beside a velocity-controlled cart. *Arch Phys Med Rehabil* 51:78-87, 1970.
9. Davis JA: Anaerobic threshold: Review of the concept and directions for future research. *Med Sci Sports Exer* 17:6-18, 1985.
10. Deboe LL, Witt PL, Kadaba MP, Reyes R, Cochran GV: An alternative to conventional prosthetic devices. *Arch Phys Med Rehabil* 66:264-266, 1983.
11. Durnin JV, Passmore R: *Energy, Work and Leisure.* Heinemann Educational Books, London, 1967.
12. Falls HB, Humphrey LA: Energy cost of running and walking in young men. *Med Sci Sports* 8:9-13, 1976.
13. Finley FR, Cody KA: Locomotive characteristics of urban pedestrians. *Arch Phys Med Rehabil* 51:423-426, 1970.
14. Gonzalez EG, Corcoran PJ, Reyes RL: Energy expenditure in below-knee amputees: Correlation with stump length. *Arch Phys Med Rehabil* 55:111-119, 1974.
15. Hash D: Energetics of wheelchair propulsion and walking in stroke patients. In

"Energetics: Application to the study and management of locomotor disabilities." *Orthop Clin Nor Amer* 9:351-377, 1978.

16. Hjeltnes N: Oxygen uptake and cardiac output in graded arm exercise in paraplegics with low level spinal lesions. *Scand J Rehab Med* 9:107-113, 1977.

17. Holloszy JO, Coyle EF: Adaptations of skeletal muscle to endurance exercise and their metabolic consequences. *J Appl Physiol* 56:834-838, 1984.

18. Hunt AK: in Waters RL, Perry J, Chambers R: Energy expenditure of amputee gait. In *Lower Extremity Amputation*, Philadelphia, W. B. Saunders, (in press).

19. Hussey RW, Stauffer ES: Spinal cord injury: requirements for ambulation. *Arch Phys Med Rehabil* 54:544-547, 1973.

20. Inman VT, Ralston HJ, Todd F: *Human Walking*. Baltimore, MD, Waverly Press, 1981.

21. Joseph J: *Man's Posture: Electromyographic Studies. Springfield, Illinois, Charles C. Thomas, 1960.*

22. Lerner-Frankeil M, Vargas S, et al.: Functional community ambulation: what are your criteria. *Clin Man PT* 6:12-15, 1986.

23. McArdle WD, Katch FI, Katch VL: *Exercise Physiology.* Philadelphia, Lea and Febiger, 1986.

24. Nowrozzi F, Salvanelli ML: Energy expenditure in hip disarticulation and hemipelvectomy amputees. *Arch Phys Med Rehabil* 64:300-303, 1983.

25. Passmore R, Durnin JUGA: Human energy expenditure. *Physiol Rev* 35:801-840, 1953.

26. Peat M, Hyman I: Electromyographic temporal analysis of gait: Hemiplegic locomotion. *Arch Phys Med Rehabil* 57:421-425, 1976.

27. Perry J, Antonelli D, Ford W: Analysis of knee joint forces during flexed knee stance. *J Bone Joint Surg* 57A:961-967, 1975.

28. Ralston HJ: Comparison of energy expenditure during treadmill walking and floor walking. *J Appl Physiol* 15:1156, 1960.

29. Ralston HJ: Energy-speed relation and optimal speed during level walking. *Int Z Angew Physiol Einschl Arbeitsphysiol* 17:277-283, 1958.

30. Rueter K, Pierre M: Energy cost and gait characteristics of flexed knee ambulation. In Waters RL, Lunsford BR: Energy expenditure of normal and pathologic gait: application to orthotic prescription. *Atlas of Orthotics*, St. Louis, C. V. Mosby Co., 1985.

31. Saltin B, Blomqvist G, Mitchell JH, Johnson RL, Jr, Wildenthal K, Chapman CB: Response to submaximal and maximal exercise after bedrest and training. *Circ 38* (suppl. 7), 1968.

32. Steinberg FU, Garcia WJ, Roettger RF, Shelton DJ: Rehabilitation of the geriatric amputee. *J Am Geron Soc 22:62-66, 1974.*

33. Thorstensson A, Roberthson HR: Adaptations to changing speed in human locomotion: Speed of transition between walking and running. *Acta Physiol Scand* 131:211-214, 1987.

34. Traugh GH, Corcoran PF, Reyes RL: Energy expenditure of ambulation in patients with above-knee amputations. *Arch Phys Med Rehabil* 56:67-71, 1975.

35. Wainapel SF, March H, Steve L: Stubby prostheses: An alternative to conventional prosthetic devices. *Arch Phys Med Rehabil* 66:264-266, 1985.

36. Waters RL, Barnes G, Husserl T, Silver L, Liss R: Comparable energy expenditure following arthrodesis of the hip and ankle. *J Bone Joint Surg* 70:1032-1037, 1988.

37. Waters RL, Campbell J, Perry J: Energy cost of three-point crutch ambulation in fracture patients. *J Orthop Trauma* 1:170-173, 1987.

38. Waters RL, Campbell J, Thomas L, Hugos L, Davis P: Energy cost of walking in lower extremity plaster casts. *J Bone Joint Surg* 64:896-899, 1982.

39. Waters RL, Hislop HJ, Perry J, Antonelli D: Energetics: application to the study and management of locomotor disabilities. *Orthop Clin N Amer* 9:351-377, 1978.
40. Waters RL, Lunsford BR, Perry J, Byrd R: Energy-speed relationship of walking: standard tables. *J Orthop Res* 6:215-222, 1988.
41. Waters RL, Lunsford BR: Energy cost of paraplegic ambulation. *J Bone Joint Surg* 67(A):1245-1250, 1985.
42. Waters RL, Lunsford BR: Energy expenditure of normal and pathologic gait: application to orthotic prescription. *Atlas of Orthotics*. St. Louis, C. V. Mosby Co., 1985.
43. Waters RL, Perry J, Antonelli D, Hislop H: The energy cost of walking of amputees—Influence of level of amputation. *J Bone Joint Surg* 58(A):42-46, 1976.
44. Waters RL, Perry J, Conaty P, Lunsford B, O'Meara P: The energy cost of walking with arthritis of the hip and knee. *Clin Orthop* 214:278-284, 1987.
45. Waters RL: Physiological rationale for orthotic prescription in paraplegia. *Clin Pros Orthot* 11:66-73, 1987.
46. Waters RL, Yakura JS, Adkins R, Barnes G: Determinants of gait performance following spinal cord injury. *Arch Phys Med Rehabil* 70:811-818, 1989.
47. Waters RL, Yakura JS: The energy expenditure of normal and pathological gait. *Critical Reviews in Physical and Rehabilitation Medicine* 1:187-209, 1989.
48. Yakura JS, Waters RL, Adkins RH: Changes in ambulation parameters in SCI individuals following rehabilitation. *Paraplegia* 28:364-370, 1990.

Abbreviations and Acronyms

ADD LONG	adductor longus
ADP	adenosine diphosphate
AFO	ankle-foot orthosis
AK	above knee
AMI	ambulatory motor index
ANK	ankle
AP	anterior-posterior
ASIS	anterior superior iliac spine
ATIB	anterior tibialis
ATP	adenosine triphosphate
BFLH	biceps femoris long head
BFSH	biceps femoris short head
BK	below knee
BMR	basal metabolic rate
bpm	beats per minute
BW	body weight
BWLL	body weight leg length
C	contraction
cal	calorie (gram)
CC	calcaneocuboid
C/G	center of gravity
cm	centimeter

CO_2	carbon dioxide
CP	creatine phosphate
C/P	center of pressure
C_7	seventh cervical vertebra
CTO	contralateral toe-off
CVA	cerebral vascular accident
CWS	customary/comfortable walking speed
db	decible
DF	dorsiflexion/dorsiflexes/dorsiflexor
EDL	extensor digitorum longus
EHL	extensor hallucis longus
EMG	electromyograph(y)
F	force
FCT	fibrous connective tissue
FDL	flexor digitorum longus
FHL	flexor hallucis longus
FTSW	foot switch
FWS	fast walking speed
g	gram
GAST	gastrocnemius
GC	gait cycle
GMax	gluteus maximus
GMax L	gluteus maximus, lower
GRAC	gracilis
GRF	ground reaction force
GRFV	ground reaction force vector
H	heel
HAT	head, arms and trunk
HD	hip disarticulation
Hg	mercury
H1-5	heel, first and fifth metatarsal
HP	hemipelvectomy
Hz	hertz
IC	initial contact
IEMG	integrated electromyography
ILIAC	iliacus
IM	isometric
ISw	initial swing
IT	iliotibial
ITB	iliotibial band
ITO	ipsilateral toe-off

KAFO	knee-ankle-foot orthoses
kcal	kilogram-calorie
kg	kilogram
KPa	kilo pascal
LA	limb advancement
LA	lever arm
LGMax	lower gluteus maximus
LL	leg length
LR	loading response
L_3	third lumbar vertebra
m	meter
M Ham	medial hamstring
min	minute
ml	milliliter
ML	medial-lateral
mm	millimeter
MMT	manual muscle test
M OHM	meg ohm (10 ohms)
MP	metatarsophalangeal
ms	millisecond
MSt	mid stance
MSw	mid swing
MT	midtarsal
Mt5	fifth metatarsal
MtP	metatarsophalangeal
MU	motor unit
mv	millivolt
MVC	maximum voluntary contraction
Nm	newton meter
O_2	oxygen
OPP FS	opposite foot support
PAL	peak axial load
PB	peroneus brevis
PF	plantar flexion/flexes
pH	hydrogen ion concentration
PL	peroneus longus
psi	pounds per square inch
PSIS	posterior superior iliac spine
PSw	pre-swing
PTB	patellar tendon bearing
PTIB	posterior tibialis

r	correlation coefficient
REF FS	reference foot support/switch
RER	respiratory exchange ratio
RF	rectus femoris
RF SURF	rectus femoris surface
RLAMC	Rancho Los Amigos Medical Center
RQ	respiratory quotient
SACH	solid ankle, cushion heel
SCI	spinal cord injury
SD	standard deviation
sec	second
SI	sacroiliac
SMEMB	semimembranosis
SOL	soleus
SLS	single limb support
ST	subtalar
S$_2$	second sacral vertebra
SWS	slow walking speed
T	torque
TA	tibialis anterior
TAMP	time adjusted mean profile
3D	three-dimensional
THA	total hip arthroplasty
TK	through knee
TL	thoracolumbar trunk
TN	talonavicular
TO	toe-off
TP	tibialis posterior
TPE	triaxial parallelogram electrogoniometer
TSt	terminal stance
TSw	terminal swing
T$_{10}$	tenth thoracic vertebra
μ	micron
uv	microvolt
V	velocity
VI	vastus intermedius
VL	vastus lateralis
VML	vastus medialis longus
VMO	vastus medialis oblique
VO$_2$	volume of oxygen
WA	weight acceptance

systems that use

alignment and

e physiological

canal that extend

force within the

brain injury near

its force.
a loss of normal

he right and left

arily assumed.
n.

Deterioration of
ttributed to wear

lsy classification.
rface of the tibia

tion signals dur-

nb secondary to

ransformed into

on.

from the midline of the

that measures acceleration,
.
vides the effective force.
the midline of the body.
ls such as crutches, canes,

cess that uses oxygen.
n of the bilateral muscle
x, abd, ext) and knee (ext

e used to enlarge the myo-

portion of the limb.
process without the use of

e ankle that contributes to

f joint motion.
A system that senses and
t operator intervention.

Automated video systems—Operator-free motion recording video as the medium.

Bilateral—Involving right an left limbs (sides of the body).

Body weight vector—Force line that indicates the mean magnitude of body weight relative to the joint of interest.

Burn—Tissue injury from excessive heat.

Cadence—step rate per minute.

Calcaneus gait—The major weight-bearing area is the heel.

Calcaneograde—calcaneal gait, walking on the heel.

Calorimetry—The measurement of body heat to determi energy expenditure.

Cauda equina—The group of spinal roots within the vertebral below the spinal cord.

Center of pressure—The location of the mean weight-bearing foot (base of the vector).

Cerebral palsy—Non-progressive paralysis resulting from a the time of birth.

Concentric contraction—Shortening of the muscle as it create

Contracture—Fibrous connective tissue shortening that cause joint range.

Contralateral—The opposite side of the body; the other limb.

Coronal plane—The longitudinal plane that passes between sides of the body, parallel to the coronal suture in the skul

Customary walking speed—The rate of walking that is volun

Deceleration—Slowing or inhibition of the prior rate of moti

Deformity—A fixed (static) malalignment of the bone or join

Degenerative arthritis—An older synonym for osteoarthritis the joint cartilage and bone of nonspecified etiology, often and tear from overuse or malus.

Digitigrade—Walking on one's toes.

Diplegia—Paralysis involving both lower limbs; a cerebral p

Dorsiflexion—Movement of the foot towards the anterior s while bending the ankle.

Double stance—Stance with both feet in contact with the floc

Drop foot—Passive equinus, excessive ankle plantar flexion.

Dynamic—Underactive muscular control.

Dynamic electromyography—Recording of the muscle activ ing functional activities.

Dysvascular amputee—An individual with the loss of a li circulatory impairment.

Efficiency—The percentage of physiological energy that is useful work.

Effort—The exertion of a force to either inhibit or create moti

Elastic contracture—Fibrous tissue restraint of motion that partially stretches with body weight or a very vigorous manual force.

Electrode—The devices used to capture the myoelectric signals (eg. wire, needle, disc).

Electrogoniometer—A device attached to the limb to record joint motion.

Electromyography—A system for recording the myoelectric signals.

Energy—The capacity to perform work.

Energy conservation—Functional measures used to reduce the energy cost of activity.

Equinus—A toe-down position of the foot, in which the forefoot is lower than the heel.

Eversion—Outward turning of the foot.

Extension—A straightening of the limb in which the bones comprising the joint move to a more parallel alignment.

Extensor thrust—Rapid backward motion at the knee that does not create overt hyperextension.

Flexed-knee gait—Gait in which the knee remains bent throughout stance.

Flexion—Bending the joint, ie. the distal segment rotates towards the proximal segment.

Filtration (electronic)—Electronic exclusion of waveform with a designated frequency.

Foot flat—Floor contact by both the heel and forefoot.

Foot support patterns—The different combinations of floor contact by the heel, medial and lateral metatarsal heads and great toe.

Footswitch—A device that measures the time of floor contact by the designated area of the foot.

Force—Any influence that causes a change in position or alters the direction or speed of motion.

Force plate—A platform set on or into the floor that is instrumented to measure the forces imposed on it.

Forefoot contact—Impact of the forefoot with the floor.

Forefoot rocker—Progression of the limb (and body) while the forefoot is the pivotal area of support.

Fracture—Broken bone.

Free gait—Walking at one's own spontaneous rate of travel.

Frequency (electronic)—A quality of an electronic signal relative to its sine wave content.

Gait analysis—A method for diagnosing the way people walk.

Gait Cycle—A single sequence of events between two sequential initial contacts by the same limb.

Gait phases—The divisions in the walking cycle that represent specific functional patterns.

Ground reaction forces—The forces recorded by a force plate generated by falling body weight or muscle action as the person walks across that area of the floor.

Ground reaction force vector—The mean directional and magnitude sum of the force imposed on the ground (floor) for that sample.

Hamstrings—The posterior thigh muscles extending from the pelvis to the shank (semimembranosis, semitendinosis and long head of the biceps femoris).

HAT—Head, arm, neck and trunk segments that comprise the passenger unit that rides atop the locomotor system.

Heel rocker—Progression of the limb (and body) while the heel is the pivotal area of support.

Heel strike—Floor contact with the heel; the normal mode for initiating stance.

Hemiplegia—Paralysis of the arm and leg and trunk on the same side of the body (right or left).

Hyperextension—Posterior angulation of the joint beyond neutral excessive extension.

Iliotibial band—A length of dense fascia on the lateral side of the thigh that extends from the pelvis (crest of the ilium) to the anterior, proximal margin of the tibia.

Inertia—Tendency to remain at rest; inability to move spontaneously.

Initial Contact—First impact with the floor, the event that begins stance.

Initial double stance—The beginning of stance when both feet are on the floor, equivalent to initial contact and loading response.

Initial swing—The first phase of limb advancement of the foot is lifted from the floor.

Instrumented walkway—A length of flooring that contains sensors to record the floor contact events.

Inversion—Turning in of the foot.

Ipsilateral—On the same side of the body, or limb.

Isokinetic contraction—Muscle action occurring while there is a consistent rate of joint motion.

Isometric contraction—Muscle action that occurs while all joint motion is inhibited.

Lean—Tilt of the trunk away from vertical position (eg. forward, backward or to the side).

Ligamentous skeleton—The ligament retained to preserve the natural connections between the bones of the body (or a segment).

Limb advancement—Forward movement of the unweighted limb, a function of swing.

Loading response—The first phase of motion during the gait cycle; a period of initial double limb support.

Locomotor unit—The two lower limbs and the pelvis that provide the mechanics of walking.

Lordosis—Posterior angulation of the spine in the sagittal plane.

Low heel contact—Floor impact by the heel with the forefoot very close to the floor thus providing a limited heel rocker.

Markers—Balls or disks applied to the skin over designated anatomical landmarks used to designate the segments for remote motion analysis.

Mid stance—The first portion of the single limb support interval.

Moment—The rotational potential of the forces acting on a joint, also called torque.

Momentum—The tendency to remain in motion unless an opposing force is applied.

Motion analysis—A system to define the movement of the different body segments during walking and other functional activities.

Motor unit—The functional neuromuscular unit consisting of the peripheral neuron (cell body, axon, end plate), myoneural junction and the muscle fibers controlled by the branches of that axone.

Muscle grade—The strength of the muscle designated by the manual muscle test on a scale of 0 to 5 (normal).

Muscular dystrophy—An inherited, progressive disease of the muscle that causes increasing weakness and contracture formation.

Myelodysplasia—A congenital form of paralysis resulting from a spinal cord malformation characterized by failure of neural tube closure.

Neuron—A single nerve fiber consisting of a cell body, axon and terminal junction.

Normalization (EMG)—Relationship of the raw EMG of an activity to a basic reference EMG (manual muscle test, maximum in gait).

Observational gait analysis—Visual definition of an individual's limb and trunk motions during walking.

Optoelectrical recording—Automated motion analysis using electronic signals (lights) as the landmarks.

Orthosis—An eternal device to provide support, limit or assist motion.

Osteoarthritis—Progressive deterioration of the joint cartilage and bone of nonspecific etiology. (In some cultures there is a genetic factor. Wear and tear of an abnormal joint is another cause.)

Oxygen cost—The amount of oxygen used per meter walked (millimeters/kilogram of body weight/meter walked).

Oxygen pulse—The ratio between the amount of oxygen used per minute and heart rate.

Oxygen rate—The amount of oxygen used per minute (millimeters/kilogram/minute).

Pantalar fusion—Surgical arthrodesis of the ankle, subtalar, and midtarsal joints.

Parallelogram electrogoniometer—A device to measure joint motion that has rectangular shaped arms consisting of four linked segments for free shape changes to accommodate the change in joint axis location.

Paraplegia—Paralysis of the two lower limbs. With cerebral palsy, the term diplegia is used.

Passenger unit—The composite body mass comprised of the head, arm, neck and trunk segments that rides atop the locomotor system.

Passive—The structure has no means of generating a force. The motion results from an outside source.

Pass-retract—Excessive hip flexion (pass) followed by rapid extension (retract) to provide terminal swing knee extension in the absence of an adequate quadriceps.

Pathokinesiology—The science of defining the function of persons with physical impairments.

Pathological gait—An abnormal walking pattern.

Patterned movement—Mass extension or flexion of the limb by primitive locomotor control.

Peak axial load—The maximum vertical force registered during walking.

Pelvic drop—Descent of one side of the pelvis below the neutral axis (zero line).

Pelvic hike—Elevation of one side of the pelvis above the neutral axis (zero line).

Pelvic tilt—Angulation of the pelvis from neutral alignment in the sagittal plane.

Percent gait cycle—The one-hundreth part within one sequence of walking mechanics.

Perimalleolar muscles—The posterior muscles that pass close to the medial and lateral malleoli of the ankle as they extend from their origins on the tibia and fibula to their insertions within the foot (tibialis posterior, flexor hallucis longus, flexor digitorum longus, peroneus longus, peroneus brevis).

Plantar flexion—Movement of the foot away from the anterior surface of the tibia, straightening the ankle joint.

Plantigrade—Simultaneous floor contact by the forefoot and heel.

Poliomyelitis—Paralysis caused by a viral invasion of the motor nerve cells in the anterior horn of the spinal cord.

Power—The rate at which work is performed.

Premature heel rise—Elevation of the heel from the floor prior to the onset of terminal stance (30% GC).

Pre-swing—The last phase of stance that also is the second period of double limb support.

Primitive locomotor control—A simple voluntary source of motion that uses mass extension and mass flexion of the limb joints. It is a extrapyramidal control system.

Progression—Advancement along the sagittal plane when walking.

Quadriplegia—Paralysis of both upper and both lower extremities.

Reciprocal gait—Alternate function of the right and left limbs.

Relative effort—Percent of the baseline maximum muscular effort displayed by normalized EMG.

Repetition rate—The number of action potentials occurring per second.

Respiratory quotient—The ratio of carbon dioxide production to oxygen consumption.

Rheumatoid arthritis—A systemic inflammatory disease that attaches the joints.

Rigid contracture—Fibrous tissue restraint of joint motion that does not yield under body weight or forceful manual stretching.

Rotation—Motion about a center point (axis) in which the distal end of the segment travels further than the proximal end.

Sagittal plane—The longitudinal plane of the body that extends from front to back, parallels the sagittal suture of the skull.

Sarcomere—The intrinsic contracting (force) unit within a muscle fiber.

Scoliosis—Lateral curvature of the spine.

Selective control—Voluntary control that allows individual muscle activation for the appropriate duration and intensity that is functionally required.

Shock absorption—Muscle action that lessens the impact of limb loading by allowing controlled joint motion.

Shear—Sliding displacement parallel with the surface of the joint.

Single axis—Joint movement in one plane.

Single limb support—Total weight-bearing on one lower extremity.

Spasticity—A hyper reactive response to stretch.

Spirometry—Measurement of the amount of air the respiratory system can move (inhale and exhale).

Stability—The body center of gravity is over the base of support.

Stance—The period in walking when the foot is in contact with the floor.

Static—Stationary, nonmoving.

Steady state—Each cycle of function is the same, being free of accelerations or decelerations.

Step—The interval in the gait cycle between initial contact with one foot and then the other foot (ie. right to left).

Step length—The distance between the sequential points of initial contact by the two feet.

Stiff knee gait—Significantly limited swing phase knee flexion.

Stride—The interval in the gait cycle between two sequential initial contacts with the same foot (ie. right to right).

Stride length—The distance between the sequential points of initial contact by the same foot.

Stride characteristics—Measurement of the time and distance qualities of the person's walk.

Surface electrode—Disks applied to the skin surface to sense the underlying EMG.

Swing through gait—A form of crutch walking that alternates support by both crutches and then by both feet. Progression occurs as the two limbs swing through during the crutch support period.

Symphysis down—Anterior tilt of the pelvis that places the symphysis below the neutral resting position.

Symphysis up—Posterior tilt of the pelvis that raises the symphysis above the neutral resting position.

Swing—The period in the gait cycle when the foot is not in contact with the floor.

Terminal double stance—The last phase of stance when both feet are in contact with the floor. The functional name for this period is pre-swing.

Terminal stance—The last half of the single limb support period.

Terminal swing—The last third of the limb advancement interval.

Time-adjusted EMG quantification—The mean EMG profile is located within the mean onset and cessation time of a series of strides.

Toe drag—Advancement of the limb is accompanied by continuing floor contact by the toe.

Torque—The rotational potential of the forces acting on a joint (also called moment).

Transverse plane—The horizontal plane of the body.

Trauma—Tissue injury by a force.

Treadmill—A device with a belt on rollers that allows locomotion (walking or running) in place.

Trendelenberg Limp—Trunk lean to the same side as the hip pathology ipsilateral lean).

Triaxial—Movement by a joint in three planes.

Triple arthrodesis—Surgical fusion of the hind foot (subtalar, calcaneocuboid and talonavicular joints).

Unguligrade—tip-toe walking.

Valgus—Lateral angulation of the distal segment of a joint, turning the foot out (a clinical synonym for eversion).

Varus—Medial angulation of the distal segment of a joint, turning the foot in (a clinical synonym for inversion).

Vector—The mean weight-bearing line of the body with both magnitude and directional qualities.

Velocity—The speed of walking in a designated direction.

Visible video recording—A record of a subject's function that allows observational analysis.

Weight acceptance—The initial period in the gait cycle when body weight is dropped onto the limb. The phases of initial contact and loading response are involved.

Wire electrode—A pair of fine nylon coated wires (50u) with 2mm bared tips that are inserted within the designated muscle to record the intensity and timing of function.

Wolf's Law—The basic bony structure will be modified by the weight-bearing and muscular forces it experiences.

Work—The product of a force times the distance the force acts.

Index

Page numbers in *italics* denote figures; those followed by "t" denote tables.